STUDIES IN NEUROPSYCHOLOGY

Studies in Neuropsychology

SELECTED PAPERS OF ARTHUR BENTON

Edited by

LOUIS COSTA, Ph.D, *and*

OTFRIED SPREEN, Ph.D

University of Victoria
Victoria, B.C.

New York   Oxford
OXFORD UNIVERSITY PRESS
1985

Oxford University Press

Oxford   New York   Toronto
Delhi   Bombay   Calcutta   Madras   Karachi
Kuala Lumpur   Singapore   Hong Kong   Tokyo
Nairobi   Dar es Salaam   Cape Town
Melbourne   Auckland

and associated companies in
Beirut   Berlin   Ibadan   Mexico City   Nicosia

Library of Congress Cataloging in Publication Data
Benton, Arthur Lester, 1909–
  Studies in neuropsychology.
  Bibliography: p.
  Includes index.
  1. Neuropsychology—Collected works.
  I. Costa, Louis.   II. Spreen, Otfried.   III. Title.
QP360.B49   **1985**   616.89   85–8768
ISBN 0–19–503636–0

Printing (last digit): 9 8 7 6 5 4 3 2 1

Printed in the United States of America

Preface

At dinner one evening in October 1983 during a meeting of the Orton Dyslexia Society in San Diego, the editors of this volume pressed Arthur Benton, as they had done in the past, to write a history of neuropsychology. As usual he demurred. Perhaps because of his eclecticism or because of a keen perception that it was too early or because of his modesty, he had never produced a general comprehensive work on neuropsychology. The following morning he approached us with a compromise. He would not write a history, but he would provide us with a selection of his historical, theoretical, and empirical papers if we wished to edit them. We promptly agreed.

Most of us are familiar with only a few of Arthur Benton's seminal papers pertaining to a field of special interest. Looking at his complete bibliography, however, shows a staggering array of contributions to neuropsychology—from early childhood to old age and from experimental studies of the phi phenomenon to clinical case studies and psychometrics. Only after reading the large array of diverse works does a unifying theme of Benton's work emerge. Here is a man who is in command of all aspects of neuropsychology, one who appreciates the classical past and reconceptualizes it in the methodology and technology of the present.

We wish to thank Arthur Benton for graciously letting us associate ourselves with what is substantively his book. The opportunity to read this collection of papers and discuss them with him in the context of his career has been most rewarding. We wish also to acknowledge our debt to Kerry deS. Hamsher who kindly made available to us the manuscript of his 1983 American Psychological Association presentation, "The Iowa Group" (*International Journal of Neuroscience*, in press). It was of much help in writing the introductory chapter of this volume. Thanks are due to the original publishers of Benton's articles who permitted us to reprint them. Finally, we would like to acknowledge the very special support of Jeffrey House of Oxford University Press who made it clear from the very beginning that, for him, this was not just another book.

Victoria, B.C.   L. C.
February 1985   O. S.

Contents

STUDIES IN NEUROPSYCHOLOGY

1.

Introduction*

The publication of two new papers in this volume marks 51 years since Arthur Benton's first published work in psychology. Yet, with the publication of well over one hundred articles, chapters, books, and tests in the field of neuropsychology, his work is, paradoxically, among the best and least well known in the literature. Although he writes fluently and well and does not shrink from complex theoretical evaluation, Benton's thoroughgoing empiricism has led him to resist simplistic and often premature characterizations of brain-behavior relations. Always willing to look at and integrate good data, he has remained unbeguiled by attractive overgeneralization. A producer of a number of carefully constructed and documented clinical test instruments in neuropsychology, he does not as an eclectic advocate the use

of a fixed test battery. Rather, his clinical approach to patients is grounded in careful observation and the application of psychometrically sound tests, as appropriate, to individual cases.

As a scientist-practitioner, Benton is equally comfortable with classical neurological, experimental, and clinical psychometric approaches to neuropsychological inquiry. He makes clear both in his writing and in his professional behavior that all three approaches are essential to the assessment of patients and the understanding of brain and behavior. He has served as a significant role model for generations of his own students, his associates, and many other professionals.

In a newly emergent field in which tests and theories are often taken up concretely as panaceas or literal truths, Benton reminds us that solid scientific inquiry is built on historical understanding. It involves careful observation and operationalization of an experimental or psychometric nature. As a professional, he has had little patience with those who would argue for the supremacy of either

* *Editors' note*: Reference to Benton's work cited in the introductory chapter may be found in the Bibliography. Other references are cited at the conclusion of the introduction. Reference lists for each of Benton's articles have been retained as they appeared in the original publication.

an experimental or a clinical approach at the expense of the other.

Perhaps because of his empirical-eclectic leanings or because of a predilection for working intensively in a diversity of problem areas in neuropsychology, Benton has never published a comprehensive textbook. Although a series of syntheses related to significant topics in neuropsychology does exist, the reader seeking to explore Benton's work fully must make use of a diversity of sources often not easily available, even in a well-equipped library. The purpose of this work is to provide the reader with a collection of Benton's major articles over the years in order to facilitate an overview of his contribution to neuropsychology.

Let us briefly examine Arthur Benton's professional career. He was born in New York City in 1909 and, except for some time in Europe with his father, a physician, he completed his primary and secondary education in New York. He attributes some of his concern for both experimental rigor and historical context to his training at Oberlin College where he earned his baccalaureate in 1931 and his master's degree in 1933. His work was largely in the area of experimental (behavioristic) psychology, although a master's-level practicum in the treatment of stuttering stimulated an interest in clinical work.

It was 1933 that saw the real beginnings of his career as a clinician. He returned to New York to pursue graduate work at Columbia University (Ph.D. 1935) and at that time was given an assistantship at the New York State Psychiatric Institute. It was there that he gained experience in psychometric testing of psychiatric patients, psychophysical experimentation, and personality-test construction. During this period of daily contact with patients and the psychiatric and neurological staff, his basic interest in clinical problems grew substantially.

After a short time as a counselor in a Civilian Conservation Corps (CCC) camp in 1936, Arthur Benton was appointed to the position of psychologist at the Payne Whitney Clinic of New York Hospital-Cornell Medical Center. He saw a variety of child and adult patients and published a series of articles on children's test performance that culminated in 1940 in a critical review of the literature on the mental development of prematurely born children. While working in the library of the New York Academy of Medicine one day in the late 1930s, he came upon an article in an obscure medical journal that dealt with the Gerstmann syndrome. He resolved to investigate this problem by means of operational techniques. This research was postponed because of World War II, but he returned to it several times later in his career. In 1939, he accepted appointments as attending psychologist at the New York Hospital-Westchester Division and as a counselor in the Student Personnel Office of the College of the City of New York; early in 1941, he volunteered for service in the medical corps of the U.S. Navy. During the war, he served as a psychologist at several naval installations. At the Naval Hospital in San Diego, he came into contact with Morris Bender who was chief of the hospital's neurological section. It was in this context that the first version of the Visual Retention Test was developed. Contact with Bender fostered Benton's interest in the phenomenon of extinction to simultaneous stimulation, which led to subsequent historical and experimental research.

In 1946, Benton left the navy and became an associate professor of psychology in the Department of Psychiatry of the University of Louisville School of Medicine. Shortly thereafter, in 1948, he accepted the post of professor of psychology and director of the clinical training program at the University of Iowa, which was then known for its outstanding graduate program in experimental psychology. In the company of Harold Bechtoldt and Judson Brown, he worked in an environment where clinical research was tested rigorously.

Arthur Benton has remained at Iowa since 1948. He has supervised at least 45 doctoral dissertations and 24 master's theses. In 1958, after a research leave, which he spent working in the Department of Neurology at Iowa, Benton relinquished the directorship of the clinical training program to accept a joint appointment as a professor of psychology and neurology. In 1978, he attained the status of emeritus and has continued to pursue an active research and writing career. Among the number of honors awarded him, the presidencies of the American Orthopsychiatric Association and the International Neuropsychological Society as well as the Award for Distinguished Professional Contributions by the American Psychological Association should be mentioned.

One of the editors (O. S.) spent several years with Arthur Benton at Iowa in the early 1960s and offers this reminiscence of him and his laboratory that is best told in the first person.

I have collaborated with Arthur for over 25 years. Recollections about this collaboration may perhaps illustrate better than general descriptions how he has stimulated and influenced so many others. Having produced a German translation of the Visual Retention Test, I met Arthur early during my first year as a postdoctoral fellow in St. Louis. I was immediately invited to Iowa City and was welcomed by him and his family like a personal friend. At the same time that three-day visit produced a plan for two studies of simulation on the Visual Retention Test (Spreen & Benton 1961, 1963). Those studies readily combined Arthur's interest in test development and my interest in exaggeration and simulation during psychological examinations for compensation purposes. Beyond that, he took an active interest in the problems of my test translation. At the same time, he impressed upon me the wide range of investigations of others in the field.

After several stimulating meetings in Iowa City and in Europe, where I was introduced to many of the best known researchers of that time, he invited me to join the Iowa Laboratory in 1962. The four years in Iowa provided continuous stimulation. All, even obscure, ideas were discussed and often immediately developed into experimentation. Problems in stimulus selection for an aphasia battery found me referred to a psycholinguistics course with Rudolph Schulz. Every patient referred to the laboratory provided new questions to be explored experimentally. This included a patient with sound agnosia but minimal aphasia (Spreen, Benton, & Fincham 1965), and one with what appeared to be a modality specific naming problem (Spreen, Benton, & Van Allen 1966). Visitors for short or extended stays were constantly introduced as old friends. I often learned later that they had worked with Arthur in circumstances similar to mine. In fact, we felt that anyone working in neuropsychology would be seen at Iowa sometime or other, if one stayed there long enough. The collaboration with members of the Neurology Department was close and resulted in a number of papers that Benton published with Robert Joynt, Maurice Van Allen, and Richard Fincham. Across the river, Benton's closest friend and collaborator in the Department of Psychology was Harold Bechtoldt.

Arthur's gentle and cordial manner minimized divisiveness. "Schools" of neuropsychology were meaningless to a man who could absorb such a variety of interests and personalities as those of Amiram Carmon, Ralph Reitan, Mariusz Maruszewski, and Henri Hécaen. A "midwestern" round-table conference from Madison (Kløve and Matthews), Minneapolis (Meier), and Iowa City met regularly and attracted numerous guests from other parts of the country and the world. Even Arthur's most critical papers (e.g., "The fiction of the Gerstmann syndrome," 1961) did not create enmity but stimulated numerous and ultimately useful discussions about the meaning of a syndrome. A widely quoted paper on cutoff scores and hit rates (Spreen & Benton 1965) perhaps gradually convinced many in the profession that much effort was wasted in "diagnosing" brain damage with psychological tests when other aspects of clinical research deserved more of our efforts.

Such research was always forthcoming from Benton's laboratory. Most often the pattern started with clinical observation and absorption of relevant literature and then moved through careful operational definition of the phenomena under investigation (e.g. the Gerstmann syndrome, aphasia, or face recognition), the construction of standardized psychometric instruments, and the application of these in psychometric research. Benton's temperament and curiosity did not enable him to dwell inordinately on any single technique or theory. Receptive to the interests of his colleagues and students— among them Donald Shankweiler, Harvey Levin, and Kerry Hamsher—he collaborated on research in a diversity of areas. The majority of the works collected in this volume are, appropriately, written by Benton alone. Perusal of his bibliography and Hamsher's "The Iowa Group" (1985) will reveal, however, that the work included here represents only a fragment of the contribution that Benton and his collaborators have made to neuropsychological investigation.

This book is arbitrarily divided into nine sections, each dealing with a problem area. As any such division must do violence to the continuity of themes evident across problem areas, we have endeavored to identify such themes in the section descriptions.

The topic of aphasia, dealt with in Section I, has been of continuing interest for Benton. Clinical examinations of brain-damaged patients fostered this interest well before his first publication on the topic. As with so many other topics, he approached aphasia from a historical point of view. His command of French and German allowed him to explore the original versions of many of the works cited in "Early descriptions of aphasia" (1960). This article was followed by a paper on three pioneers in the study of aphasia (1963) and by studies that focused on aphasia in children (1964), on Johann Gesner (1965), and on the development of two aphasia instruments—the Neurosensory Center Comprehensive Examination for Aphasia (1969, 1977) and the Multilingual Aphasia Examination (1974, 1983). Individual patients with atypical symptomatology triggered the development of new tests for sound recognition and tactile naming and for careful experimental studies of auditory agnosia (1965) and stimulus-specific anomia (1966). Each study was preceded by a historical review of the topic. The second paper in Section I, "Bergson and Freud on aphasia: a comparison," is a recent work not previously published, "Hemispheric dominance before Broca" (1984), which appears in Section II, deals with historical aspects of aphasia in the context of laterality.

Section II contains articles dealing with cerebral localization and hemispheric dominance. Five of the six papers are historical in nature and, taken together with those in Section I, expand our knowledge of early neuropsychology. Spatial, somesthetic, visual, and language functions are dealt with in the context of localization and dominance. "The 'minor' hemisphere" (1972) deals primarily with the relatively scant literature, from the time of Hughlings Jackson to World War II, on the contribution of the right hemisphere to linguistic and visual spatial functions. This was a period when the left hemisphere was, indeed, considered by most to be the major hemisphere for all cognitive functions. Benton pointed to contrary evidence that existed in the literature of the time and that eventually stimulated postwar investigators to restructure their conceptualizations of hemispheric role.

This theme is carried further in "Hemispheric cerebral dominance and somesthesis" (1972), where the role of careful methodological investigation in attenuating the doctrine of contralateral innervation is outlined.

The one empirical research study in Section II, "Tactile perception of direction in normal subjects" (1973), illustrates Benton's recognition that experimental variables—in this case, exposure duration—play a significant role in elucidating or masking hemispheric differences. A careful investigation resulted in right-hemisphere superiority on a tactile-spatial task. The authors, however, in contrast to many investigators of laterality in the early 1970s, went beyond significance tests to ascertain the number of individuals who showed or failed to show the predicted pattern.

"The interplay of experimental and clinical approaches in brain lesion research" (1978) documents the influence of early animal lesion studies on the thinking of neurologists investigating visual processes. Some of Benton's own empirical work on hemispheric dominance for vision can be found in the three studies in Section VIII. "Focal brain damage and the concept of localization of function" (1981) is a historical and theoretical paper in which Benton espouses an intermediate position that, like many contemporary views, owes a great debt to Hughlings Jackson. The final paper in Section II concerns the failure of physicians in the century before 1860 to identify clearly the association between left-hemisphere lesions and aphasia. The case materials of

three who failed to find the relationship and one who did are reviewed.

Benton's collaboration with Morris Bender during World War II in San Diego stimulated further the continued exploration of normal and abnormal tactile perception illustrated in Section III. The method of double stimulation of the patient (e.g., simultaneous stimulation on both arms), which was introduced by Oppenheim into the neurological examination in 1885, was first dealt with by Benton in 1956. "Jacques Loeb and the method of double stimulation" (1956) identifies the origins of the approach in nineteenth-century animal research. Benton's own empirical study with Harvey Levin, "An experimental study of 'obscuration' " (1972) is also reprinted in Section III.

Benton's interest in somesthesis produced numerous studies of finger localization and resulted in a series of papers with Amiram Carmon that investigated tactile thresholds, tactile perception of direction, and the general review of somesthesis that is reprinted in Section II.

Constructional apraxia and its relation to visual, spatial, and linguistic deficit is the focus of Section IV. By 1962, Benton had explored the use of the Visual Retention Test as a measure of constructional praxis and with his graduate student Max Fogel developed both a two-dimensional and a three-dimensional construction test that utilized matchsticks and blocks (Benton & Fogel 1962; Fogel 1962). "Constructional apraxia and the minor hemisphere" (1967) deals with the intercorrelations of these three tests and the block designs of the Wechsler Adult Intelligent Scale (WAIS). The test intercorrelations are low, suggesting that the construct is, indeed, a complex one. A significant number of patients with mild constructional apraxia and left-hemisphere lesions are identified. Further work in this area was done by another of Benton's students (Dee 1970); in 1973 Benton published the second paper in this section: "Visuoconstructive disability in patients with cerebral disease: its relationship to side of lesion and aphasic disorder." In this empirical study, the relationship of linguistic deficit to dyspraxia in patients with left-sided lesions is examined. The final selection, "Spatial thinking in neurological patients: historical aspects" (1982) is a recent book chapter in which Benton presents a theoretical review of research in the area since 1864. At least 14 studies from his laboratory are cited and integrated into the main body of the review.

The reaction-time method dates to the beginnings of experimental psychology in the nineteenth century. Rarely, however, was the technique employed with nonpsychotic brain-damaged patients before the study by Benton and his student Blackburn in 1955. This was followed by additional papers in the late 1950s. The article by Benton and Joynt in Section V "Reaction time in unilateral cerebral disease" (1959) investigated differences in performance of the hands ipsilateral and contralateral to the site of injury as well as the complexity of the decision-making task. An investigation of "The crossmodal retardation in reaction time of patients with cerebral disease" (1962) was based on a technique developed originally by Benton's collaborator Samuel Sutton. Speed of decison making was studied by Dee and Van Allen (1973). Finally Benton reported a study of "Interactive effects of age and brain disease on reaction time" in 1977. This study should also be considered together with the last two articles in Section IX that reflect his interest in the neuropsychology of aging.

Section VI contains articles related to the Gerstmann syndrome. During the 1950s, Benton's interest focused on somesthetic disorders, including stereognosis and finger agnosia, which led up to his book on right-left discrimination and finger localization. It is easy to see how this interest would lead to an investigation of the combination of four different deficits (right-left disorientation, dyscalculia, finger agnosia, and dysgraphia), both in brain-damaged adults and in normal and mentally handicapped schoolchildren. His first paper described the Gerstmann symptoms after electroshock treatment (1952). Typically, there followed a historical paper, "Early description of the Gerstmann syndrome" (1956), that traced Badal's research (1888). But the question arose: Was it a syndrome? Benton (1961) argued cogently that, to be described as a syndrome of clinical value, the four symptoms should be more closely associated with each other than with other parietal lobe symptoms, such as constructional dyspraxia, dyslexia, or disorders of visual memory. Benton presented correlational data showing that the association among the Gerstmann symptoms was about as strong as with any other combination of four of these deficits. In addition, he argued that, in patients who do show the Gerstmann configuration of symptoms, cerebral localization of lesion was quite diverse, thus throwing doubt on the focal lesion significance. His paper, provocatively titled "The fiction of the 'Gerstmann syndrome' " (1961), aroused considerable discussion about the meaning of neuropsychological syndromes. Benson and Geschwind (1969) maintained that the Gerstmann syndrome remained meaningful as an indicator of dominant parietal lesions, even in "partial" form or in combination with other symptoms, and they extended the term to refer to a "developmental" form in children as a type of learning disability. Poeck and Orgass (1966) doubted the meaningfulness of the syndrome and found an association with manifest or latent aphasic symptomatology. Heimburger, DeMyer, and Reitan (1964) stated that they had never encountered the Gerstmann syndrome in isolation. Benton reviewed the theoretical and practical import of the discussion in the final paper of Section VI, "Reflections on the Gerstmann syndrome" (1977).

Section VII contains three articles on hemispheric dominance and vision. They provide a sample of the research in vision that has been conducted in Benton's laboratory since the late 1960s. Following a study by Carmon and Bechtoldt (1969), "Stereoscopic vision in patients with unilateral cerebral disease" (1970) was written with Hécaen and confirmed right-hemisphere superiority for this function. Further work on stereopsis was done by Hamsher (1978).

Perception of line direction was also shown to be mediated primarily by right-hemisphere mechanisms. Building on an earlier study of identification of orientation of tachistoscopically exposed lines in normals (Fontenot & Benton 1972), Benton, Hannay, and Varney presented a more complicated version of the task to patients with lateralized lesions and controls, which is reported in "Visual perception of line direction in patients with unilateral brain disease" (1975). It is interesting to speculate, although the authors did not, on the role of double stimulation (see Section III) in enhancing deficit performance on some trials of the task used. The last article in Section VII is an original review, "Facial recognition, 1984," which integrates clinical research on face recognition and prosopagnosia, including the work done in Benton's laboratory with tachistoscopic laterality studies of face recognition in normals.

Many of Benton's studies, although originating from observations on adult brain-damaged patients, were extended into childhood and old age because of the need for normative data in these age ranges. Beyond this, however, he took a direct interest in specific developmental problems, particularly mental handicap and dyslexia in children and, more recently, dementing disorders in the elderly. Section VIII includes a seminal paper, "The concept of pseudofeeble-mindedness" (1956), in which a then-popular term is carefully analyzed and its usefulness seriously questioned. The second selection provides a wide, sweeping view of "Interactive determinants of mental deficiency" (1970), one that even now has not been fully appreciated by workers in the field who continue to prefer a simple causative model. The third paper, "Dyslexia: evolution of a concept" (1980), again takes a historical approach to the concept of dyslexia and analyzes its genetic, cognitive, neurological, emotional, educational, and social components in modern usage, enlarging and revising Benton's integrative summary in the Benton and Pearl (1978) book. The overviews presented here were the product of years of direct studies with dyslexics and mentally retarded children. The final selection "Child clinical neuropsychology: retrospect and prospect" (1982) provides a survey of child clinical neuropsychology as a developing discipline. Two papers at the other end of the spectrum, old age, are included in Section IX because they address more methodological issues.

The final section contains three articles grouped together because of their focus on methodological issues. Benton's classic article, "Problems of test construction in the field of aphasia" (1967), deals both with historical approaches to the testing of mental abilities in neurological patients and with the methods used in the construction of the Neurosensory Center Comprehensive Examination for Aphasia.

"Normative observations on neuropsychological test performances in old age" (1981) contrasts performance of younger and older normal subjects on nine tests in use in Benton's laboratory, seven of which originated or were first standardized there. In this work, as in so many others reprinted here, his preference for presenting the number of subjects who show, operationally defined, deficit performance is evident. The reader is not encumbered by tests of significance illustrating small-group differences that may be useless in clinical decision making or by matrices of correlations with little practical value. In this respect, Benton's clinical work has an elegant simplicity.

"Problems and conceptual issues in neuropsychological research in aging and dementia" (1984), written with his daughter Abigail Sivan, is a methodological treatment of significant issues in this emerging research area.

A final word to the reader to suggest ways in which this book may be read: the historical material found in the frankly historical papers as well as in many of the longer experimental papers and theoretical reviews, provides a topic-oriented, eclectic, history of neuropsychology. The empirical research itself contains much of significance for contemporary thought. And for the reader wishing to focus on and assess the contributions of Arthur Benton to modern neuropsychology, these reprinted articles provide an introduction to his work.

REFERENCES

Badal, J. (1888). Contribution à l'étude des cécités psychiques: alexie, agraphie, hémianopsie inférieure, trouble du sens de l'espace. *Archives d'Ophtalmologie, 8*, 97–117.

Benson, D. F., & Geschwind, N. (1969). Developmental Gerstmann syndrome. *Neurology, 20*, 203–208.

Carmon, A., & Bechtoldt, H. P. (1969). Dominance of the right cerebral hemisphere for stereopsis. *Neuropsychologia, 7*, 29–39.

Dee, H. L. (1970). Visuoconstructive and visuoperceptive deficit in patients with unilateral cerebral lesions. *Neuropsychologia, 8*, 305–314.

Dee, H. L., & Van Allen M. W. (1973). Speed of decision-making processes in patients with unilateral cerebral disease. *Archives of Neurology, 28*, 163–166.

Fogel, M. L. (1962). The Gerstmann syndrome and the parietal symptom complex. *Psychological Record, 12*, 85–99.

Hamsher, K. deS. (1978). Stereopsis and unilateral brain disease. *Investigative Ophthalmology and Visual Science, 17*, 336–343.

Hamsher, K. deS. (1985). The Iowa Group. *International Journal of Neuroscience, 25*, 295–305.

Heimberger, R. F., DeMyer, W. C., & Reitan, R. M. (1964). Implications of Gerstmann's syndrome. *Journal of Neurology, Neurosurgery and Psychiatry, 27*, 52–57.

Poeck, K., & Orgass, B. (1966). Gerstmann's syndrome and aphasia. *Cortex, 2*, 421–427.

I.
Aphasia

2.

Early Descriptions of Aphasia*

INTRODUCTION

One of the features of the spirited and prolonged discussion that followed Paul Broca's famous pathological demonstrations before the Académie de Médecine of Paris in 1861 was the "exhumation," to use the caustic term of Desiré Bernard, of ancient and long-forgotten descriptions of aphasia. Thus, Jules Falret,[1] in his analysis of the various clinical forms of aphasia, mentioned case reports by Johann Gesner (1770) and Alexander Crichton (1798) as being among the earliest in the field. Trousseau[2] went farther back, citing the anecdotes of the elder Pliny as evidence that aphasia was known as early as the first century A.D., and quoting the comments of Schenck von Grafenberg (1585) to the effect that he had observed patients who were unable to speak because of loss of memory.

The discovery of "prehistoric" case reports and references dealing with aphasia continued through the latter decades of the century and into the present century. Coupland,[3] Jastrowitz,[4] and Ebstein[5] called attention to Goethe's description in "*Wilhelm Meisters Lehrjahre*" (1795), and Ogle[6] to the still earlier self-description of Samuel Johnson. Kulz[7] presented a German translation of Linné's (1745) brief but most interesting account of expressive aphasia; later, Hultgren[8] discussed it at some length. Bernard[9] pointed out that Johann Schmidt's description of alexia in 1676 compared quite favorably with later reports. Soury[10] cited the very early references to traumatic aphasia by Nicolò Massa (1558) and Francisco Arceo (1588). Gans[11] (1914) presented a German translation of the description by Rommel (1683) of a case of what he regarded as "transcortical" motor aphasia.

That the early history of aphasia continues to be of considerable interest to neurologists is evidenced by the recent contributions to it by a number of

* A. L. Benton and R. J. Joynt, *Archives of Neurology*, 1960, 3, 205–222. Copyright 1960, American Medical Association.

authors. In 1943, Viets,[12] possibly unaware of the German translation of Külz, published an English translation of the case report of Linné. More recently, Antoni,[13] apparently unaware of the contributions of both Külz and Viets, again called attention to it and indicated his feeling that it has been unjustly neglected in historical surveys of the field. Some years ago, Riese[14] cited Goethe's account as being the "first description containing basic features of aphasia," an opinion with which many students would not agree. In 1950, Eliasberg[15] called attention to the descriptions of Spalding (1783) and Herz (1791) which appeared in the *Magazin für Erfahrungsseelenkunde.* Most recently, Hoff, Guillemin, and Geddes[16] have provided an account of the self-description in 1787 by the French scientist, Grandjean de Fouchy, of his transitory aphasia.

Since the early history of aphasia has claimed our own interest, we believe that it would be of value to assemble in systematic fashion all the older allusions and case reports which have been cited by various authors at various times and places. In making this collation, we have depended almost completely upon references in the literature to guide us to the original writings and have not undertaken an independent examination of original sources which might contain hitherto undiscovered material. The survey is not altogether nonevaluative in nature. Some descriptions are obviously more adequate than others and deserve to be recognized as such. At the same time, there is no doubt that some students have read into certain writings a much greater import than they actually possess, and these misinterpretations warrant correction. On the whole, the facts are clear enough and speak for themselves. The period covered in this survey extends from the possible references to aphasia in the Hippocratic Corpus to the end of the eighteenth century.

ANCIENT DESCRIPTIONS

Hippocratic Corpus (ca. 400 B.C.). There are many references to "aphonia" in the Hippocratic writings, usually in the adjectival form *aphōnos* (Aphorisms, Epidemics, Sacred Disease, Coan Prognosis). The term is used to designate one of the features of apoplexy or epilepsy and also occurs in descriptions of the course of protracted, usually fatal, illnesses. It is rendered in the English translations of Adams[17] and Jones[18] as "speechless," "loss of speech," or "loss of power of speech." However, the new translation by Chadwick and Mann[19] usually gives it as "aphonia" or "loss of voice," although in some places it is rendered as "speechless" or "aphasia."

It is sometimes remarked that Hippocrates "must" have appreciated the distinction between aphasia and aphonia, since in one case description (Epidemics III, Case 3) it is noted that the patient was *anaudos* ("without voice or utterance, speechless"), as well as *aphōnos.* In their translation of the passage, Chadwick and Mann render *anaudos* as "aphasia," *aphōnos* as "aphonia." Adams and Jones, since they have consistently translated *aphōnos* as "speechless" or the equivalent, are obliged to break the rule in the translation of this passage. Both now render *anaudos* as "speechless" and utilize another term for *aphōnos.* Adams gives it as "loss of articulation"; Jones, as "voiceless."

There is no doubt that the physicians of the Hippocratic School observed aphasic or aphasia-like manifestations in patients with cerebral disease or dysfunction. So must have generations or physicians before them. The distinction of the

School in this respect lies in the very frequent specific references to these conditions. However, it is usually impossible to judge exactly what was meant by the terms *aphōnos* and *anaudos*. That they were distinguished from one another is suggested by the use of both terms in the case description cited above. On the other hand, the varying contexts in which the descriptive term *aphōnos* appears suggest that sometimes it meant aphasia, sometimes anarthria, sometimes loss of voice. In one passage (Coan Prognosis, No. 315 in the Chadwick-Mann translation), the term *hypaphōnon* ("partial loss of speech or dumbness") is used. It is probable that, as in our own day, the same term was used by different writers to mean different things.

There is a passage in the Coan Prognosis (No. 353 in the Chadwick-Mann translation) which associates temporary speechlessness (*anaudiē*) following convulsions "with paralysis of the tongue, or of the arm and right side of the body." When this is combined with the observation that "an incised wound in one temple produces a spasm in the opposite side of the body" (Coan Prognosis, No. 448 in the Chadwick-Mann translation), it is seen that the essential ingredients for relating aphasia to a lesion of the left hemisphere were present in the Hippocratic writings. But, of course, there is no evidence that the correlation was actually made.

Valerius Maximus (ca. A.D. 30).[20] This Latin author and commentor notes that a learned man of Athens, after being struck in the head by a stone, lost his memory of letters, to which he had been particularly devoted, but retained his memory of everything else. This is perhaps the earliest reference to a traumatic alexia to be found in Western literature.

Pliny (A.D. 23–79).[21] In his *Clinique Médicale*, Trousseau[2] quoted Pliny to illustrate the thesis that "the physiological conditions of aphasia" were not unknown in antiquity. The relevant lines, which come after an account of some wondrous feats of memory, are as follows:

And yet there is not a thing in man so fraile and brittle againe as it, whether it be occasioned by disease, by casual injuries and occurrents, or by feare, through which it faileth sometime in part, and otherwhiles decaieth generally, and is cleane lost. One with the stroke of a stone, fell presently to forget his letters onely, and could read no more; otherwise his memory served him well ynough. Another, with a fall from the roufe of a very high house, lost the remembrance of his own mother, his next kinfolke, friends, and neighbours. Another, in a sicknesse of his forgot his owne servants about him: and *Messala Corvinus* the great Oratour, upon the like occasion, forgot his owne proper name.

From a perusal of this charming passage, the reader may decide for himself the extent to which Pliny understood "the physiological conditions of aphasia." In any event, the passage does make clear reference to a case of traumatic alexia, quite possibly the same "very learned man of Athens" mentioned by Valerius Maximus.

Soranus of Ephesus (A.D. 98–135). The treatises on acute and chronic diseases by Soranus, chief exponent of the Methodist sect, are known to us through the writings of Caelius Aurelianus, who flourished about A.D. 450.[22] In his discussion of "paralysis" ("On Chronic Diseases," Book II), in which he distinguished between sensory and motor impairment and between flaccid and spastic paralysis, Caelius points out that while paralysis of the tongue leads to faulty articulation of speech, such paralysis "may be distinguished from cases of loss of speech resulting from some other disease. For in these latter cases, the tongue does not change color or the condition of its surface, or lose sensation or mobility, or change position." According to Creutz,[23] most of the medical writers of this period made the same distinction between impairment of speech or of the voice due to paralysis of the tongue and that due to other causes. The nature of the speech impairments which were referable to other factors remains an open question. No doubt it included aphasia but it may also have had reference to loss of voice from localized peripheral affections. In this respect, it is noteworthy that, directly after making the distinction between loss of speech due to paralysis of the tongue and that due to other causes, Soranus makes an apparently analogous distinction between "paralytic" anosmia and other types. "When the organ of smell is paralyzed, it can no longer detect odors. But this paralysis is to be distinguished from the disease of the nostrils called 'ozaena.' "

Sextus Empiricus (ca. A.D. 200).[24] The great skeptic philosopher finds a place in this review because he is commonly supposed to be among the first to use the term *aphasia*. It need only be pointed out that Sextus had in mind a particular philosophic position of the Skeptics, namely, "nonassertion," which referred not at all to the clinical condition of aphasia.

We explain Aphasia as follows: The word *phasis* is used in two ways, having a general and a special signification. According to the general signification, it expresses affirmation or negation, as "It is day" or "It is not day"; according to the special signification, it expresses an affirmation only. . . . Now Aphasia is the opposite of *phasis* in its general signification, which, as we said, comprises both

affirmation and negation. It follows that Aphasia is a condition of mind, according to which we say that we neither affirm nor deny anything.

One cannot help but remark that Hughlings Jackson's conception of aphasia as "a loss of power to propositionise" approaches this use of the term by the Greek Skeptics. From such a point of view, Trousseau's choice of it acquires an aura of prescience. However, whatever may be the relations in a deeper sense between modern concepts of aphasia and its technical meaning in ancient philosophy, it must be conceded that Sextus Empiricus has no real place in the early history of aphasia.

RENAISSANCE DESCRIPTIONS

Antonio Guainerio (?–1440).[25] Guainerio's references to aphasia are perhaps the earliest of the Renaissance descriptions. Pointing out that when too much phlegm accumulates in the posterior ventricle "the organ of memory can retain little or nothing," he mentions: "I had under my care two old men, one of whom did not know more than three words. . . . The other . . . rarely or never recalled the right name of anyone. When he summoned someone, he did not call him by name." From this brief description and Guainerio's interpretation of the disorder as being essentially one of memory, it might be guessed that the first patient suffered from a motor aphasia, the second from an amnestic aphasia.

Baverius de Baveriis (ca. 1480).[26] Among the *Consilia* of Baverius of Imola is one (No. 65) dealing with a patient, "an excellent young man," who suffered from "inability to move one side of the body with inability to speak, much sleeping, and weakness of nerves." The inability to speak, which is not further described, is ascribed to "weakness of the seventh pair of nerves, by which the tongue is moved." The side of the body affected is not specified. Whether the patient was dysphasic or dysarthric can hardly be determined from these few lines. In another *Consilium* (No. 2), a pregnant woman is described as "having a cramp in the vertebrae of the neck, so that she cannot raise herself up, and also having a cramp in the tongue so that it impedes her speech."

Paracelsus (1493–1541). Ebstein[27] has called attention to the fact that this formidable figure of Renaissance medicine, who apparently was well aware of the relationship of paralysis and speech disturbances to disease of the brain, also pointed out that centrally determined deficits of speech, as well as of hearing and vision, could occur in the absence of paralysis. The relevant passage in *Der grossen Wundartzney* . . . (cited by Ebstein) runs as follows:

Wounds of the head which cause sudden death or epilepsy. . . . It should be recognized that when the chambers of vision, hearing or speech are affected; this is not stroke or paralysis; these are wounds in and of themselves which do not heal completely unless they be very slight.

Ebstein infers from this passage that Paracelsus recognized that focal symptoms, particularly speech disturbances, could occur as a consequence of head injuries.

Nicolò Massa (?–1569).[28] Massa, one of the great anatomists and syphilologists of his day, describes a case of traumatic aphasia or anarthria which he cured by surgical intervention.

Also restored to health by my efforts was a handsome young man, Marcus Goro, who was wounded by the sharp point of a spear having on one side an axe and on the other a sword, which they call a halberd. There was a fracture not only of the cranial bone but also of the meninges and the brain substance extending to the basal bone. Because this was protruding, a silver tube, which extended to the basal bone and exerted pressure on it, was placed in the wound. In addition to all his other misfortunes, the young man was speechless for eight days. Asked by many distinguished officials, I came there and noted that . . . the fracture of the bone was about the length of the external ear, a half-finger deep and equally wide. . . . Since the doctors declared that they had seen no bone, I concluded that the reason for the loss of voice was that part of the bone was lodged in the brain. I took an instrument from a certain surgeon who was in attendance and extracted the bone from the wound, whereupon the patient began to speak at once, saying, "Praise God, I am cured." This drew much applause from the doctors, nobles, and attendants who were present.*

Francisco Arceo (1493–1573?).[29] In citing Massa's case report, Soury[10] mentions that a similar experience was also related by the Spanish surgeon Arceo, who describes quite briefly the condition of a workman who was struck on the head by a falling stone. Parts of the skull were depressed into the brain, and for several days after the accident the patient was "not onely speechles, but lay without moving." Arceo reflected the bone fragments back into place and, in doing this, observed that the meninges were inflamed. Three days later, "he spake, yet unfecklie, and as men of troubled minde are wonte to doe." In due time, the patient recovered completely and "married a wife. For he was then a young man."

---

* Translated by Mrs. Lillian C. Nelson.

Johann   Schenck   von   Grafenberg (1530–1598).[30] As we have mentioned, Trousseau (1931) cited Schenck von Grafenberg as being one of the early physicians who appreciated the essential nature of aphasia. In his lectures, the following passage from Schenck's *Observationes* is quoted:

I have observed in many cases of apoplexy, lethargy, and similar major diseases of the brain that, although the tongue was not paralyzed, the patient could not speak because, the faculty of memory being abolished, the words were not produced.

SEVENTEENTH-CENTURY DESCRIPTIONS

In the seventeenth century there appeared two case reports, one by Schmidt, the other by Rommel, which attained a level of description that was significantly above anything which had hitherto appeared. Both cases are described in sufficient detail so that not only is there no doubt that the patients were truly aphasic but also the type of language disability which was manifested is made clearly evident. Since, to our knowledge, English versions of these reports are not available, full translations of them will be presented.

Johann Schmidt (1624–1690).[31] In 1673, Schmidt made observations on a case of aphasia which were published three years later in the *Miscellanea* of the Academia Naturae Curiosorum of Leipzig. They concerned a patient who suffered from a motor aphasia following a stroke. In due time, the aphasia receded but the patient remained completely alexic.

On Loss of Reading Ability Following Apoplexy with Preservation of Writing*

A leading citizen among us, Nicholas Cambier, an old man of 65 years, was seized with a very

* Translated by Mrs. Lillian C. Nelson.

severe attack of apoplexy which all his attendants feared would lead to his death. Many remedies were applied, including copious venesection, irritating enemas to stimulate the sleeping faculties, cupping with deep incisions of the scapular and nuchal regions, together with inunction of the neck, forehead and nose and, from time to time, essences and spirits for the head to the degree that his condition would permit.

Upon his return home, it was evident that his right side was paralyzed and that he had difficulty in speaking. He muttered a good deal but was incapable of expressing the feelings of his mind; he substituted one word for another so that his attendants had difficulty in determining what he wanted. He then developed epilepsy with severe convulsions; this disappeared and he returned to his former state. Thus was the wretched man tortured. Finally, by the goodness of God, these terrible enemies were overcome. At no time had they carried the threat of immediate death.

A final evil remained to be overcome. He could not read written characters, much less combine them in any way. He did not know a single letter nor could he distinguish one from another. But it is remarkable that, if some name were given to him to be written, he could write it readily, spelling it correctly. However, he could not read what he had written even though it was in is own hand. Nor could he distinguish or identify the characters. For if he were asked what letter this or that was or how the letters had been combined, he could answer only by chance or through his habit of writing. It appeared that he wrote without deliberation. No teaching or guidance was successful in inculcating recognition of letters in him.

It was otherwise with a certain stone cutter in our country. Wilhelm Richter came to see me after his apoplexy receded because he was not able to read at all or to recognize letters. However, he learned the alphabet elements of the language again in a short time. He then combined them and attained perfection in his reading.

This case report of Schmidt, dating back almost three centuries, is indeed a remarkable one. It provides, so far as we are aware, the first unmistakable descriptions of paraphasia and alexia. Moreover, as Desiré Bernard[9] pointed out, Schmidt took pains, by a comparison of his two cases, to show that the course of an acquired impairment in reading could vary. In his brief discussion following the case reports, Schmidt mentions the patient's inability to read script which he himself had just written as being the most "memorable" feature of his first case. This phenomenon has been repeatedly observed since his time and its significance is still a subject of lively interest.

Peter Rommel (1643–1708).[32] Rommel (1683), who designated his case a "rare aphonia," described a patient with motor aphasia and incapacity for repetition but with considerable retention of capacity for serial speech and for understanding of oral and written language. A translation of his report reads as follows:

On a Rare Aphonia*

The wife of Senator H., of the imperial city of Laufen, a highly respected lady 52 years of age, fell ill seven years ago, after which she was bled without medical consultation, as unfortunately is so often the case. After a fairly strenuous walk which she took after dinner, she suffered a mild delirium and apoplexy with paralysis of the right side. At the same time, she lost all speech with the exception of the words, "yes" and "and." She could say no other word, not even a syllable, with these exceptions: the Lord's Prayer, the Apostles' Creed, some Biblical verses and other prayers, which she could recite verbatim and without hesitation but somewhat precipitously. But it is to be noted that they were said in the order which she was accustomed to saying them for many years and, if this regular sequence were interrupted and she were asked to recite a prayer or Biblical verse not in its accustomed

place, she either could not do it at all or only after a long interval and with great difficulty. I tried this test myself and was astonished to hear her reciting some prayers. However, when I requested her to repeat a prayer she had already recited she could not do it even after great effort, until her maid, who had long been familiar with the order of the prayers, would recite it. Then she would recite the requested prayer, although with some difficulty. Similarly, I asked her to repeat some words in the order in which I said them, e.g., "God will help." Stimulated to effort, she tried several times, but was unsuccessful. Overcome with misery, she burst into tears. Then we tried to determine whether she could repeat very short sentences consisting of the same words found in her prayers. However, she was also unsuccessful in this.

Nevertheless, her memory was excellent. She grasped and understood everything that she saw and heard and she answered questions, even about events in the remote past, by affirmative or negative nods of the head. In her own way, she showed censure or approval of things done badly or well in her household. She attended church, listened to the sermons and claimed that she received great comfort from them. At home she even read the Holy Writ and other theological books but complained that what she read impressed her less and was forgotten more readily than what she heard. The fingers of her right hand were contracted and the whole arm was deprived of movement and warmth but not, however, of feeling.

Otherwise, she has been in excellent health, has a very good appetite, sleeps well and, in spite of her age, menses are regular. Indeed she states that in general she is healthier than she was before. She has given up all medication, since she took a variety of drugs prescribed by the most eminent physicians with her condition remaining the same. She now lives content with her lot.

This case report must be considered to be outstanding. The defects and preserved capacities of the patient are clearly delineated; indeed, the description of her

* Translated by Mrs. Lillian C. Nelson.

language disorder compares favorably with that to be found in most contemporary clinical reports. In referring to his case as one of "rare aphonia," Rommel had in mind, of course, what he considered to be the striking feature of the clinical picture, namely, the discrepancy between the patient's impairment in spontaneous verbal expression and in repetition and her retained capacity for serial speech. Thus he must be given credit for presenting the first descriptive analysis of this commonly encountered aphasic profile.

EIGHTEENTH-CENTURY DESCRIPTIONS

As might be expected, many descriptions of aphasia or allusions to it appeared during the eighteenth century. A number of them are outlined below. No doubt systematic examination of the medical literature of the period would disclose additional instances.

Duc de Saint-Simon (1675–1755).[33] A note by Cullerre[34] called attention to a brief description of an aphasic, in the memoirs of the Duc de Saint-Simon, which possesses a feature of special interest. Among the entries for the year 1718 the following statement about the diplomatist and military leader, the Duc d'Harcourt, appears:

Marshall d'Harcourt finally died on 19 October, at the age of only 55 years. Having been reduced by several apoplectic attacks to the point where he could not utter a single syllable, he would indicate with a pointer the letters of a large alphabet which was set before him and which an ever watchful secretary would accordingly write and form into words. He would do this with all the impatience and despair imaginable.

Cullerre points out that this visual use of the letters of the alphabet to form words is, in a sense, a precursor of the diagnostic test of movable letters employed by Trousseau and other clinicians to determine the status of "internal language" in their aphasic patients. He also remarks that the brief allusion to the intense affective state of the Duc as he coped with the difficulties of expressing his thoughts foreshadows the more detailed observations of Trousseau on this aspect of aphasic behavior.

Gerard van Swieten (1700–1772).[35] Van Swieten's oft-quoted reference to aphasia reads as follows:

I have seen many patients whose cerebral functions were quite sound after recovery from apoplexy, except for this one deficit: In designating objects, they could not find the correct names for them. These unfortunate people would try with their hands and feet and an effort of their whole body to explain what they wanted and yet could not. This disability often remained incurable for many years.

Brief as this description is, it points clearly to the type of aphasic deficit shown by these patients, and one seems to be on safe ground in considering it to be an unmistakable allusion to amnestic aphasia.

Carl Linné (1707–1778).[36] In 1745, Linné published a case report describing the condition of an educated man who, in conjunction with a "sleeping sickness" (cataphora), showed markedly disordered speech. Initially he showed paraphasic disturbances, speaking "as it were, a foreign language, having his own names for all words, e.g., to drink *To Ti*, etc." After this, it was found that he was incapable of writing any name, even his own or those of his wife and children. If a name which he was apparently trying to say was spoken to him, he would say "yes," but he could not repeat the word, saying "cannot." Yet he seemed to be able to read names with understanding, and "when he wanted to mention the names of any of his colleagues, he pointed to the *Catalogum Lectionum* in which the name was found." The aphasia receded shortly before his death. Linné remarks that the patient had thus lost "first, the memory of all nouns and, second, the ability to express nouns."

An English translation of Linné's report has been published by Viets[12] and a German translation by Külz.[7] As Nils Antoni[13] has pointed out, Linné presents a fairly clear, if brief, description of a paraphasia followed by severe expressive aphasia, including loss of capacity for repetitive speech. The patient retained some capacity for reading. The exact extent to which he could understand oral speech remains questionable; apparently considerable understanding of spoken language was retained. According to Hultgren,[8] the learned patient was Arvid Arrhenius, Professor at the University of Uppsala.

Olof Dalin (1708–1763).[37] In their papers, both Hultgren and Antoni called attention to the fact that, directly proceeding Linné's communication in the proceedings of the Royal Swedish Academy of Science, there is another description of aphasia by the historian and litterateur Olof Dalin. It reads as follows:

On a Mute Who Can Sing*

Jon Persson, a farmer's son from Ofvankihl, in the parish of Juleta in Sörmanland, born in 1703, brought up in the usual simple way to know his Christianity and to read; in 1736, after he had been married for three years, he had an attack of a violent illness which resulted in paralysis of the entire right side of the body and complete loss of speech. After almost half a year in bed, he began to move to

* Translated by Prof. Arthur A. Wald.

some degree but he limped and carried his right arm in a sling.

For two years he went to a mineral spring at Juleta parsonage which many people had found to be helpful. However, he did not note any improvement except that he was able to walk more steadily and to pronounce correctly the small but often important word, "yes." However, he gained one advantage, which was later observed and which is the occasion for his present notoriety. He can sing certain hymns, which he had learned before he became ill, as clearly and distinctly as any healthy person. However, it should be noted that at the beginning of the hymn he has to be helped a little by some other person singing with him. Similarly, with the same type of help, he can recite certain prayers without singing, but with a certain rhythm and in a high-pitched, shouting tone. Yet this man is dumb, cannot say a single word except "yes" and has to communicate by making signs with his hands.

To be sure, he has always been somewhat simple-minded and naïve. Yet now, as in the past, he is quite normal in his own way, in his ability to hear and understand, and he is God-fearing, quiet and well behaved.

The vicar of Juleta parish, Joh. Ihering, whose personal and signed statement is the source of my information, has kept him in the vicarage for eight years and has made every effort to determine whether this is a deception or illusion on the part of the man for the purpose of providing himself with food more easily. However, the vicar has found the case to be completely genuine. Parishioners of higher and lower rank offer the same testimony. I have also personally seen this man and have heard him sing.

The strange and varied effects that accompany a stroke are only too familiar. I wish to add nothing to this account other than to make the comment that people who stammer are able to sing without impediment and quite distinctly although they cannot utter ten whole words in succession when they speak.

Why Dalin, who was primarily an important literary figure, should have concerned himself with this case and taken the trouble to report it to the Academy becomes understandable when one considers his background. Hultgren points out that he intended to become a physician and actually studied medicine for a time. Exactly why he abandoned his medical studies is not known. The attitude of therapeutic nihilism expressed by his teacher, Stobaeus, may have operated to reduce his interest. His esthetic and emotional sensitivity may have been a determining factor. In all probability, the change was dictated more by an intense love for literature than by any animus against medicine, for Dalin maintained his interest in science and medicine throughout his life. He was elected a member of the Academy of Science in 1742 and served as its president in 1749.

Dalin's description is of interest in demonstrating, as did the earlier case report of Rommel, that the capacity for serial speech may be obtained by a patient with motor aphasia even when he has lost all other aspects of expressive language. It is of particular interest because of the specific reference to singing, which is, in essence, melodic serial speech. Apparently the patient retained understanding of spoken language to a considerable degree, but here, as in so many case reports, it is impossible to judge whether there was a significant loss in this area as well. Dalin's remarks about the ability of stammerers to sing with fluency suggests that this phenomenon had been observed before and that he was merely calling it to the attention of the reader.

Giovanni Battista Morgagni (1682–1771).[38] Morgagni's great De Sedibus ... , published in 1762, includes numerous brief descriptions of cases of speechlessness associated with apoplexy, head injury, and cerebral disease in which autopsy study disclosed injury or disease of the brain. They possess three noteworthy features. The first is the frequency

with which Morgagni took pains to point out that, although the patient could not talk, he was able to understand spoken language.

But before the thirtieth day, the fever came on again with a coldness: and to this was added, about the thirty fourth day, an apoplectic affection, with a loss of speech, and a privation of motion in the whole right side of the body, though the sense remained at the same time. However, she show'd by nods and signs that she understood what was said.

· · ·

But many errors in diet being committed, and some febrile accessions having already preceeded, about the eleventh day a very violent epileptic convulsion attack'd him: and when this remitted, the patient did not speak: although he signified that he understood what others said.

· · ·

... he scarcely spoke at all, and when he did, he stammer'd; but he answered in such a manner, by nods and signs, to those who ask'd him questions, that you might perceive his internal senses to be strong and perfect.

The second noteworthy feature of Morgagni's work is that, as would be expected in the De Sedibus, his clinical descriptions are supplemented by the findings of autopsy. These examinations showed that various types of cerebral lesion—trauma, vascular accident, and tumor—could be associated with paralysis and motor speech impairment.

The third characteristic of his observation which deserves mention is the frequency with which motor speech disorders are described in concurrence with right hemiplegia and subsequent autopsy evidence of disease or injury of the left cerebral hemisphere. Morgagni amassed considerable clinicopathologic evidence in support of the association between paralysis of one side of the body and the presence of disease in the opposite cerebral hemisphere, and he discussed the matter at some length. On the basis of this, Ebstein[27] concluded that Morgagni (and his master, Valsalva) had established the relationship between aphasia, right hemiplegia and disease of the left cerebral hemisphere. He writes: "These extracts are quite sufficient to indicate that not only does clinical and autopsy observation of contralateral innervation originate with Valsalva and Morgagni but also the association of right hemiplegia with speech disorders. In the future we can speak frankly of the Valsalvi-Morgagni doctrine or law."

There seems to be little doubt that Ebstein overstates the case for Morgagni. Incidental description without interpretation does not amount to discovery. Despite the frequency with which motor speech disorder and right hemiplegia appear together in his descriptions and his clear appreciation of crossed innervation, there is no evidence whatever that Morgagni actually correlated aphasia with right hemiplegia or with lesions in the left cerebral hemisphere. Possibly the best evidence that he drew no conclusions about the relationship between aphasia and right hemiplegia (or left hemisphere disease) is the fact that, although the *De Sedibus* was one of the most widely used medical works for several decades after its publication, not only in the original Latin but also in English, French, and German translations, it does not seem to have suggested this relationship to its many readers.

Morgagni's descriptions are typically brief, and the exact nature of the expressive speech disorders which he mentions is never quite clear. In our search, we have encountered no description of a deficit in the understanding of speech which is sufficiently specific to suggest sensory aphasia.

Johann Gesner (1738–1801).[39] Gesner

devoted a section of about 75 pages to the subject of "Die Sprachamnesie" in the second volume (1770) of his *Samlung von Beobachtungen aus der Arzneygelahrtheit*. In it he presents a number of descriptions of aphasic patients, based on either his personal observations or those of older writers, as well as a discussion of the psychopathology of these conditions.

The first case (later cited by Crichton[40] and Falret[1]) is one of jargon aphasia. A 73-year-old man had a seizure in which he experienced a cramp in the muscles of the mouth and at the same time "an itch like the crawling of ants which he tried to eliminate by rubbing." About two weeks later there was a sudden onset of a confusional state which was accompanied by "a very peculiar impairment of speech." He articulated fluently but uttered incomprehensible neologisms. He had no paralysis but did show a slight unsteadiness in gait. He also wrote jargon and his written words corresponded phonetically to the words as pronounced. He could not write his name nor could he read. Nevertheless, it was evident that he was not grossly demented and retained his understanding of objects in the environment. He was aware of the fact that he was speaking jargon.

The second case report summarizes a description by Wepfer of a middle-aged man, who showed a pronounced impairment in memory immediately following a sleeping sickness of nine days' duration. He seemed to have forgotten past events and for a period of some weeks failed to recognize his wife and children. He could not read, although his vision was unimpaired. In due time, however, he recognized his family, was able to recite the Lord's Prayer and the Psalms and to read some words, being more successful in Latin than in German. He would often write whole lines and paragraphs in an elegant hand, but what he wrote made no sense. By means of gestures and isolated words he was able to convey that he recognized his friends, but he could not call them by name. He was concerned about household affairs and would offer "advice" to his wife in the form of many meaningless words. Often he would start a conversation, speaking reasonably and clearly, and then falter in the middle of it. All other abilities were found to be unimpaired.

The third case report describes the condition of an abbot who, just as he was about to give some instructions to a peasant, found himself unable to do so. The impairment lasted for three days. He could recognize objects but could not read. There were no sensory or motor deficits. He improved gradually, but as late as the eighth day it was noted that he would still use inappropriate words in conversation. He could recite the Lord's Prayer fluently but faltered when he attempted longer psalms or songs. In due time, he partially regained the ability to read, the degree of recovery being greater for Latin than for German. He himself felt that he had suffered some decline in judgement, in the ability to calculate, and in the capacity for understanding the speech of others.

The next case is one taken from the writings of Friedrich Hoffmann. A man found himself afflicted with a sudden loss of memory. He could not speak, read, or write but was able to understand what others said to him. He retained his memory for past events and was able to indicate that a physician should be sent for.

There follows a description of an elderly patient whose tongue became paralyzed. After a day of treatment (Spanish flies and venesection) he began to speak again, "but he used the same words to name various objects, words that seemed to come from a foreign language." During the course of the next few weeks he improved to the point that he could read newspapers with understanding. However, he could not read aloud.

The final case report concerns a patient who was personally observed by Gesner. After a severe stroke, a teacher found that, although he recognized letters and words, he invariably misspoke when he read them aloud. He was aware of the deficit, remarking: "I know this letter and realize that I have seen and spoken it countless times; yet when I want to say it aloud, I say something else. This has made me so disturbed and bitter that I do not like to attempt it any more." Nevertheless, his understanding of what was said or read aloud to him seemed to be completely intact.

Gesner's discussion of the psychopathology of these conditions is quite lengthy, has many interesting features, and deserves more detailed consideration than can be given it here. Very briefly stated, he attributes the language deficits not to general intellectual decline or to a loss of memory "in general," as was the habit of some older writers, but to a specific impairment in verbal memory. This impairment in memory consists in the inability to associate images or abstract ideas with their expressive verbal symbols. Paraphasic substitutions occur when the idea which the patient has in mind is a vivid one and he has a strong need to express it. Thus, when a patient utters a neologism or an inappropriate word, he is manifesting a forgetting of speech and not a disorder in thinking or understanding. The basic cause of these language deficits is disease of the brain which reflects itself in a weakness or inertia of the relationships between the different parts of that organ.

It is evident that Gesner's contribution to the clinical and theoretical aspects of aphasia was a major one. His case descriptions indicated clearly that expressive aphasia could not be interpreted as merely a paralysis of the tongue or any other organ. He showed that jargon aphasia was typically accompanied by jargon agraphia and that there could be a phonetic correspondence between the two modalities of expression. As in the previous case reports of Rommel and Dalin, it is noted that the capacity for serial speech may be retained by a patient who shows gross impairment in the other aspects of expressive language. That one deals here with distinctive language deficits, and not with a generalized disorder in thinking, is repeatedly emphasized.

Gesner's theoretical analysis also represented a major advance in thinking about aphasia. He was the first to advance the idea that the basic psychopathology of these disorders consists in a failure to associate image or idea with linguistic sign. This concept was destined to become the basic idea underlying the views of most nineteenth century clinicians concerning aphasia.

Jean Paul Grandjean de Fouchy (1707–1788).[41] Hoff, Guillemin, and Geddes[16] have called attention to this early self-observation of a transitory paraphasia. At the time of the incident (1783), de Fouchy, a man of broad interests and many talents, was 76 years old. The directly pertinent lines in his account, which is translated in full by Hoff, Guillemin, and Geddes, read as follows:

Toward the end of dinner, I felt a little increase of pain above the left eye, and in that very instant I became unable to pronounce the words that I wanted. I heard what was said, and I thought of what I ought to reply, but I spoke other words than those which would express my thoughts, or if I began them I did not complete them, and I substituted other words for them. I had nevertheless all movements as freely as usual. . . . I saw all objects

clearly, I heard distinctly what was being said; and the organs of thought were, it seemed to me, in a natural state. This sort of paroxysm lasted about a minute.

Johann Joachim Spalding (1714–1804).[42] This description, by an eminent German theologian, of his experiences during an episode of paraphasia and dysgraphia was reported in 1783. A translation of it appeared in Alexander Crichton's "Inquiry into the Nature and Origin of Mental Derangement"[40] and was reprinted in Forbes Winslow's "On the Obscure Diseases of the Brain and Disorders of the Mind."[43] In 1950, Eliasberg[15] presented a fresh English translation in a paper on the "prehistory" of aphasia.

Spalding relates how, after a rather busy morning, he had begun to write a receipt for some monies received and discovered that he could not continue after having written the first two words, "for I could not recollect the words which belonged to the ideas I had in mind." Exerting every effort, he started to write again slowly and deliberately, only to find that he was writing words other than those intended. Turning to the person who was waiting for the receipt, he could not express himself clearly but managed by a combination of monosyllables and gestures to get him to understand that he was not to wait fot the receipt. There followed "a tumultous disorder in my senses, in which I was incapable of remarking anything in particular, except that one series of ideas forced themselves involuntarily on my mind. . . . I endeavoured to speak, in order to discover whether I was capable of saying anything that was connected, but although I made the greatest efforts of attention, and proceeded with the utmost caution, I perceived that I uniformly spoke other words than those I intended. My mind was as little master of the organs of speech, as it had been before of my hand in writing."

According to Spalding's estimate, this state of affairs lasted about half an hour and was followed by a period of about the same duration during which he felt constrained to speak slowly and deliberately. By afternoon he was sufficiently recovered to be able to write the description which was subsequently published.

Spalding's self-description is an extremely interesting one but did not add anything that was essentially new to the fund of existing knowledge. As Eliasberg has pointed out, a theoretical explanation of the deficits was attempted by the philosopher, Moses Mendelssohn.[44]

Samuel Johnson (1709–1784).[45] Ogle[6] was probably the first medical writer to call attention to Dr. Johnson's description of the aphasic and agraphic disturbances accompanying his stroke, which occurred about 3 o'clock in the morning of June 17, 1783. In a letter (June 19, 1783) to Mrs. Thrale, he wrote:

On Monday the 16. I sat for my picture and walked a considerable way without inconvenience. In the afternoon and evening I felt myself light and easy, and began to plan schemes of life. Thus I went to bed, and in a short time waked and sat up as has long been my custom, when I felt a confusion and indistinctness in my head which lasted, I suppose about half a minute; I was alarmed and prayed God, that however he might afflict my body he would spare my understanding. This prayer, that I might try the integrity of my faculties I made in Latin verse. The lines were not very good, but I knew them not to be very good, I made them easily, and concluded myself to be unimpaired in my faculties.

Soon after I perceived that I had suffered a paralytick stroke, and that my Speech had been taken from me. I had no pain, and so little dejection in this dreadful state that I wondered at my own apathy, and considered that perhaps death itself when it should come, would

excite less horror than seems now to attend it. . . .

I then wrote a card to Mr. Allen, that I might have a discreet friend at hand to act as occasion should require. In penning this note I had some difficulty, my hand, I knew not how nor why, made wrong letters. . . . I have so far recovered my vocal powers, as to repeat the Lord's Prayer with no very imperfect articulation. My memory, I hope, yet remains as it was.

Johnson seems to have recovered quickly from these impairments in speech and writing. However, examination of printed versions of the letters which he wrote after the stroke shows occasional repetition of words, suggesting that recovery from the dysgraphia may not have been complete. That his ability to write varied from time to time may be inferred from a letter written (in a clear hand) on May 10, 1784, to June Langton, which begins: "I am sorry that your pretty Letter has been so long without being answered: but when I am not pretty well, I do not write plain enough for young ladies." Critchley's[46] detailed analysis of Johnson's writing, which is based on photocopies of his letters before and after the stroke, should clarify this question.

Ryklof Michel van Goens (1748–1810).[47] Van Goens, a philologist and classical scholar, contributed a description of a case of paraphasia to Volume VII (1789) of the *Magazin für Erfahrungsseelenkunde*. The report was subsquently summarized by Crichton[40] and Forbes Winslow.[43] The patient, who was the wife of the professor of mathematics at the University of Utrecht, was herself a mathematician and astronomer. The pertinent passages in van Goens' report[47] are as follows:

After an illness, she suddenly was afflicted with a forgetting, or, rather, an incapacity or confusion of speech. ... If she desired a chair, she would ask for a table; if she wished to have a book she would ask for a glass. If one said to her the desired word, for which she had substituted another, she could not repeat it.

Sometimes she herself had perceived that she misnamed objects; at other times, she was annoyed when a *fan*, which she had asked for, was brought to her, instead of the *bonnet*, which she thought she had requested. This unusual disorder persisted for several months.

Her speech was generally confused and rather clumsy, but her amnesia applied only to certain words. Otherwise, her memory was sufficiently intact that she continued to manage the household. She was able even to show her husband the position of the stars on a chart as correctly as when she had been completely well. She recovered gradually and has enjoyed the full use of her mental powers for several years.

Marcus Herz (1747–1803).[48] This case report by Herz, a prominent physician and intellectual figure of his time in Berlin, was published in 1791 and was quoted by Crichton[40] and Forbes Winslow.[43] It was summarized by Eliasberg,[15] who interpreted the patient's disorders as being due to a "combination of subcortical aphasia with conduction aphasia." The English version in Crichton's book (which we have compared with the original and found to be essentially accurate) runs as follows:

In August 1785, I was called to an officer of the artillery, a man about 40 years old, who, as I was informed, was seized with a palsy in consequence of cold and violent anger. His tongue, hands, and feet were lamed by the attack. He was under the care of one of our first physicians, at whose desire I was consulted concerning the propriety of using electricity. From the time that this remedy was first employed until the following year, I never saw him; but then he sent for me again, as his own physician, he said, had deserted him.

I found him so much recovered as to have the complete use of his feet; his hands were

also much stronger; but in regard to his speech, the following very remarkable circumstance was to be observed. He was unable to articulate distinctly any words which either occurred to him spontaneously, or when they were slowly and loudly repeated to him. He strenuously exerted himself to speak, but an unintelligible kind of murmur was all that could be heard. The effort he made was violent and terminated in a deep sigh. On the other hand, he could read aloud with facility. If a book, or any written paper, was held before his eyes, he read so quickly and distinctly, that it was impossible to observe that there was the slightest fault in his organs of speech. But if the book or paper was withdrawn, he was then totally incapable of pronouncing one of the words which he had read the instant before. I tried this experiment repeatedly, not only in the presence of his wife, but of many other people. The effect was uniformly the same.

It is difficult to see how this patient's condition can be accounted for by postulating a "combination of subcortical motor aphasia with conduction aphasia." We doubt the justification of considering him a case of aphasia at all. Taking all the recorded facts into consideration—the bilateral paralysis and "paralysis of the tongue" which followed some kind of emotional upset, which lasted for a year, and which was apparently cured in large part by "electricity," together with the peculiar combination of absolute incapacity for spontaneous or repetitive speech, and complete fluency in reading aloud—we think that the weight of evidence favors a diagnosis of hysteria.

Johann Wolfgang von Goethe (1749–1832).[49] Goethe's description of motor aphasia, which appears in "*Wilhelm Meisters Lehrjahre*" has been cited and quoted many times (cf. Coupland,[3] Jastrowitz,[4] Ebstein,[5] Riese[14]). The novel was first published in 1795, and it is surmised that Goethe's experience with aphasia was based on the fact that his maternal grandfather, Johann Wolfgang Textor, had a stroke with right hemiplegia and aphasia as residuals. The relevant passage reads in one English translation[49] as follows:

But, unfortunately, this happiness was but of short duration; my father was suddenly seized with palsy, which attacked his right side, and deprived him of the power of speech. We were obliged to guess at everything he wanted, for he never expressed the words which he intended to utter. Oftentimes this was to me fearfully distressing, particularly upon occasions when he insisted upon being left alone with me—he would signify, by violent gestures, that every other person should retire; but when we were left together, he found himself unable to express his thoughts. His impatience then became extreme, and his distress was deeply afflicting. This much seemed certain—that there was something which he was anxious to confide to me of the utmost importance to myself. I cannot express the anxiety which I felt to know it. Formerly I could see his wishes in his eyes—but this was no longer the case. His eyes no longer spoke.

This brief description of motor aphasia is sufficiently specific to identify the disorder as such. The incapacity of the patient to express himself, his emotional reaction to his disability, and his use of gesture to communicate are presented clearly enough. However, in the light of what we know about earlier descriptions of aphasia, it seems obvious that Goethe's account is no way outstanding and hardly worthy of being singled out for special mention. It is certainly incorrect to claim any priority for it as the first adequate or near-adequate description of aphasia or to suggest that Goethe might be "actually considered the discoverer of the speech center."[50]

Alexander Crichton (1763–1856).[40] In his book, Crichton discusses what he calls "a very singular defect of memory,"

which "ought rather to be considered as a defect of that principle, by which ideas, and their proper expressions, are associated, than of memory; for it consists in this, that the person, although he has a distinct notion of what he means to say, cannot pronounce the words which ought to characterize his thoughts." In addition to citing Gesner's first case as an illustration of the deficit, Crichton also reports a personally observed case of paraphasia.

The first case of this kind which occurred to me in practice was that of an attorney, much respected for his integrity and talents, but who had many sad failings, to which our physical nature too often subjects us. Although nearly in his 70th year, and married to an amiable lady much younger than himself, he kept a mistress whom he was in the habit of visiting every evening. The arms of Venus are not wielded with impunity at the age of 70. He was suddenly seized with a great prostration of strength, giddiness, forgetfulness, insensibility to all concerns of life, and every symptom of approaching fatuity. His forgetfulness was of the kind alluded to. When he wished to ask for any thing, he would constantly make use of some inappropriate term. Instead of asking for a piece of bread, he would probably ask for his boots; but if these were brought, he knew they did not correspond with the idea he had of the thing he wished to have, and was therefore angry; yet he would still demand his boots or shoes, meaning bread. If he wanted a tumbler to drink out of, it was a thousand to one he did not call for a certain chamber utensil; and if it was the said utensil he wanted, he would call it a tumbler or a dish. He evidently was conscious that he pronounced wrong words for when the proper expressions were spoken by another person, and he was asked if it was not such a thing he wanted, he always seemed aware of his mistake, and corrected himself by adopting the appropriate expression. This gentleman was cured of his complaint by large doses of valerian, and other proper medicines.

Crichton's description of paraphasia is clear enough but added little to the knowledge already gained from older case reports. However, it is noteworthy that, like Gesner (with whose work he was familiar), Crichton characterized the deficit as being one not merely of memory but, rather, of the associative bonds between ideas and their linguistic expression.

COMMENT

In the elucidation of clinical phenomena, accurate recognition and adequate description usually precede formulations about causation and pathogenesis. Aphasia is no exception to this rule. As this historical survey shows, the published literature on aphasia before 1800 was primarily, but not exclusively, descriptive. Taken in its totality, the literature constitutes what was "known" about aphasia in 1800, i.e., what a well-informed student *would* know about aphasia. This body of knowledge may be analyzed from three standpoints—the clinical manifestations of aphasia, conceptions of its essential psychopathology, and ideas about its neuropathologic basis.

Clinical manifestations

As we have seen, the oldest descriptions referred merely to "speechlessness," usually complete, sometimes partial. From a reading of these descriptions, it is usually not possible for one to be confident that the described conditions represented forms of motor aphasia rather than of anarthria. Perhaps the first clear (but extremely brief) reference to aphasic disorders is that of Guainerius (1481), with his citation of one patient who knew only three words, and of another, who rarely could recall the names of people, although presumably he could talk. The first unmistakable description of a motor aphasia (in the form of paraphasia) seems to be that

of Schmidt (1673). This was soon followed by Rommel's (1683) superb account of a patient who was incapable of spontaneous or repetitive speech but who could recite prayers and verses. The earliest unmistakable allusion to amnestic aphasia is that of van Swieten (1742). The coincidence of aphasia and agraphia was observed by Linné (1745). Gesner (1770) contributed the first adequate descriptions of jargon aphasia, showed that it could be accompanied by jargon agraphia, and described differential impairment in reading in patients who knew Latin as well as their native language. Alexia was mentioned by Valerius Maximum and Pliny, but was first adequately described by Schmidt. The case reports of Dalin (1745), van Goens (1789), and Crichton (1798) provided descriptions of various clinical features of aphasia, such as unawareness of the disability and the intense affective reactions to frustration which are so often observed. A number of interesting self-descriptions, most notably that of Spalding (1783), had been published.

In brief, almost all the clinical forms of aphasia—complete motor aphasia, paraphasia, jargon aphasia, agraphia, and alexia—had been described before 1800. The unawareness of defect which may accompany paraphasia and jargon aphasia had been noted, as well as the coincidence of aphasia and agraphia. Retention of capacity for serial speech (in the form of recital of prayers and of singing) when spontaneous, conversational, and repetitive speech was gravely impaired had been remarked. Differential impairment in reading one language as compared with another and characteristic frustration reactions had been described.

The one major form of aphasia which seems to have been missed is sensory aphasia in the form of impairment in comprehension of oral speech. To be sure, Gesner mentioned the self-evaluation of one of his patients to the effect that he had suffered some impairment in understanding the speech of others. However, beyond this, there is no mention of specific impairment in speech comprehension in the early literature. Indeed, quite often emphasis was placed on the patient's retained capacity for understanding spoken language within the setting of defective expression of speech (cf. Rommel, Morgagni, Dalin, Gesner).

A number of possible reasons may be suggested for this failure to identify sensory aphasia as such. Gross lack of comprehension of oral language was probably interpreted either as a manifestation of dementia or as a loss of hearing. Less severe impairment in comprehension possibly went unrecognized because of the patient's retained capacity to respond appropriately to simple questions and requests. On the basis of our current understanding of jargon aphasia, it must be assumed that the patients of Gesner and Crichton did in fact have receptive deficits which escaped attention. It may be noted that sensory aphasia remained virtually unrecognized as a specific language deficit for another three-quarters of a century, until the appearance of Wernicke's monograph, in 1874.

The milder forms of agrammatism or syntactic aphasia, as manifested in telegraphic speech, alterations of intonation, and syntactical poverty, are also not mentioned in the early literature.

Psychopathologic conceptions

The earliest interpretation of severe motor aphasia was that it was due to paralysis of the tongue. In cases of expressive language deficit, in which it was obvious that the action of the tongue and the other peripheral speech organs were unimpaired, recourse was had to a global explanation of "loss of memory." Alexia

was interpreted as a partial loss of memory, one that was restricted to letters. Linné characterized his patient's paraphasia and subsequent Broca-type aphasia as a loss of memory for nouns and an inability to express them.

Gesner's (1770) more specific conception that paraphasia and jargon aphasia were due to an interruption in the connections between an image or an idea and its expressive linguistic sign constituted a notable advance in theorizing about expressive aphasic disorders. The same idea was presented by Crichton (1798). Developed in greater detail, this conception formed the basis for the classical theory of aphasia which was developed in the nineteenth century and which, it must be said, still guides the thinking of many clinicians, despite the cogent criticisms of such men as Jackson, Head, Pick, and Goldstein.

Neuropathology

From the earliest times it was recognized that aphasic disorders were due to disease or injury of the brain or, at least, of the ventricles. The differentiation of such centrally determined speech deficits from those caused by peripheral factors seems to have been made quite early (e.g., by Soranus), although one cannot be absolutely certain on this point. At any rate, the distinction was clearly made by Renaissance physicians. In due time it was observed that aphasic disturbances were often asociated with stroke or convulsions and that they could occur as a consequence of trauma, fever, vascular accident, or tumor. The clinicopathologic correlations of Morgagni provided incontrovertible evidence of these relationships.

The association of aphasia with right hemiplegia was not remarked, despite the repeated incidental observation of the clinical combination of aphasia and dextral paralysis. This relationship escaped the notice of even so keen and careful a student as Morgagni, who had had the opportunity of observing so many instances of this concurrence. The failure to make this correlation was not, of course, peculiarly distinctive of medical observation before 1800. Scores of aphasic patients with dextral paralysis must have been observed during the first 60 years of the nineteenth century. Yet, with the exception of Marc Dax, no clinician noted the association until Broca's demonstrations in 1861 forced recognition of it.

When one asks why this relationship, which now seems so obvious to us, escaped the attention of earlier observers, a reasonable answer would appear to be that such a correlation did not make "sense." Nor does it make "sense" even today. In spite of the theoretical speculations which have been advanced to explain the association, it remains a "low-order" relationship, established by empirical observation and admittedly of tremendous clinical importance. Yet its basic psychoneurologic significance still eludes us.

Nor, with one exception, did the early workers attempt neuropathologic localization of aphasia along the anterior-posterior dimension of the brain—a question which only a short time later Gall and Bouillaud were to raise so forcefully. The exception is represented by the few remarks of Guainerius (1481), who ascribed the aphasia of his elderly patients to an excessive accumulation of phlegm in the posterior ventricles, deducing this from the premise that the "organ of memory" was in this region.

In conclusion, this analysis of the literature on aphasia from the Hippocratic writings to 1800 shows that the early contributions to the subject were not quite as few as is often assumed to be the case. A substantial amount of clinical knowledge had been gained by the beginning of the nineteenth century. This body of knowledge, which was created for the most part by contributions in the seventeenth and eighteenth centuries, was elaborated and augmented in the first half of the nineteenth century, as clinical information accumulated and an interest in the problem of localization developed. However, it does not appear that the *basic* character of this body of knowledge was altered by the contributions of the first half of the nineteenth century. Instead, there seems to have been a continuous and gradual development of the field until the latter half of the nineteenth century, when the intense interest in aphasic disorders which followed Broca's discovery introduced new conceptions and created an incomparably richer corpus of knowledge.

SUMMARY

This survey of the literature on aphasia from the Hippocratic writings to 1800 indicates that:

1. Most of the clinical forms of aphasia (e.g., motor aphasia, jargon aphasia, amnestic aphasia, alexia, agraphia) had been described and certain common features of aphasic disorders (e.g., retention of capacity for serial speech, concurrence of jargon aphasia and jargon agraphia, unawareness of disability) had been noted. However, sensory aphasia had not been recognized as a specific entity.

2. It was known that aphasia could occur as a consequence of various diseases of the brain, but no important ideas about localization had been advanced.

3. The thesis that the basic psychopathology of aphasic disorders was an interruption in the connections between images or ideas and their linguistic signs had been advanced.

4. The outstanding early contributions appear to be those of Johann Schmidt (1673) on alexia, of Peter Rommel (1683) on motor aphasia, and of Johann Gesner (1770) on jargon aphasia and the theory of aphasic disorders.

REFERENCES

1. Falret, J.: Des troubles du language et la mémoire des mots dans les affections cérébrales, Arch. gén. med. 3: 336–354, 591–609, 1864.
2. Trousseau, A.: Clinique médicale de l'Hôtel Dieu de Paris, Ed. XII, Paris, J.-B. Baillière et Fils, 1931.
3. Coupland, S.: Description of Aphasia by Goethe, Brit. M.J. 1: 19, 1874.
4. Jastrowitz, M.: Historische Notiz über Aphasie, Berl. klin. Wchnschr. 12: 323, 1875.
5. Ebstein, E.: Goethes Anteil an der Lehre von der Aphasie, Ztschr. ges. Neurol. u. Psychiat. 17: 58–64, 1913.
6. Ogle, J. W.: Part of a Clinical Lecture on Aphasia, Brit. M.J. 1: 163–165, 1874.
7. Külz, E.: Zur Geschichte der Aphasie, Berl. klin. Wchnschr. 12: 699, 1875.
8. Hultgren, E. O.: Historiska Notiser i Afasiläran, Svenska läk.-sällsk. Förhandl. 42: 1022–1037, 1916.
9. Bernard, D.: De l'aphasie et de ses diverses formes, Paris, Lecrosnier et Babé, 1889.
10. Soury, J.: Le système nerveux central: structure et fonctions: histoire critique des théories et des doctrines, Paris, Carré et Naud, 1899.
11. Gans, A.: Über einen im Anfang des 18. Jahrhunderts von Dr. Peter Rommel klassisch beschriebenen Fall von transcorticaler motorischer Aphasie, Ztschr. ges. Neurol. u. Psychiat. 24: 480–482, 1914.
12. Viets, H. R.: Aphasia as Described by Linnaeus and as Painted by Ribera, Bull. Hist. Med. 13: 328–329, 1943.
13. Antoni, N.: "En lärd man i Upsala," Opuscu. med. 2: 153–160, 1957.
14. Riese, W.: The Early History of Aphasia, Bull. Hist. Med. 21: 322–334, 1947.
15. Eliasberg, W.: A Contribution to the Prehistory of Aphasia, J. Hist. Med. 5: 96–101, 1950.
16. Hoff, H. E., Guillemin, R., & Geddes, L. A.: An 18th Century Scientist's Observation of His Own Aphasia, Bull. Hist. Med. 32: 446–450, 1958.
17. Adams, F.: The Genuine Works of Hippocrates, Baltimore, Williams & Wilkins Company, Inc., 1939.
18. Jones, W. H. S.: Hippocrates, New York, G. P. Putnam's Sons, 1923–1931.
19. Chadwick, J. & Mann, W. N.: The Medical Works of Hippocrates, Oxford, Blackwell Scientific Publications, 1950.
20. Kempf, K.: Valerii maximi factorum et dictorum memorabilium libri novem, Leipzig, B. G. Teubner, 1888.
21. Holland, P.: The Historie of the World, Commonly Called the Natural Historie of C. Plinius Secundus, London, 1601.
22. Drabkin, I. E.: Caelius Aurelianus: On Acute Diseases and on Chronic Diseases, Chicago, University of Chicago Press, 1950.
23. Creutz, W.: Die Neurologie des 1–7. Jahrhunderts nach Chr., Leipzig, Georg Thieme, 1934.
24. Patrick, M. M.: Sextus Empiricus and Greek Scepticism, Cambridge, Deighton Bell & Co., 1899.
25. Guainerio, A.: Opera medica, Pavia, Antonius de Carcano, 1481.
26. Baverius de Baveriis: Consiliorum de re medica sive morborum curationibus liber, Argentinae, Libraria Balthasari Pistoris, 1543.
27. Ebstein, E.: Das Valsalva-Morgagnische Gesetz: ein Beitrag zur Vorgeschichte der Aphasie, Deutsche Ztschr. Nervenh. 53: 130–136, 1915.
28. Massa, N.: Epistolarum medicinalium tomus primus, Venetiis, ex Officina Stellæ Iordani Zilleti, 1558.
29. Arceo, F.: A Most Excellent and Compendious Method of Curing Woundes in the Head, London, Thomas East for Thomas Cadman, 1588.
30. Schenck a Grafenberg, J.: Observationes medicæ de capite humano, Lugduni, 1585.
31. Schmidt, J.: De oblivione lectionis ex apoplexia salva scriptione, Miscellanea curiosa

medico-physica Academiae naturae curiosorum 4: 195–197, 1676.

32. Rommelius, P.: De Aphonia Rara, Miscellanea curiosa medico-physica Academiae naturae curiosorum 2(Ser. 2): 222–227, 1683.

33. Saint-Simon, L.: Mémoires, Paris, Gallimard, 1958.

34. Cullerre, A.: Un aphasique au XVIIIe siècle, Chronique Médicale, 13: 300, 1906.

35. Van Swieten, G.: Commentaria in Hermanni Boerhaave Aphorismos, de cognoscendis et curandis morbis, Lugduni, J. & H. Verbeek, 1742–1746.

36. Linnaeus, C.: Glömska of alla substantiva och isynnerhet namn, K. Swenska Wetensk. Acad. Handlungen 6: 116–117, 1745.

37. Dalin, O.: Berättelse om en dumbe, som kan siunga, K. Swenska Wetensk. Acad. Handlingar 6: 114–115, 1745.

38. Morgagni, G. B.: The Seats and Causes of Diseases Investigated by Anatomy, translated by Benjamin Alexander, M. D., A. Millar & T. Cadell, London, 1769.

39. Gesner, J. A. P.: Samlung von Beobachtungen aus der Arzneygelahrtheit und Naturkunde, Nördlingen, C. G. Beck, 1769–1776.

40. Crichton, A.: An Inquiry into the Nature and Origin of Mental Derangement, Comprehending a Concise System of the Physiology and Pathology of the Human Mind and a History of the Passions and Their Effects, London, T. Cadell, Jr., and W. Davies, 1798.

41. Grandjean de Fouchy, J. P.: Observation anatomique, Histoire de l'Académie Royale des Sciences, Mémoires, 399–401, 1784.

42. Spalding, J. J.: Ein Brief an Sulzern über eine an sich selbst gemachte Erfahrung, Magazin für Erfahrungsseelenkunde, 1(Pt. 1): 38–43, 1783.

43. Winslow, F.: On the Obscure Diseases of the Brain, and Disorders of the Mind, Ed. 4, London, John Churchill & Sons, 1868.

44. Mendelssohn, M.: Psychologische Betrachtungen auf Veranlassung einer von dem Herrn Oberkonsistorialrat Spalding an sich selbst gemachten Erfahrung, Magazin für Erfahrungseelenkunde 1(Pt. 3): 46–75, 1783.

45. Chapman, R. W.: The Letters of Samuel Johnson, with Mrs. Thrale's Genuine Letters to Him, Oxford, Clarendon Press, 1952.

46. Critchley, M.: Dr. Johnson's Aphasia, Medical History, 6: 27–44, 1962.

47. van Goens, R. M.: Einige Beispiele von Geistes- oder Gedächtnissabwesenheit, Magazin für Erfahrungsseelenkunde 7(Pt. 3): 77–80, 1789.

48. Herz, M.: Wirkung des Denkvermögens auf die Sprachwerkzeuge, Magazin für Erfahrungseelenkunde 8(Pt. 2): 1–6, 1791.

49. Goethe, J. W.: Wilhelm Meister's Apprenticeship, translated by R. Dillon Boylan, London, Bell and Daldy, 1871.

50. Bryk, O.: Entwicklungsgeschichte der reinen und angewandten Naturwissenschaft im XIX Jahrhundert, Leipzig, J. A. Barth, 1909.

3.

Bergson and Freud on Aphasia: A Comparison*

In this paper I plan to outline the views that Henri Bergson and Sigmund Freud advanced about the nature of aphasic disorders in the 1890s, to consider how their views differed from prevailing concepts, and to assess the impact that their positions had on subsequent thinking about aphasia. To begin with, we need to review the status of aphasia theory in 1890, that is, what was known about the aphasic disorders and what ideas about their basic nature were generally accepted.

That loss of speech could follow injury to the brain was known at the time of ancient Greek medicine and probably even before then. Through the centuries, a fairly substantial literature describing the features of the speech disorders associated with brain disease accumulated (see Benton & Joynt, 1960; Benton, 1964, 1981). By 1850, most of the aphasic syndromes familiar to us today had been described,

for example, expressive aphasia with relative preservation of the capacity to understand speech, amnesic aphasia with word-finding disturbance, jargon aphasia and jargon agraphia, and isolated loss of the ability to read. The distinction between a fluent type of aphasic disorder (characterized by disordered speech) and a non-fluent type (characterized by poverty of speech and difficulty in articulation) had also been made. The lack of awareness of defect shown by some patients with jargon speech and the unequal loss of proficiency in different languages in polyglot patients had been noted. Impairment of speech with preserved ability to sing had been described, too. Franz Joseph Gall had postulated the existence of centers for speech articulation and word memory in the frontal lobes and his localization was the subject of rather acrimonious debate during the first half of the nineteenth century.

Still aphasia was scarcely a subject of great interest to either practicing physicians or medical scientists. The disorder had no specific diagnostic significance,

* Paper presented by A. L. Benton at the Interdisciplinary Conference on Bergson and Modern Science, University of Texas Medical Branch, Galveston, Texas, February 9–11, 1984.

nor was it possible to correlate it in any meaningful way with brain function. But when, in the early 1860s, Paul Broca established the association between expressive speech disability and focal lesions in and around the third frontal gyrus of the left hemisphere, aphasia became a major topic in neurological medicine. To physicians, Broca's discovery demonstrated that a specific disability could have specific implications about the condition of the brain and, hence, that it could possess a specific diagnostic significance. To physiologists, the association between a behavioral deficit and a limited cerebral lesion suggested that the brain could, indeed, be divided into defined areas, each with its distinctive functional properties. And it was this possibility that provided a powerful impetus for intensive experimental study of localization of brain function in the 1870s and 1880s.

Broca coined the term *aphemia* to designate the nonfluent expressive speech disorder that he had correlated with left frontal lobe disease. He contrasted it with the fluent speech disorder that was then know as word amnesia and that had as its most prominent feature word-finding difficulty and paraphasic utterances, that is, the incorrect use of words. Aphemic patients understand what is said to them and are not devoid of ideas. However, because of an impairment in the coordination of the movements of speech, they cannot express their ideas in words. Amnesic patients are also not devoid of ideas, but they have lost knowledge of the conventional relations between ideas and words. Because they have lost their appreciation of the symbolic value of words, they cannot understand what is said to them and use words inappropriately in their own speech. However, neither form of aphasic disorder involves a disturbance of thinking as such, and both should be

distinguished from mental deterioration in which condition patients are speechless because, as Broca phrased it, "of a lack of ideas to express."

Broca himself was not greatly concerned with the neurological mechanisms underlying speech and its disturbance. It was left to a younger physician, Carl Wernicke, to develop a mature theory of the nature of aphasic disorders. In a monograph that appeared in 1874, Wernicke demonstrated that fluent aphasic disorder, characterized by impaired understanding of speech and disordered expressive speech, was specifically associated with disease in the territory of the posterior temporal lobe of the left hemisphere. Like Broca, he conceived of aphasia as a disorder of the sign function of language. He denied that aphasic patients were necessarily impaired in intellect, even though, as a clinician, he knew that many aphasics (perhaps a majority) did, in fact, show cognitive defects that extended beyond the realm of language. But he insisted that "nothing could be worse for the study of aphasia than to consider the intellectual disturbance associated with aphasia as an essential part of the disease picture."

However, Wernicke went beyond his empirical discovery and his restriction of aphasia to a disorder of the sign function of language to create a model of the neurological mechanisms, derangements of which produced aphasic disorder. His model—and the revisions of it developed by other neurologists—postulated the existence of interconnected cerebral centers of speech in which memory-images of the different modalities of speech were stored. A center for memory-images of the movement patterns of expressive speech was located in Broca's area in the posterior frontal region. A center for auditory memory-images of words was located in Wernicke's area in the posterior temporal lobe. A center for visual memory-images of words was located farther back in the angular gyrus. Whether or not there was a specific center for memory-images of the movement patterns of writing was a subject of debate. Those who believed in the existence of such a center placed it either in the second frontal gyrus above Broca's area or in the supramarginal gyrus close to the center for visual memory-images of words.

The diverse symptom-pictures of aphasia encountered in clinical practice were explained in terms of either a lesion in one or more centers (i.e., the central aphasias) or a lesion in the connections between them (i.e., the conduction aphasias). A lesion in Broca's area resulted in a loss of motor memory-images and, hence, produced a primarily expressive aphasia with preservation of the capacity to understand speech. A lesion in Wernicke's area resulted in a loss of auditory-verbal memory-images and, hence, produced impairment in the understanding of speech. A lesion in the connections between Wernicke's area and Broca's area resulted in a distinctive symptom-picture in which patients were able to understand speech (because the center for auditory-verbal memory-images was intact), but their speech was disordered and they were unable to repeat what was said to them (because there was defective transmission of information from the auditory-verbal center to the motor speech center). And so on.

This was the dominant theory of the nature of aphasic disorder that was almost universally accepted by neurologists in the 1890s. Aphasia was a disturbance in the utilization of words as signs of ideas with no necessary impairment in intellect. The neurological basis of speech and language consisted of specific cortical areas in which verbal memory-images were stored. Aphasia was pro-duced by lesions in these areas or in the connections between them.

In later years, these models of the neurological basis of language and its disorders were derided as empty diagram making that bore no relationship to clinical reality. In fact, they were not as unreal or sterile as their critics made them out to be. They achieved some notable successes in deducing the existence of aphasic symptom-pictures that were not known at the time but that were later validated by clinicopathologic study. Moreover, despite their limitations, they exemplified a scientific approach to aphasia that generated empirically testable hypotheses. Thus, Lichtheim (1885), a leading diagram maker, wrote " . . . whether our interpretations are correct or not will be determined by further observations . . . we must not hesitate to draw the consequences deducible from our hypotheses. The more we do so the sooner we will gain information to correct them, or if necessary, abandon them, if this is what the findings indicate. An erroneous view may be of value."

But the models did encounter serious difficulties. Many observations on aphasia and its neurological basis could not be accommodated by them. And they were unacceptable on a more fundamental level. They purported to elucidate the neural mechanisms underlying normal speech and language by postulating the existence of limited cortical areas, the cells of which were the repository of memory-images or representations of word sounds and speech movements. This seemed incomprehensible to some thoughtful students of the nervous system who refused to believe that the neural elements comprising these limited cortical areas could be endowed with such extraordinary capacities. It was not that they believed in the functional equipotentiality of all parts of the cerebral hemispheres. Nor did they deny the facts of clinical localization of brain lesions. But they were convinced that the model builders had fallen into the error of confusing a symptom with a function. The British neurologist, Hughlings Jackson, made this point succinctly when he warned that "to locate the lesion which destroys speech and to locate speech are two different things."

Jackson was one of the few neurologists in the 1870s and 1880s who opposed the assumptions, formulations, and conclusions of the associationist theory held by the leading neurologists of the time—Wernicke in Germany, Charcot in France, and Bastian in England. First, he denied that aphasia could be defined as a loss of words, instead, it was an impairment in the utilization of words in thinking. He distinguished between two levels of speech: automatic (or emotional) speech and intellectual speech. Typical aphasics retain their capacity for automatic speech (e.g., as reflected in oaths and recurring meaningless utterances). At the same time, they lose the capacity to make meaningful verbal statements (propositions, Jackson called them) either to others or to themselves. Jackson held that the basic unit of language is not the word, as was assumed by the associationists, but the proposition, the meaningful statement. It is at this level that speech becomes "a *part* of thought," and it is at this level that aphasic defect manifests itself. Consequently, he said, those forms of thought that require, or are facilitated by, inner verbalization will of necessity be impaired in the aphasic patient.

Thus Jackson opposed the prevailing associationist theory at every major point. There were no cortical centers of language but only focally situated lesions that impaired language. Aphasia was not a loss of words as signs of thought but a disturbance in verbal thinking itself. Aphasic patients have words at their disposal, but they can use them only at the lower level of automatic speech, not at the higher level of propositional speech.

For a number of reasons, Jackson's views did not attract much attention, even in Britain, and Continental neurologists scarcely knew of their existence. However, one person who did read Jackson's papers with interest and appreciation was a young Viennese neurologist by the name of Sigmund Freud.

Freud was 35 years old when he wrote his monograph *The Interpretation of the Aphasias* in 1891. This was two years before he and Josef Breuer presented their preliminary communication on hysteria and four years before publication of the famous Breuer/Freud monograph on hysteria. With the possible exception of a brief unsigned entry on aphasia in a medical encyclopedia (Villaret, 1888), Freud had not written on the topic before. This did not deter him from undertaking to write a major critique of the dominant theory of the nature of aphasia as reflected in the work of its most authoritative proponents, Carl Wernicke and Ludwig Lichtheim. In so doing, he followed the recommendation of Lichtheim. He examined the clinical facts of aphasia and compared them with the deductions emerging from centrist theory. Finding that the deductions did not fit the facts, he proposed a different formulation.

Having outlined Wernicke's original model and Lichtheim's more elaborate models, Freud developed his critique. His first point was that although the models predict aphasic performance patterns in which a specific function is completely lost and other functions are completely intact, in fact, the typical clinical picture is one in which all the different speech functions are impaired to a greater or lesser degree. A second weakness of the models, he said, was that they fail to account satisfactorily for certain aphasic symptom-pictures that are encountered in clinical practice. Here, Freud cited an example that had been offered by Lichtheim himself, namely, the fact that motor aphasics are often alexic, that is, they show a specific impairment in understanding what they read.

He then went on to deny the validity of the fundamental distinction between central aphasias and conduction aphasias postulated in the models. Influenced by physiological evidence that isolation of a central area from the rest of the brain produces the same effect as excision of that area, he concluded that "the destruction of a so-called center comes about only through simultaneous interruption of several fiber tracts." As had previous authors, he criticized the concept of a center as a specific central area in which memory-images were stored and pointed out the confusion engendered by this mixing of anatomic and psychic entities. He concluded that all aphasic disorders were conduction aphasias, not in the restricted Wernicke/Lichtheim sense but in the broader sense that they were produced by interruptions in the neural connections within the brain.

Freud did not deny that lesions in the so-called centers, that is, Broca's area, Wernicke's area, and the angular gyrus, produced different aphasic symptom-pictures. But the reason for this specificity was not a peculiar functional endowment of these areas but the circumstance that they were intimately related to specific cortical sensory and motor regions: Broca's area with motor cortex, Wernicke's area with auditory cortex, and the angular gyrus with visual cortex. It was, thus, understandable that lesions in these areas could lead to distinctive aphasic syndromes.

At the same time, Freud laid great stress on a functional, as opposed to a purely morphological, approach to apha-

sia. He cited Bastian's (1887) schema of three levels of reduced excitability of cortical areas: the least severe being one in which the area responds to direct sensory stimulation as well as stimulation from other areas but not to volitional influences; the most severe being one in which the area is completely unresponsive. He went on to postulate that the functional state of all areas of the brain entered into the determination of aphasic symptom-pictures, and he adopted "as a guiding principle Hughlings Jackson's doctrine that all these modes of reaction represent instances of functional retrogression (dis-involution) of a highly organized apparatus, and therefore correspond to earlier states of its functional development. This means that under all circumstances an arrangement of associations which, having been acquired later, belongs to a higher level of functioning, will be lost, while an earlier and simpler one will be preserved." And he linked Bastian's three levels of excitability to the Jacksonian doctrine.

Thus, Freud's basic conception was that the neural mechanism of speech was located in a definite but continuous cortical region that was bounded at one end by the auditory and visual receptive fields and at the other end by the frontal motor areas. Therefore, disease or injury in this region destroys communication between various parts of it as well as with the rest of the brain. A limited number of aphasic symptom-pictures occur, depending on the locus and severity of injury. Above all, Freud said, aphasic disorders result not from a loss of memory-images but from impairment of the speech apparatus as a whole.

Every point that Freud made already had been made by one or another earlier writer. The concept of centers of speech had been criticized by Hughlings Jackson. The significance of the intimate anatomic relationship of Broca's area, Wernicke's area, and the angular gyrus territory to the primary motor and sensory areas of the cortex had been pointed out as early as 1869 by the British physician, Moxon. Trousseau (1864, 1877) and Finkelnburg (1870) as well as Jackson had insisted that aphasia involved an intellectual change that transcended the mechanisms of speech expression and reception. Freud's real achievement was to organize all these points into a coherent, carefully reasoned critique that could be used to formulate an alternative conception of the basis and nature of aphasic disorder.

Henri Bergson was 37 years old when he addressed the nature of aphasic disorder in his book *Matière et mémoire*, which was published in 1896. Thus, he was about the same age as Freud when the latter wrote his monograph on the topic. However, Freud as a neurologist was interested in aphasia for its own sake, whereas Bergson as a philosopher was interested in the disorder primarily as a source of empirical data that could be used in understanding the relationship between mind and matter or, more specifically, between the mind and the brain. Thus, Bergson approached aphasia from the vantage point of his rejection of psychophysical parallelism in its absolute form; his insistence on the unity of memory, perception, and action; and his view that the brain constitutes a mechanism for the initiation of purposeful motor action rather than being a storehouse of "pure" or "real" memories.

He mounted an eloquent attack on the concept that the brain is a storehouse of memory images and on the explanation of aphasic "forgetting" in terms of a loss of these memory-images from destruction of the cortical centers in which they are stored. Pointing out that the same word is pronounced differently by different speakers and, hence, that there must be countless memory-images of it in the brain, he asks readers whether they can really believe that all these memory-images are stored there. He reminds readers that these memories are conceived as fixed entities and, thus, that it is difficult to imagine how the brain might select a single one for storage and, if it does, how it matches a new perception of a word with its memory-image. Thus, in Bergson's view, the explanation of aphasia as a loss of memory-images is quite untenable.

Citing the familiar clinical observation that aphasics have maximal difficulty in producing proper names and least difficulty in producing verbs, with common nouns occupying an intermediate position in this hierarchy of difficulty, he advanced his own concept of the nature of aphasic disorder, namely, that it is a functional disturbance, an impairment in the capacity to actualize memories. To be recalled, memories (which are never lost) require a mental attitude in intimate connection with a bodily attitude. Because verbs generally express actions, their recall is facilitated by physical effort and aphasic patients can engage in such an effort in their attempts to produce them. In contrast, proper nouns are fairly remote from bodily activity and physical effort cannot facilitate their recall. The influence of bodily activity is also seen when patients who are unable to produce the name of an object describe its mode of action.

Above all, verbal understanding is an active, selective process. It is primarily concerned with sentences (i.e., Jackson's propositions), which have structure and carry meaning, and not with isolated words. The failure of aphasic patients to understand what they hear or see is a failure in function. It is a failure to achieve a complete perception, which by definition includes a coalescence with past experience. Such a complete perception is the product of intellectual effort, for it involves reconstructing the continuous flow of speech into a meaningful message. Thus, there is an intrinsic intellectual component in the aphasic patient's failure to understand speech. On the expressive side, aphasia is not a mere failure to utilize words as signs of thought but, instead, a specific arrest in thinking that leads to a verbal deficiency.

Bergson's thought coincides with that of Freud on a number of major points. It is obvious that both writers rejected the notion that the cerebral cortex serves as a repository of memory-images and that aphasia results from a destruction of these memory-images by organic disease. Both maintained that the clinical facts of the localization of the lesions causing aphasia do not justify localizing normal language processes in limited cortical areas. Both viewed aphasia from a functional standpoint as reflecting a breakdown in the efficient operation of a complicated neural mechanism. Both insisted that perception and memory (association in Freud's terminology) form a single process.

There is, however, a fundamental difference in the conceptions of the nature of aphasia held by the two men. Freud did not lay great stress on the role of intellectual factors in the disorder, except that, by definition, aphasia had to be considered a specific cognitive disability. To Bergson, aphasia was above all an expression of a basic impairment in intellectual activity, of an incapacity to engage the body in the realization of intentions.

It is clear that Bergson's concepts had a significant influence on subsequent thought about aphasia in France. In 1906, that is, ten years after the publication of *Matière et mémoire*, the French neurologist, Pierre Marie, wrote a series of papers under the title, "Revision of the Question of Aphasia." In these papers, he attacked the prevailing notions about the lesional localization of aphasic disorders as well as the pluralistic concept of discrete types of aphasia. Maintaining that, in fact, there was only one basic aphasic disorder, he insisted that it always involved an impairment of intelligence. Marie was not very specific about the characteristics of the aphasic patient's defect in intelligence; apparently, what he had in mind was an inability to cope with diverse tasks that were outside the sphere of language, an intellectual passivity and a lack of initiative.

Marie's papers created a furor in French neurological circles and over the next few years a series of spirited, at times, rancorous debates took place. In the end, Marie's views won a large following, and the idea that at least the major forms of aphasic disorder involved some degree of impairment of intelligence was generally accepted. This was scarcely Bergsonism, but it was an important fragment of it. Jules Dejerine, the other major figure in French neurology at the time, also came to accept the proposition that aphasia involves a defect in intelligence. So far as I am aware, neither Marie nor Dejerine mentioned Bergson in their writing. But *Matière et mémoire* was widely read, and some commentators have classified Marie as "the neurological disciple" of Bergson (see Ombredane, 1951; Hécaen & Angelergues, 1965). Aspects of Bergson's thought were later reflected in the writing of a number of neurologists such as Van Woerkom (1921, 1923), Mourgue (1920–1921), Goldstein (1924), and J. Lhermitte (1938), all of whom emphasized impairment in intellectual functions, particularly spatial thinking and abstract reasoning, as a cardinal feature of the symptom-picture of aphasia.

The influence of Freud's 1891 monograph is problematic. It is stated that only 257 copies were sold over a ten-year period, and that the book was totally neglected (see Jones, 1953). If this is so, there is an odd fact associated with the monograph that calls for explanation. In discussing the necessity for distinguishing between failure to name an object and failure to recognize it, Freud coined the term *agnosia* to denote the failure in recognition, and he proposed its use. Not many years passed before his suggestion was generally adopted and agnosia replaced older terms such as mindblindness, psychic blindness, and psychic deafness to designate the disability. Thus, Freud's monograph could not have been completely overlooked. In any case, the views he expressed are certainly found in later writing on aphasia.

Henri Bergson was scarcely a specialist in the field of aphasia. He was not a physician, he had no firsthand experience with aphasic patients, and his knowledge of the field came entirely from his analysis of the literature. Surprisingly, to a considerable degree, the same can be said of Sigmund Freud. Although he was a neurologist, it does not appear that he had had much actual experience with aphasic patients. His monograph contains no descriptions of patients he had personally examined and cared for. Thus, like Bergson, he based his formulation entirely on his analysis of the literature. Would firsthand experience with aphasic patients have caused either to modify his conclusions? The chances are that it would not. What a clinician sees, or at least deems worthy of note, in his assessment of aphasic patients is determined, in large part, by his own preconceptions. In any case, despite whatever possible handicap may have been imposed by their lack of clinical experience, their superb intellectual gifts enabled Bergson and Freud to make contributions that have a secure place in the history of clinical neuropsychology.

REFERENCES

Bastian H. C. On different kinds of aphasia. *British Medical Journal* 1887, 2, 931–936, 985–990.

Benton A. L. Contributions to aphasia before Broca. *Cortex* 1964, 1, 314–327.

Benton A. L. Aphasia: historical perspectives. In *Acquired aphasia* (M. T. Sarno, ed.). New York, Academic Press, 1981.

Benton A. L. and Joynt R. J. Early descriptions of aphasia. *Archives of Neurology* 1960, 3, 205–222.

Bergson H. *Matière et mémoire*. Paris, Alcan, 1896.

Broca P. Remarques sur le siège de la faculté du langage articulé, suivies d'une observation d'aphémie. *Bulletin de la Société Anatomique* 1861, 6, 330–357.

Broca P. Localisation des fonctions cérébrales: siège du langage articulé. *Bulletin de la Société d'Anthropologie* 1863, 4, 200–203.

Broca P. Du siège de la faculté du langage articulé. *Bulletin de la Société d'Anthropologie* 1865, 6, 337–393.

Finkelnburg F. C. Niederrheinische Gesellschaft: Sitzung vom 21. März in Bonn. (Also published as Finkelnburg's 1870 lecture on aphasia with commentary, R. J. Duffy & B. Z. Liles [Trans.] *Journal of Speech and Hearing Disorders* 1979, 44, 156–168.

Freud S. *Zur Auffassung der Aphasien*. Leipzig und Wien, Deuticke, 1891. (Also published as *On aphasia*, E. Stengel [Trans.] New York, International Universities Press.

Goldstein K. Das Wesen der amnestischen Aphasie. *Schweizer Archiv für Neurologie und Psychiatrie* 1924, 15, 163–175.

Hécaen H., & Angelergues R. *Pathologie du langage*. Paris, Larousse, 1965.

Jackson J. H. On affections of speech from disease of the brain. *Brain* 1878, 1, 304–330.

Jones E. *The life and work of Sigmund Freud*. New York, Basic Books, 1953.

Lhermitte, J. Langage et mouvement. *Encéphale*, 1938, 33, 1–26.

Lichtheim L. On aphasia. *Brain* 1885, 7, 433–485. (Originally published in *Deutsches Archiv für klinische Medizin* 1885, 36, 204–268.)

Marie P. Revision de la question de l'aphasie: la troisième circonvolution frontale gauche ne joue aucun rôle spécial dans la fonction du langage. *Semaine Médicale* 1906, 26, 241–247.

Marie P. Revision de la question de l'aphasie: que faut-il penser des aphasies sous-corticales (aphasies pures)? *Sémaine Medicale* 1906, 26, 493–500.

Marie P. Revision de la question de l'aphasie: l'aphasie de 1861 à 1866: essai de critique historique sur la genèse de la doctrine de Broca. *Sémaine Medicale* 1906, 26, 565–571.

Mourgue R. Aphasie et psychologie de la pensée. *Encéphale* 1920, 15, 649–664; 1921, 16, 26–33, 85–91.

Moxon W. On the connexion between loss of speech and paralysis of the right side. *British and Foreign Medical Chirurgical Review* 1866, 74, 481–489.

Ombredane A. L'aphasie et l'elaboration de la pensée explicite. Paris, Presses Universitaires de France, 1951.

Trousseau A. De l'aphasie, maladie décrite récemment sous le nom impropre d'aphémie. *Gazettes des Hôpitaux* 1864, 37, 13–14, 25–26, 37–39, 48–50.

Trousseau A. *Clinique médicale de l'Hôtel-Dieu de Paris*, Ed. 5. Paris, Baillière et fils, 1877.

Van Woerkom W. La signification de certains éléments de l'intelligence dans la genèse des troubles aphasiques. *Journal de Psychologie Normale et Pathologique* 1921, 18, 730–751.

Van Woerkom W. Sur l'état psychique des aphasiques. *Encéphale* 1923, 18, 286–304.

Villaret A. *Handwörterbuch der gesamten Medizin*. Stuttgart, Enke, 1888.

Wernicke C. Der Aphasische Symptomenkomplex. Breslau, Cohn and Weigert, 1874.

II.
Cerebral Localization and Hemispheric Dominance

4.

The "Minor" Hemisphere*

The purpose of this paper is to sketch the early development of the idea that the "minor" hemisphere in man (i.e., the right hemisphere in right-handed persons) possesses distinctive functional properties with respect to the mediation of behavior in analogy to the predominant role of the left hemisphere with respect to language. The idea of a minor hemisphere derives, of course, from the broader concept of "cerebral dominance" which arose as a consequence of the discovery by Broca of a specific association between motor aphasia and disease of the left frontal lobe.[1] Soon after the validity of Broca's correlation was confirmed, it became evident that other forms of aphasic disorder, such as impairment in language understanding, disturbances in naming, and loss of reading ability, were related to disease of the left temporal and parietal areas. Inferring the positive from the negative, students of human cerebral function readily concluded that, at least in right-

handed persons, language behavior was mediated primarily (if not necessarily exclusively) by neural mechanisms located in the left hemisphere.

The concept of left hemisphere dominance was applied at first only to language functions. However, as continuing clinical study indicated that the left hemisphere apparently subserved a number of other aspects of mentation and cognition, the concept was broadened considerably. To begin with, there was the observation that many aphasic patients showed impairment in intellect which clearly extended beyond their language disabilities. This was a point made by Trousseau as early as 1864,[2] and its confirmation fostered the conception (held by many authorities in the field) that "true" aphasia always involved a particular impairment in mentation, an impairment principally involving abstract reasoning and the use of symbols in thought. Thus Hughlings Jackson spoke of the aphasic patient as being "lame in his thinking,"[3] Pierre Marie of a defect in higher-level intellectual skills,[4] and Kurt Goldstein of a loss of the

* A. L. Benton, *Journal of the History of Medicine and Allied Sciences*, 1972, 27, 5–14.

capacity for "categorical behavior."[5] Acceptance of this generalization led inevitably to the conclusion that the left hemisphere must be "dominant" with respect to these distinctively human capacities for reasoning and symbolic thinking as well as for language functions in the strict sense.

A further extension of the concept of left hemisphere dominance took place at the beginning of the twentieth century when the Berlin neurologist Hugo Liepmann established apraxia as a distinctive category of behavioral deficit that might be shown by patients with cerebral disease.[6] In addition to his analysis of these disturbances in the execution of purposeful movement-sequences, Liepmann was able to show that at least one major type which he had described, ideomotor apraxia, resulted from lesions of the left hemisphere. Some twenty years later, Karl Kleist described the form of visuoconstructive disability which he called "constructional apraxia";[7] he localized the responsible lesion in the posterior parietal area of the left hemisphere, a region in which visual and proprioceptive information was presumably integrated so that visual guidance of action was made possible.

In the 1920s, Josef Gerstmann described "finger agnosia," i.e., inability to recognize or name the fingers of either hand.[8] Combining this rather peculiar deficit with three other types of behavioral impairment (right-left disorientation, agraphia, and acalculia) into a syndrome, he maintained that his syndrome could occur as a consequence of focal cerebral disease, its locus being in the region of the angular gyrus of the left hemisphere. His explanation was that certain aspects of the bilateral body image find their cerebral representation in the parieto-occipital area of the dominant hemisphere.

These diverse observations coalesced to emphasize the specific importance of the left hemisphere in providing the neural substrate not only for language behavior but also for conceptual thinking, higher-level praxis and orientation to one's body. At the same time, they fostered the idea that the left hemisphere was the "major" hemisphere insofar as the mediation of higher-level cognitive behavior was concerned.

The designation of the left hemisphere as "major" implied, of course, that the right hemisphere was the minor hemisphere. In this context, the term "minor" evidently had a number of interrelated meanings. First, it indicated that, in accord with the doctrine of contralateral innervation, the right hemisphere mediated motion and sensation on the opposite side of the body; in this respect, it was functionally equivalent to the left hemisphere. Secondly, it meant that the right hemisphere was subordinate to the left in subserving language performances. This was not to say that the right hemisphere did not participate at all in language, but rather that under normal conditions, the left hemisphere was the "leading" hemisphere with the right hemisphere playing the role of a minor (and for the most part silent) partner.

The latter conclusion was derived primarily from observation of the language behavior of aphasic patients. It had been noted that, although these patients were incapable of truly propositional language, they did produce automatic, interjectional, and emotional speech; these positive features of an aphasic's language behavior were interpreted as reflecting the operation of mechanisms in his unaffected minor hemisphere. The observation was also made that under special conditions (e.g., in a stressful situation) an aphasic patient might produce perfectly intelligible propositional speech which he could not utter under ordinary circumstances. It was presumed that this speech was produced by the minor hemisphere. This meant that, in the course of language learning, verbal engrams were laid down in the right hemisphere as well as in the left. These minor hemisphere engrams remained inactive because of the specialization of the major hemisphere for language.

The same explanation was applied to account for recovery from aphasic disorder, the assumption being that the right hemisphere had taken over the function of mediating language performances. Since recovery often took place over the course of a few weeks or months, it seemed clear that the minor hemisphere must have participated in the original learning of language. In short, the study of aphasic patients brought forth facts which appeared to be consonant with the idea that the dominance of the left hemisphere for language was of a relative rather than absolute nature. Thus the designation of the right hemisphere as "minor" seemed quite appropriate.

Finally, the term "minor," as applied to the right hemisphere, implied that it had no distinctive functions. It shared certain functional properties with the left hemisphere but, at least with respect to higher-level performances, whatever it could do, the left hemisphere could do better.

However, almost from the very birth of the concept of hemispheric cerebral dominance, there were clinicians who opposed the prevailing opinion that the right hemisphere was merely a weaker version of the left and who insisted that it also possessed distinctive functional properties. The evolution of this trend of thought, as reflected in the publications of the relatively few neurologists, ophthalmologists, and psychologists who advanced the idea over a period of about seventy years (from 1874 to 1941), will be sketched.

The pioneer figure in this movement to give the right hemisphere its due was the British neurologist Hughlings Jackson. In 1874 he published a paper in which he surmised that, while the left hemisphere was specialized with respect to expressive speech functions, the posterior area of the right hemisphere played a crucial role in visual recognition and visual memory.[9] He conceded that the evidence for his generalization was not strong. However, two years later, he was more sure of his ground when he published a case report describing a patient with a tumor in the temporo-occipital region of the right hemisphere.[10] "I diagnosed tumour, and tumour of the right posterior lobe, I may here remark, from the following facts—the kind of mental defect and from its preceding the hemiplegia, from the hemiplegia being left-sided, and because the arm suffered less than the leg" (p. 434).

The "kind of mental defect" shown by Jackson's patient consisted in visual disorientation, failure to recognize persons and dyspraxia for dressing. He designated this constellation of disabilities as "imperception" and argued that it was as specifically characteristic of disease of the posterior right hemisphere as impairment in expressive speech was of disease of the anterior left hemisphere.

Some thirty years later, the German neurologist Conrad Rieger, in all probability unaware of Jackson's thinking, advanced roughly the same idea. In a monograph which appeared in 1909 he postulated the existence of two distinct and interacting "apparatuses" (as he called them) in the brain, one subserving verbal-conceptual functions and the other subserving spatial-practical functions.[11] Pursuing this idea, his student Martin Reichardt concluded from clinico-pathological observations that the spatial "apparatus" was located primarily in the posterior right hemisphere while the verbal "apparatus" was, of course, located in the left hemisphere.[12]

During the same period there were observations in the field of ophthalmology which pointed to the possibility that the right hemisphere played a particularly important role in subserving certain aspects of visual perception. In the 1880s and 1890s, disturbances in spatial orientation, as reflected in loss of geographical memory, difficulty in locating objects in space, and inability to find one's way from one place to another, were topics of considerable interest to ophthalmologists.[13] The fact that this disability might be shown by patients suffering from focal cerebral disease and with intact central visual acuity indicated that it was a "higher-level" disorder and not simply an expression of sensory defect or significant intellectual impairment. The classic case report of Foerster in 1890, describing a patient who first showed a right homonymous hemianopia without complicating disturbances following a stroke and who, after a second stroke, showed a double hemianopia and spatial disorientation with preservation of central vision and intellect, did much to establish the prevailing trend of thinking about the necessary and sufficient conditions for the appearance of visuospatial disorientation, namely, that it could be caused by a focal occipital lesion, but only one which was bilateral in nature and which therefore entailed a loss of visual memory images.[14]

However, this view was challenged by a few ophthalmologists who were impressed by the frequency with which impairment in topographic memory appeared to be associated with disease of the right hemisphere. The first to do so was Thomas D. Dunn who described a patient with a double hemianopia, intact central vision, and "loss of the sense of

location" but without impairment in other aspects of visual memory, such as the recognition of faces.[15] Dunn therefore rejected the hypothesis that a general "loss of recollection of optical images" was the underlying disability. The circumstance that his patient showed defects in topographical orientation only after a second stroke which resulted in a left hemianopia being superimposed on a preexisting right hemianopia led him to postulate "a centre (which may, for convenience, be named the geographic centre) on the right side of the brain for the record of the optical images of locality, analogous to the region of Broca for that of speech on the left side in right-handed persons" (p. 54). Dunn's hypothesis did not fare well in the hands of the eminent ophthalmologist De Schweinitz, who discussed his paper when it was presented at a meeting of the College of Physicians of Philadelphia.[16] In fact, De Schweinitz did not even deign to mention it but instead advanced the view

that the loss of orientation, which has been a marked feature in fully 50 per cent. of the cases of double hemianopsia thus far reported, may be, and, indeed, has been, explained by the greatly contracted visual field, the patient being unable properly to locate landmarks within the field of his vision and thus aid his judgment in forming an opinion as to his relation to his surroundings. (p. 55)

A year later, Peters described two patients with visual disorientation, both of whom had only a left homonymous hemianopia.[17] Thus a double hemianopia did not appear to be a necessary precondition for the appearance of an orientation defect. Significantly, Peters remarked that he was at first inclined to ascribe a greater influence to the right hemisphere than to the left in the production of disturbances of orientation. However, he was dissuaded from reaching this conclusion by the circumstance that there were case reports in the literature which were not in accord with it. Some ten years later the problem was taken up again by Lenz in a comprehensive study of hemianopic defects.[18] Emphasizing that visual disorientation was by no means a rare feature of the hemianopias following stroke (12 per cent of his case material), he pointed out that no less than seven of his eight cases of homonymous hemianopia with visual disorientation had a left field defect, i.e., involved a lesion of the right hemisphere. Recalling Peters's earlier observations, Lenz also raised (in a rather diffident way) the question of whether "the right occipital lobe is perhaps more strongly related to orientation than the left."

A rather different line of evidence pointing to the possibility of distinctive properties of the minor hemisphere was initiated by Babinski's description in 1914 of anosognosia in the specific form of unawareness (or denial) of left hemiplegia.[19] As he and other clinicians observed additional cases showing an apparently specific association between this peculiar partial defect of awareness and disease of the right hemisphere,[20] they were led to raise the question of whether a "center" for the integration of somatosensory information with somesthetic memory images might not exist in that hemisphere.

As has been mentioned, it was in the early 1920s that Kleist described constructional apraxia as a distinctive form of behavioral impairment resulting from disease of the left hemisphere.[21] His conception was a fairly precise one. Separating constructional apraxia from other forms of visuoconstructive disability that occur as an expression of impairment in visual perception, he defined it as a disturbance in constructional activity shown by a patient who at the same time has adequate visual form perception and discrimination

and preserved ability to localize objects in visual space. He considered that, in its pure form, the disability was neither perceptual nor motor in nature but rather an impairment in translating intact visual perceptions into appropriate motor action and he conceived of a rupture between visual and proprioceptive processes as providing the basis for its appearance.

The broad descriptive aspects of Kleist's concept were readily accepted by subsequent workers and constructional apraxia became recognized as a type of behavioral deficit which might be shown by a brain-damaged patient. However, his precise formulation of the nature of the disability as being neither perceptual nor motor but instead "connectional" in nature was either denied or ignored and the term "constructional apraxia" was used to designate any visuoconstructive disability, regardless of whether or not it appeared within a setting of impairment of visual perception. A number of clinicians in the late 1920s and early 1930s then made the observation that constructional apraxia in this broad sense was shown by patients with lesions of the right hemisphere and indeed with at least as high a frequency as by those with disease of the dominant hemisphere.[22] They also noted that related visuospatial disabilities occurred with impressively high frequency in patients with right hemisphere disease.[23]

Many of these observations were utilized by the French neurologist Dide in a paper which emphasized the importance of the right hemisphere in the mediation of perceptual and motor performances.[24] Dide outlined what he called the "syndrome of the right parietal area," the cardinal features of which were certain types of sensory and motor impairment, the anosognosia of Babinski, constructional apraxia, and spatial disorientation. He also discussed the question of the cerebral representation of musical abilities as reflected in singing, musical performance, and the recognition of melodies. The prevailing opinion was that, together with language, musical capacities were mediated by mechanisms in the left hemisphere. Nevertheless, over the decades a few clinicians had raised the question of the importance of the right hemisphere for musical functions. Dide allied himself with this group and advanced the view that musical functions depended upon the integrity of the superior temporal gyrus of the right hemisphere, in analogy to the dependence of language functions on Wernicke's area in the left hemisphere.[25] He also insisted that a distinctive type of bilateral somesthetic impairment could result from disease of the right hemisphere.

There were two contributions of a psychometric nature during this early period. The monumental study of aphasia by Weisenburg and McBride included consideration of the performances of a group of nonaphasic patients with right hemisphere disease as well as normal control subjects and the target group of aphasic patients.[26] They found that the right hemisphere patients showed a distinctive pattern of performance with significant impairment in some nonverbal performances while verbal abilities were close to the normal level. They made no explicit inferences but did feel impelled to call attention to the qualitative differences between these patients and both the normal and aphasic groups. In 1939 Hebb described the pattern of test performance of a patient who, after having undergone a large excision in the right temporal lobe, showed superior verbal intelligence but markedly defective performance on visuoperceptive and visuoconstructive tests as well as on a test of tactile form recognition.[27] Contrasting the results with his previous findings on patients with left frontal lobe excisions, Hebb concluded that impairment in both visual and tactile form perception may well be a specific consequence of right temporal lobe defect.

One last clinical contribution in this early period deserves mention. In 1941 Russell Brain published a detailed description of spatial disorientation in patients with massive lesions of the right parietal lobe and concluded "that certain syndromes, notably anosognosia, are seen exclusively or almost exclusively as a result of lesions in the right hemisphere."[28].

DISCUSSION

Viewed in retrospect and taken in their totality, these clinical contributions would seem to have produced at least suggestive evidence for the view that the right hemisphere should not be considered simply as a minor hemisphere with no distinctive functional properties. Yet it is clear that at the time they had no significant effect on prevailing conceptions of hemispheric cerebral dominance. One can conjecture about the probable reasons for this lack of impact. First, the contributions were scattered over a period of seventy years, sometimes with decades intervening between them; consequently they had little cumulative effect. At the same time, a counteractive influence may have been exerted by the much larger body of literature pointing to the paramount importance of the left hemisphere for thinking and perception, as well as for language. Secondly, some reports were not widely disseminated; for example, Jackson's papers were published in journals that were not widely read outside of England and the contribution of Rieger was buried in a monograph with a rather limited circulation. Moreover, some authors (e.g., Peters, Lenz, Weisenburg and McBride) were not prepared to draw conclusions from their observations and such a stance was not likely to encourage others to reflect on the implications of their results. Conversely, some papers, consisting of single case reports and advancing broad generalizations that went far beyond the scanty empirical facts, scarcely constituted evidence that was strong enough to challenge well-established doctrine.

However, these early contributions were not without effect on the next generation of workers, for their influence on O. L. Zangwill and Henry Hécaen, whose studies between 1944 and 1951 initiated the modern period of investigation in this field, is fairly evident. Paterson and Zangwill,[29] in their paper in 1944 on visuospatial deficits associated with right hemisphere disease, cited both the contributions of Brain and Hebb as well as the conclusions of the German neurologist Lange that the right parietal area is of particular importance for the spatial aspects of visual perception. Similarly, in their first papers, Hécaen and Ajuriaguerra called attention to the work of Lange, Dide, and Brain in reporting their own studies of apraxic and visuoconstructive disabilities resulting from lesions of the right hemisphere.[30] Thus, although for the most part ignored at the time when they were published, these pioneer efforts to ascribe distinctive functional properties to the "minor" hemisphere did have an impact on the development of thinking about asymmetry of cerebral hemispheric function in man.

REFERENCES

1. P. Broca, "Remarques sur le siège de la faculté du langage articulé, suivies d'une observation d'aphémie," *Bull. Soc. Anat., Paris*, 1861, 6, 330–357; "Localisation des fonctions cérébrales: siège du langage articulé," *Bull. Soc. Anthrop. Paris*, 1863, 4, 200–203.

2. A. Trousseau, "De l'aphasie, maladie décrite récemment sous le nom impropre d'aphémie," *Gaz. Hôp. Paris*, 1864, 37, 13–14, 25–26, 37–39, 48–50.

3. J. Hughlings Jackson, "On the nature of the duality of the brain," *Med. Press Circ.*, 1874, 17, 19, 41, 63 (reprinted in *Brain*, 1915, 38, 80–103).

4. P. Marie, "Revision de la question de l'aphasie: la troisième circonvolution frontale gauche ne joue aucun rôle spécial dans la fonction du langage," *Sem. Médicale*, 1906, 26, 241–247.

5. K. Goldstein, "Die Lokalisation in der Grosshirnrinde," In A. Bethe, G. von Bergmann, G. Embden, & A. Ellinger, eds., *Handbuch der normalen und pathologischen Physiologie*, Bd. 10, *Spezielle Physiologie des Zentralnervensystems der Wirbeltiere* (Berlin, 1927).

6. H. Liepmann, "Das Krankheitsbild der Apraxie," *Mschr. Psychiat. Neurol.*, 1900, 8, 15–44, 102–132, 182–197.

7. K. Kleist, "Kriegsverletzungen des Gehirns in ihrer Bedeutung für die Hirnlokalisation und Hirnpathologie," In O. von Schjerning, ed., *Handbuch der ärztlichen Erfahrung im Weltkriege 1914/1918*, Bd. IV, *Geistes- und Nervenkrankheiten* (Leipzig, 1923); H. Strauss, "Über konstructive Apraxie," *Mschr. Psychiat. Neurol.*, 1924, 56, 65–124.

8. J. Gerstmann, "Fingeragnosie: eine umschriebene Störung der Orientierung am eigenen Körper," *Wien. klin. Wschr.*, 1924, 37, 1010–1012; "Fingeragnosie und isolierte Agraphie: ein neues Syndrom," *Z. ges. Neurol. Psychiat.*, 1927, 108, 152–177.

9. Jackson (n. 3).

10. J. Hughlings Jackson, "Case of large cerebral tumour without optic neuritis and with left hemiplegia and imperception." *Roy. London Ophthal. Hosp. Rep.*, 1876, 8, 434–444.

11. C. Rieger, "Über Apparate in dem Hirn," *Arb. psychiat. Klin. Würzburg*, 1909, 5, 176–197.

12. M. Reichardt, *Allgemeine und spezielle Psychiatrie: ein Lehrbuch für Studierende und Aerzte*, 3rd ed. (Jena, 1923).

13. A brief historical account of these developments is presented by A. L. Benton,

"Disorders of spatial orientation," in P. J. Vinken & G. W. Bruyn, eds., *Handbook of clinical neurology*, vol. 3, *Disorders of higher nervous activity* (Amsterdam, 1969). Further information is given in: Macdonald Critchley, *The parietal lobes* (London, 1953); C. Faust, *Die zerebralen Herdstörungen bei Hinterhauptsverletzungen und ihre Beurteilung* (Stuttgart, 1955); J. de Ajuriaguerra and H. Hécaen, *Le cortex cérébral* (Paris, 1960); K. Gloning, *Die zerebral bedingten Störungen des räumlichen Sehens und des Raumerlebens* (Vienna, 1965).

14. R. Foerster, "Über Rindenblindheit," *Graefes Arch. Ophthal.*, 1890, *36*, 94–108; a report of the autopsy of Foerster's patient was published by H. Sachs, "Das Gehirn des Förster'schen Rindenblinden," *Arb. psychiat. Klin. Breslau*, 1895, *2*, 55–122.

15. T. D. Dunn, "Double hemiplegia with double hemianopsia and loss of geographic centre," *Trans. Coll. Phycns Philad.*, 1895, *17*, 45–56.

16. G. E. De Schweinitz, discussion of Dunn's paper (n. 15).

17. A. Peters, "Über die Beziehungen zwischen Orientierungsstörungen und ein- and doppelseitiger Hemianopsie," *Arch. Augenheilk.*, 1896, *32*, 175–187.

18. G. Lenz, *Beiträge zur Hemianopsie* (Stuttgart, 1905).

19. J. Babinski, "Contribution à l'étude des troubles mentaux dans l'hémiplegie organique cérébrale (anosognosie)," *Rev. neurol.*, 1914, *22*, 845–848.

20. J. Babinski, "Anosognosie," *Rev. neurol.*, 1918, *25*, 365–367; "Sur l'anosognosie," *Rev. neurol.*, 1923, *30*, 731–732. J. A. Barré, L. Morin, & Kaiser, "Etude clinique d'un nouveau cas d'anosognosie de Babinski," *Rev. neurol.*, 1923, *30*, 500–503; A. Barkman, "De l'anosognosie dans l'hémiplegie cérébrale: contribution clinique à l'étude de ce symptôme," *Acta. med. Scand.*, 1925, *62*, 235–254; E. Joltrain, "Un nouveau cas d'anosognosie," *Rev. neurol.*, 1924, *31*, 638–640.

21. K. Kleist (n. 7).

22. O. Pötzl, *Die Aphasielehre vom Standpunkte der klinischen Psychiatrie*, Bd. 1: *Die optisch-agnostischen Störungen* (Leipzig, 1928); B. Schlesinger, "Zur Auffassung der optischen und konstruktiven Apraxie," *Z. ges. Neurol. Psychiat.*, 1928, *117*, 649–697; J. Lange, "Fingeragnosie und Agraphie," *Mschr. Psychiat. Neurol.*, 1930, *76*, 129–188; M. Kroll & D. Stolbun, "Was ist konstructive Apraxie?" *Z. ges. Neurol. Psychiat.*, 1933, *148*, 142–158.

23. J. Lange, "Agnosien und Apraxien," in O. Bumke & O. Foerster, eds., *Handbuch der Neurologie*, Bd. VI (Berlin, 1936).

24. M. Dide, "Les désorientations temporo-spatiales et la prépondérance de l'hemisphère droit dans les agnoso-akinésies proprioceptives," *Encéphale*, 1938, *33*, 276–294.

25. The first experimental confirmation of the kernel of truth in Dide's rather rash generalization was provided some twenty years later by Brenda Milner. See B. Milner, "Psychological defects produced by temporal lobe excision," *Res. Publ. Ass. Res. nerv. ment. Dis.*, 1958, *36*, 244–257; "Laterality effects in audition," in V. B. Mountcastle, ed., *Interhemispheric relations and cerebral dominance* (Baltimore, 1962).

26. Theodore Weisenburg & Katherine McBride, *Aphasia* (New York, 1935).

27. D. O. Hebb, "Intelligence in man after large removals of cerebral tissue: defects following right temporal lobectomy," *J. gen. Psychol.*, 1939, *21*, 437–446.

28. W. Russell Brain, "Visual disorientation with special reference to lesions of the right cerebral hemisphere," *Brain*, 1941, *64*, 244–272.

29. A. Paterson & O. L. Zangwill, "Disorders of visual space perception associated with lesions of the right cerebral hemisphere," *Brain*, 1944, *67*, 331–358.

30. H. Hécaen & J. de Ajuriaguerra, "L'apraxie de l'habillage: ses rapports avec la planotopokinésie et les troubles de la somatognosie," *Encéphale*, 1945, *35*, 113–143; H. Hécaen, J. de Ajuriaguerra, & J. Massonet, "Les troubles visuoconstructives par lésion pariéto-occipitale droite," *Encéphale*, 1951, *40*, 122–179.

5.

Hemispheric Cerebral Dominance and Somesthesis*

THE CONCEPT OF HEMISPHERIC CEREBRAL DOMINANCE

The historical development of the concept of hemispheric cerebral dominance has been characterized, since its inception about 100 years ago, by both increasing breadth and increasing differentiation. As everyone knows, the concept was "born" in the 1860s with the discovery by Broca of a specific association between motor aphasia and disease of the left frontal lobe. Broca's observation was quickly confirmed. Further clinical study showed that other areas of the left hemisphere played an equally crucial role in the production of aphasic disorders, and the doctrine of the dominance of the left hemisphere for language in right-handed individuals became firmly established, at least from a pragmatic standpoint.

For a number of decades the concept of left-hemisphere dominance was applied

* A. L. Benton in M. Hammer, K. Salzinger, and S. Sutton (Eds.), *Psychopathology: Essays in Honor of Joseph Zubin*. New York, Wiley-Interscience, 1972, pp. 227–242.

only to the language functions. Extension of the concept to cover other aspects of human mentation and behavior began in the early years of the twentieth century, with the work of Liepmann (1900, 1908) establishing "apraxia" as a distinctive category of behavioral deficit shown by patients with cerebral disease. In addition to his analysis of these higher-level psychomotor disorders, Liepmann was able to show that at least one type, so-called ideomotor apraxia, resulted from lesions of the left hemisphere, a correlation that has since been fully confirmed. In the 1920s, Gerstmann (1924, 1927, 1930), having described the peculiar deficit of "finger agnosia," related it and other disabilities (such as right-left disorientation) to disease of the parieto-occipital region of the left hemisphere. Subsequent study has shown that, although Gerstmann's localization was rather too precise, its general import was basically valid in the sense that finger agnosia and associated disabilities are associated far more frequently with disease of the left hemisphere than of the right (Benton, 1959, 1961;

Heimburger, DeMyer, & Reitan, 1964; McFie & Zangwill, 1960). During the same period, there was a strong tendency on the part of such theorists as Head (1926) and Goldstein (1924) to emphasize the defects in abstract reasoning and conceptual thinking associated with aphasic disorders (and therefore, by inference, with disease of the left hemisphere).

These observations extended the concept of dominance of the left hemisphere to cover higher-level praxis, aspects of the body schema, and conceptual thinking, as well as language. At the same time, they fostered the idea that the left hemisphere was the "major" hemisphere insofar as the mediation of human conduct was concerned. Conversely, the right hemisphere was regarded as the "minor" or "subordinate" hemisphere, and indeed large regions of it were sometimes designated as "silent" areas with no obvious functional significance.

However, from the very birth of the concept in the 1860s, there were those who were skeptical of these claims for an exclusive dominance of the left hemisphere and who insisted that the right hemisphere also played a significant role in the mediation of language and other symbolic activities. Hughlings Jackson (1874), for example, placed emotive and automatic speech in the right hemisphere, and there were others who suggested that this hemisphere mediated "musical language," as reflected both in musical performance and in the recognition of melodies. Jackson (1876) was also the first to intimate that the right hemisphere had other distinctive functions, stating his belief that the parieto-occipital region of this hemisphere was particularly crucial for visual recognition and memory.

A later development of a conceptual nature was also of importance in raising the question of right-hemisphere "dominance" for certain functions. In a monograph that appeared in 1909, Rieger postulated the existence of two distinct and separately localized "apparatuses" (as he called them) in the brain, one subserving verbal-conceptual functions and the other subserving spatial-practical functions. Pursuing this idea, Reichardt (1923) surmised on the basis of clinicopathological study that the spatial "apparatus" was located primarily in the posterior right hemisphere, while the verbal "apparatus" was, of course, located in the left hemisphere. There followed a series of studies in the 1940s and early 1950s which provided strong, if not compelling, evidence that such deficits as impairment in visual space perception, constructional apraxia, so-called apraxia for dressing, and unilateral visual inattention occurred with considerably higher frequency in patients with lesions of the right hemisphere than in those with left-hemisphere disease. Thus a new dimension was added to the concept of hemispheric cerebral dominance: it was no longer concerned with a single hemisphere (i.e., the left) but rather was involved with the distinctive functions of each of the hemispheres.

Since that time, investigative work in the field of hemispheric cerebral dominance has been concerned primarily with the problem of identifying and defining the types of performance that appear to possess a differential association with the function of one or the other hemisphere. This work, which for the most part has dealt with linguistic, visual, and auditory performances, has generated a substantial body of knowledge about the role of each hemisphere in the processing of visual and auditory information of various types. Moreover, in recent years the attention of some investigators has turned to the question of whether hemispheric asymmetry in function is also demonstrable in the field of somesthesis. It is this question that is the specific topic of the present chapter.

THE DOCTRINE OF CONTRALATERAL INNERVATION

As is well known, the sensory examination is based on the doctrine of contralateral innervation, namely, that the sensory and motor functions of one side of the body are mediated by (or "represented in") the opposite cerebral hemisphere. This doctrine has a long and interesting history. The clinical facts that suggested it were known as early as 400 B.C., and the first explicit statement of the doctrine was made as early as A.D. 200 by Aretaeus of Cappodocia (Adams, 1856). However, for 1500 years thereafter, the theory was a controversial issue, many physicians preferring other explanations for the observation that a wound on one side of the brain leads to sensorimotor impairment on the other side of the body (cf. Giannitrapani, 1967). However, in the eighteenth century, the experimental demonstrations of Pourfour du Petit (1710) and the clinicopathologic correlations of Morgagni (1769) established the validity of the doctrine beyond any reasonable doubt. Its diagnostic value was then demonstrated by nineteenth-century clinicians, and it became the basis for the sensory examination in neurological diagnosis.

Nevertheless, despite the universal acceptance of the doctrine (which was, of course, fully warranted), exceptional cases that apparently did not follow the rule of contralateral innervation were reported from time to time. Oppenheim (1906), Foix (1922), and Goldstein (1927) described patients with lesions apparently confined to the left hemisphere who showed *bilateral* disturbances in stereognosis. Guillain, Alajouanine, and Garcin (1925) described a left-handed patient

with a lesion of the right hemisphere who showed astereognosis and loss of position sense on the *right* side, in the absence of disturbances of sensitivity to touch and pin prick on that side. Some of these early observers advanced the concept that, although simple sensory performances followed the rule of contralateral innervation, the left hemisphere played a special role in mediating higher-level performances (such as stereognosis and position sense) on *both* sides of the body. Thus, for example, Foix (1922) regarded the ipsilateral defects that he had observed in patients with left-hemisphere lesions as being disturbances of recognition which were of the same order as those seen in visual agnosia, rather than as elementary sensory deficits.

However, in the 1930s other observers (Bychowsky & Eidinow, 1934; Körner, 1938) reported studies of patients with unilateral lesions who showed bilateral disturbances of sensitivity to touch, pressure, pain, and vibration. Moreover, the majority of these patients had lesions of the right hemisphere (thus weakening the concept of a special role of the left hemisphere in the mediation of tactile performances on both sides of the body). The conclusion drawn by these observers was that tactile sensitivity on each side of the body is actually represented in both cerebral hemispheres rather than in only the contralateral hemisphere, as assumed by the traditional conception.

All these reports added up to a mere handful of cases and could scarcely be considered to offer a serious challenge to traditional concepts. However, it should be borne in mind that the apparent paucity of observations of bilateral or ipsilateral tactile deficit in patients with unilateral lesions may have been due to a methodological bias in the sensory examination. This bias consists in utilization of the procedure of comparing sensitivity on the side of the body suspected of being affected with that on the assumedly healthy side, and adopting the findings on the assumedly healthy side as the normative basis for judgments of the presence or absence of deficit on other side. Thus, in the conventional procedure, each patient serves as his own control and a clinical judgment is made without regard to the absolute level of performance on the assumedly healthy side, which may in fact deviate significantly from the group norm. It may be taken for granted that, in practice, gross deviations from normality on the assumedly healthy side would be noted by the examiner, in which case he would conclude that there were in fact bilateral disturbances in tactile sensitivity. But it is equally evident that relatively moderate deviations from normality on the assumedly healthy side might be missed or ignored, particularly in view of the rather crude assessment procedures employed in the typical sensory examination. In these circumstances, a decided difference in level of sensitivity between the two sides of the body would lead to the conclusion of ipsilateral sensory defect when in fact the patient suffered from bilateral disturbances of different degrees of severity on the two sides.

In his classic studies, Head (1920) did not describe bilateral sensory disturbances in any of the patients with unilateral lesions whom he discussed in such great detail. His judgments were made on the basis of a comparison of sensory performances on the two sides of the body. Yet, as Carmon (1969) has pointed out, examination of Head's data shows that, on occasion, thresholds for touch and pin prick which were classified as pathological when they were found on the hand contralateral to the lesion were considered to be normal when they occurred on the ipsilateral hand.

Thus these exceptional cases may not have been so exceptional after all. At the same time, these early observations failed to come to grips with a basic problem in this area, namely, to define tactile impairment explicitly in terms of a quantitative deviation from the expectations based on the performance of normal subjects.

RECENT STUDIES

So much for what may be called the prehistory of this topic. A new era was ushered in by the publication in 1960 of the comprehensive study by Semmes, Weinstein, Ghent, and Teuber of tactile performances in large samples of patients with unilateral lesions as well as in a group of control patients with peripheral nerve injuries involving the lower extremities. Utilizing objective assessment procedures, they examined war veterans with penetrating brain wounds involving either the left or the right hemisphere. The patients were given four somatosensory tests, namely, threshold for light pressure, two-point discrimination, point localization, and threshold for passive movement. The tactile tests were applied to the palm and the proprioceptive test to the middle finger of each hand. Since the two hands were tested independently, the sensitivity of each in the brain-lesioned group could be compared with that of the control group. On the basis of normative observations on the control group impairment was defined empirically as a performance level so poor that it could be expected to occur in the control group only 1% of the time.

Five specific findings in this major study are of particular interest:

1. Many patients with unilateral lesions showed somatosensory disturbance in the *ipsilateral* hand.
2. Ipsilateral defects occurred more frequently in patients with left-hemi-

sphere lesions than in those with lesions of the right hemisphere.

3. In the patients with left-hemisphere lesions, tactile impairment of the contralateral hand appeared to be specifically associated with lesions of the left sensorimotor and posterior parietal areas, that is, it occurred more frequently with lesions of these areas than with lesions of other areas of the left hemisphere. In contrast, no such association was found for the left hand, that is, the observed frequency of tactile impairment in the left hand was not significantly different for lesions in various parts of the right hemisphere. Moreover, this difference in hemispheric relationships held for the ipsilateral, as well as the contralateral, hand.

4. However, this differential relationship which was found for the tactile tests did not hold for the passive movement threshold. In the case of the proprioceptive test, there was a specific association between frequency of deficit and lesions in the sensorimotor area of both hemispheres.

5. On the right hand, the scores on the three tactile tests were positively and significantly intercorrelated. In contrast, the intercorrelations of the three scores on the left hand were lower and not always significant.

These results led Semmes et al. (1960; Semmes, 1968) to draw a number of conclusions.

1. Ipsilateral and bilateral somatosensory impairment can occur as a consequence of unilateral cerebral disease and is, in fact, not rare.

2. These ipsilateral and bilateral defects occur more frequently as a consequence of lesions of the left hemisphere than of the right hemisphere.

3. The representation of sensation in the left hand is more diffuse in the right hemisphere than is the corresponding representation for the right hand in the left hemisphere.

4. The patterns or combinations of tactile disturbances are different in the two hands. Specifically, dissociated impairment is more likely to be found in the left hand than in the right.

These findings of a relatively frequent occurrence of bilateral sensory deficits in patients with ostensibly unilateral lesions and their particularly high frequency in patients with left hemisphere damage were rather unexpected. It is natural to try to explain them first in a parsimonious way on the basis of some general disability such as aphasia or disturbances in attention. However, analyses of the relationship of aphasia, general mental impairment, and epileptic disorder to the sensory findings failed to disclose any significant associations between these factors and the occurrence of bilateral sensory deficit.

Since the publication of the study of Semmes et al. (1960), a number of investigations bearing directly or indirectly on its findings and conclusions have appeared. The information provided by these investigations may be considered in terms of the major conclusions of the original study. First, in regard to the question of the occurrence of bilateral or ipsilateral somatosensory defects in patients with unilateral disease, there is clear support for the generalization that such defects may be shown by patients with ostensibly unilateral disease. In this respect the relevant studies are as follows.

Vaughan and Costa (1962) found bilateral impairment of two-point discrimination in patients with both left- and right-hemisphere disease; bilateral impairment in pressure sensitivity was found only in the patients with left-hemisphere lesions.

Corkin, Milner, and Rasmussen (1964) found defects in pressure sensitivity, two-point discrimination, and point localization in patients who had undergone unilateral cortical excisions; the frequency of ipsilateral defects in point localization was particularly high.

Wyke (1966) reported that postural arm drift in the absence of vision, which is presumably determined, at least in part, by proprioceptive control, is bilaterally augmented in some patients with left-hemisphere lesions but not in those with right-hemisphere lesions.

Milner, Taylor, and Corkin (1967) found only contralateral deficit of tactile form recognition in patients with unilateral lesions.

Carmon and Benton (1969b) found bilateral impairment in the perception of the direction of punctate stimuli applied to the skin surface in patients with lesions of the right hemisphere but not in those with left-hemisphere lesions; they did not find ipsilateral deficits in the perception of the number of punctate tactile stimuli in either group of patients.

Carmon (1969) found ipsilateral impairment in two-point discrimination and in the absolute pressure threshold (but not in the differential pressure threshold) in patients with unilateral lesions.

These results are summarized in Table 1. Taken in their totality, they indicate that ipsilateral tactile and proprioceptive defects occur in patients with unilateral lesions. The specific nature of the sensory or perceptual performance appears to be a factor in the occurrence of ipsilateral deficit. Thus it is possible that two-point discrimination and point localization will prove to be the deficits most frequently observed. However, it is curious that the tactile perception of number, which would seem to be a similar task, does not show an impressive frequency of ipsilateral deficit.

With respect to the question of left-hemisphere "dominance" for the occurrence of ipsilateral somatosensory defects, inspection of Table 1 indicates that the results are less clear cut. The findings of Corkin et al. (1964) appear to be completely negative in this respect. Ipsilateral defects in pressure sensitivity, two-point discrimination, and point localization occurred with essentially equal frequency in patients with excisions in one or the other hemisphere. The findings of Carmon (1969) were also negative with respect to this question; he did find ipsilateral impairment in pressure sensitivity and two-point discrimination, but the two hemispheric groups did not differ in respect to the relative frequency of such impairment.

However, the studies of Vaughan and Costa (1962) and of Wyke (1966) support the indications of left-hemisphere "dominance" reported by Semmes et al. (1960). Vaughan and Costa found ipsilateral defects in pressure sensitivity in patients with left-hemisphere lesions but not in those with lesions of the right hemisphere. Both groups showed ipsilateral defects in two-point discrimination. Wyke found excessive drift of the contralateral arm in both groups of patients. However, excessive drift of the ipsilateral arm was shown only by the patients with left-hemisphere lesions.

Thus far, the question of hemispheric "dominance" in respect to tactile functions has been considered only with respect to a special role of the left hemisphere. However, the study by Carmon and Benton (1969b) has raised the question of whether some tactile performances may not reflect a relative "dominance" of the right hemisphere. In this study, the tactile perception of direction and number in patients with unilateral lesions was

Table 1. Occurrence of ipsilateral defects in patients with unilateral lesions[a]

	Semmes et al. (1960)	Vaughan & Costa (1962)	Corkin et al. (1964)	Wyke (1966)	Carmon & Benton (1969b)	Milner et al. (1967)	Carmon (1969)
Absolute pressure threshold	++(L) +(R)	+(L) −(R)	+(L) +(R)				+(L) +(R)
Differential pressure threshold							−
Two point threshold	++(L) +(R)	+(L) +(R)	+(L) +(R)				+(L) +(R)
Point localization	++(L) +(R)		++(L) ++(R)				
Passive movement threshold	++(L) +(R)						
Postural arm drift				+(L) −(R)			
Perception of direction					−(L) +(R)		
Perception of number					−		
Form recognition						−	−

[a] L = left-hemisphere lesions; R = right-hemisphere lesions; + = ipsilateral defect; ++ = particularly high frequency of ipsilateral defect; − = no ipsilateral defect.

investigated. The experimental procedure consisted in stimulating the palms of each hand with one to three small tactile stimuli presented in nine different combinations of direction and number (Figure 1). The patients were required to identify the presented tactile stimulus on a visual display showing all the combinations, either by pointing to it or by calling a number that was placed at the top of each square. Two types of errors were scored in evaluating performance: responses involving the incorrect identification of number, and responses involving the incorrect identification of the direction of the tactile stimulation. Thus, with the exception of the single-point stimulus, each stimulation could be scored simultaneously for these two aspects of response.

The mean error scores in the tactile perception of number and direction made by patients with left- and with right-hemispheric lesions are shown in Figure 2. The number of patients in each group (N's=30) who made defective performances (defined as a number of errors greater than that made by the poorest control patient) is shown in Figure 3. Inspection of the figures indicates clearly

that impairment in perceiving the number of tactile stimuli applied to the palms was confined to the contralateral hand in both groups of patients. However, there are hemispheric differences with respect to the tactile perception of direction. In the patients with lesions of the left hemisphere, the errors were confined to the contralateral hand. In contrast, a high proportion of patients with lesions of the

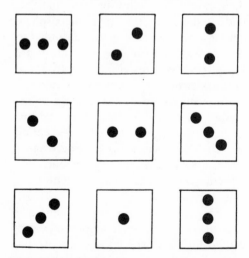

Fig. 1. Visual display on which patient identified experienced patterns of tactile stimulation. (From Carmon & Benton, 1969b.)

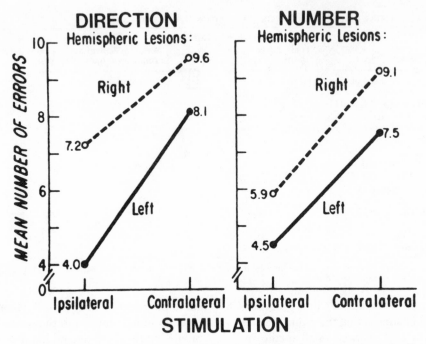

Fig. 2. Mean error scores in the tactile perception of direction and number in patients with unilateral cerebral lesions. (From Carmon & Benton, 1969b.)

right hemisphere showed defective tactile perception of direction on the ipsilateral, as well as the contralateral, hand.

Carmon and Benton (1969b) view their results as indicating that patients with lesions of the right hemisphere demonstrate the same spatial disability in this tactile performance that they are likely to show in visuoperceptive and visuoconstructive tasks. This interpretation is supported by the findings of the study by Dee (1970) that inferior performance on a test of tactile form perception was closely associated with the occurrence of visuoperceptive impairment and constructional apraxia in patients with cerebral disease.

The conclusion of Semmes and her coworkers that tactile functions are represented focally in the left hemisphere but more diffusely in the right hemisphere has not been subjected to searching empirical test. However, such work as has been

reported has not provided confirmation of this generalization. Thus Corkin et al. (1964) found that severe somatosensory defect was associated only with lesions of the postcentral gyrus, and this was true of patients with lesions of either hemisphere. Similarly, Carmon and Benton (1969a) were unable to detect any difference in the effect of intrahemispheric locus of lesion on the frequency of tactile defects shown by patients with right- and with left-hemisphere lesions.

The further conclusion that tactile deficits are more closely intercorrelated on the right hand than on the left hand also has not been confirmed by subsequent work. Vaughan and Costa (1962) found a correlation coefficient of .52 between pressure sensitivity and two-point discrimination for the contralateral (right) hand in their patients with left-hemisphere disease, a value indicative of a substantial positive relation. However, they

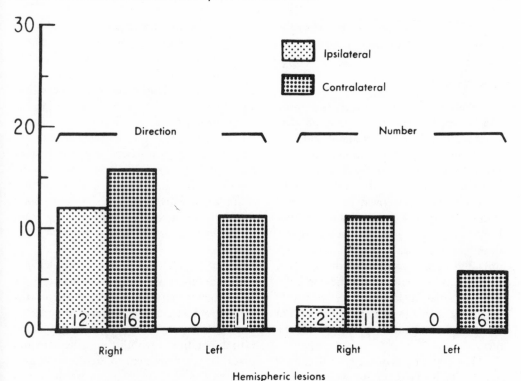

Fig. 3. Frequency of defective performance in tactile perception of direction and number. (From Carmon & Benton, 1969b.)

reported an even higher correlation coefficient (.87) for the contralateral (left) hand of their patients with disease of the right hemisphere. On their part, Carmon and Benton (1969a) did not find any impressive differences in the strength of the associations among various tactile performances in patients with left- and right-hemisphere lesions. Inspection of their results (Table 2) indicates clearly that the correlation coefficients among levels of tactile sensitivity on the contralateral hand were not higher in patients with left-hemisphere lesions than in those with lesions of the right hemisphere. The same holds for the interrelationships of the

Table 2. Correlations among tactile performances in patients with unilateral cerebral lesions[a]

	Patients with hemispheric lesions			
	Right		Left	
Performance	Ipsilateral hand	Contralateral hand	Ipsilateral hand	Contralateral hand
Absolute and differential threshold	.41[b]	.65[c]	.16	.37[b]
Absolute threshold and two-point discrimination	.48[c]	.50[c]	.30	.45[c]
Differential threshold and two-point discrimination	.36[b]	.56[c]	.45[c]	.62[c]

[a] Carmon & Benton (1969a).
[b] $p < .05$.
[c] $p < .01$.

three measures of tactile sensitivity for the ipsilateral hand.

CONCLUSIONS

This analysis of recent studies, beginning with that of Semmes et al. (1960), makes it abundantly clear that bilateral and ipsilateral somatosensory defects may be shown by patients with ostensibly unilateral disease, at least under the conditions of examination employed in the several studies. The question arises as to whether this circumstance does not merely reflect some more general mental impairment unrelated to sensory status, for example, fluctuations in attention, slowness in judgment, or aphasia. In this case, we would be dealing with a familiar phenomenon of no great theoretical or practical importance.

Although this possibility still cannot be completely excluded, the weight of evidence is against it. As has been pointed out, the analyses of Semmes et al. (1960) were negative in this respect. The findings of bilateral defect by Corkin et al. (1964) are particularly telling because their patients had rather limited cortical lesions and, from a general intellectual standpoint, were quite intact. Carmon and Benton (1969b) have also observed bilateral deficit in the tactile perception of direction in patients without the slightest evidence of general mental impairment or aphasia. Hence, even if the general explanation applies to some cases, it cannot be made to fit all of them.

Thus it is reasonable to conclude that at least some somatosensory performances on each side of the body are mediated by both the contralateral and ipsilateral hemispheres and not merely by the contralateral. As Semmes (1968) has pointed out, a substantial amount of physiological data is consonant with this concept of bilateral cerebral representation of somatosensory processes. No doubt the contribution of the ipsilateral hemisphere is generally smaller than that of the contralateral. However, it is possible that there is considerable individual variation in this respect. The implication of this conclusion for the clinical sensory examination is that the time-honored method of comparing sensitivity on the two sides of the body and using the patient as his own control has serious limitations and that the sensitivity of each side of the body should be assessed independently with reference to established normative standards.

In regard to the focal problem of whether there are differences between the two hemispheres in respect to the occurrence of bilateral or ipsilateral somesthetic defects, it seems that present findings tend to favor this possibility and yet are not sufficiently consistent to dictate a positive answer. As has been shown, some results suggest a relative dominance of the left hemisphere for certain performances, most notably for tactile pressure sensitivity and for postural arm control. However, other data do not support this trend. A crucial question here is why different investigators have obtained discrepant results. Until the reasons for these discrepancies are clarified, the hypothesis of a stronger ipsilateral representation of certain somatosensory processes in the left hemisphere must be considered rather questionable.

The other aspect of the problem is the one represented by the study of Carmon and Benton (1969b), indicating that the right hemisphere plays a particularly important role in the tactile perception of direction. The results of Corkin's (1965) study of tactile maze learning, in which she found that patients with lesions of the right hemisphere were consistently inferior to those with left lesions, support these indications of a relative dominance of the right hemisphere in the mediation of tactile performances involving a spatial component. This conclusion is not difficult to accept because it accords so well with the now widely accepted concept of a special role of the right hemisphere in the mediation of the spatial aspects of behavior. However, before accepting these findings at face value, one would like to see whether further studies, involving particularly a strict control of extent and type of lesion, will confirm them.

In conclusion, investigative work during the past decade has indicated the strong probability that bilateral and ipsilateral sensory defects are a frequent consequence of unilateral cerebral disease in man and the distinct possibility that lesions in each hemisphere have significantly different consequences in this respect. There are a number of unsettled questions which future research can be expected to answer. But the work to date has been more than sufficient to show that traditional conceptions of the somatosensory consequences of cerebral disease require considerable revision.

REFERENCES

Adams, F. *The extant works of Aretaeus, the Cappodocian.* London: Sydenham Society, 1856.

Benton, A. L. *Right-left discrimination and finger localization: Development and pathology.* New York: Hoeber Medical Division, Harper & Row, 1959.

Benton, A. L. The fiction of the "Gerstmann syndrome." *Journal of Neurology, Neurosurgery and Psychiatry,* 1961, **24**, 176–181.

Bychowsky, G., & Eidinow, M. Doppelseitige Sensibilitätsstörungen bei einseitigen Gehirnherden. *Nervenarzt,* 1934, 7, 498–506.

Carmon, A. *Contralateral and ipsilateral tactile sensitivity in patients with unilateral cerebral lesions.* (Doctoral dissertation, University of Iowa) Ann Arbor, Mich.: University Microfilms, 1969. No. 69–13, 136.

Carmon, A., & Benton, A. L. Patterns of impaired tactile sensitivity in unilateral cerebral disease: Re-examination of Head's theory. *Journal of the Israeli Medical Association,* 1969, 77, 287–290 (Hebrew, with English summary). (a)

Carmon, A., & Benton, A. L. Tactile perception of direction and number in patients with unilateral cerebral disease. *Neurology,* 1969, 19, 525–532. (b)

Corkin, S. Tactually guided maze learning in man: Effects of unilateral cortical excisions and bilateral hippocampal lesions. *Neuropsychologia,* 1965, 3, 339–351.

Corkin, S., Milner, B., & Rasmussen, T. Effects of different cortical excisions on sensory thresholds in man. *Transactions of the American Neurological Association,* 1964, 89, 112–116.

Dee, H. L. Visuoconstructive and visuoperceptive deficits in patients with unilateral cerebral lesions. *Neuropsychologia,* 1970, 8, 305–314.

Foix, C. Sur une varieté de troubles bilatéraux de la sensibilité par lésion unilaterale du cerveau. *Revue Neurologique,* 1922, 29, 322–331.

Gerstmann, J. Fingeragnosie: eine umschriebene Störung der Orientierung am eigenen Körper. *Wiener Klinische Wochenschrift,* 1924, 37, 1010–1012.

Gerstmann, J. Fingeragnosie und isolierte Agraphie: Ein neues Syndrom. *Zeitschrift für die Gesamte Neurologie und Psychiatrie,* 1927, 108, 152–177.

Gerstmann, J. Zur Symptomatologie der Hirnläsionen im Übergangsgebiet der unteren Parietal- und mittleren Occipitalwindung. *Nervenarzt,* 1930, 3, 691–695.

Giannitrapani, D. Developing concepts of lateralization of cerebral functions. *Cortex,* 1967, 3, 353–370.

Goldstein, K. Das Wesen der amnestischen Aphasie. *Schweizer Archiv für Neurologie und Psychiatrie,* 1924, 15, 163–175.

Goldstein, K. Die Lokalisation in der Grosshirnrinde. In A. Bethe, G. Bergmann, G. Embden, & A. Ellinger (Eds.), *Handbuch der normalen und pathologischen Physiologie.* Berlin: Springer, 1927.

Guillain, G., Alajouanine, T., & Garcin, R. Un cas d'apraxie idéomotrice bilatérale coïncidant avec une aphasie et une hémiparésie gauche chez une gauchère. Troubles bilatéraux de la sensibilité profonde. *Revue Neurologique*, 1925, **2**, 116–124.

Head, H. *Studies in neurology*. London: Oxford University Press, 1920.

Head, H. *Aphasia and kindred disorders of speech*. Cambridge: Cambridge University Press, 1926.

Heimburger, R., DeMyer, W., & Reitan, R. M. Implications of Gerstmann's syndrome. *Journal of Neurology, Neurosurgery and Psychiatry*, 1964, **27**, 52–57.

Jackson, H. On the nature of the duality of the brain. *Medical Press & Circular*, 1874, **1**, 19.

Jackson, H. Case of large cerebral tumour without optic neuritis and with left hemiplegia and imperception. *Royal London Ophthalmic Hospital Reports*, 1876, **8**, 434–444.

Körner, S. C. Die Beeinflussbarkeit der Sensibilität an symmetrischen Hautgebieten bei einseitiger Hirnschädigung und bei Gesunden. *Deutsche Zeitschrift für Nervenheilkunde*, 1938, **145**, 116–130.

Liepmann, H. *Das Krankheitsbild der Apraxie ("Motorischen Asymbolie")*. Berlin: Karger, 1900.

Liepmann, H. *Drei Aufsätze aus dem Apraxiegebiet*. Berlin: Karger, 1908.

McFie, J., & Zangwill, O. L. Visual-constructive disabilities associated with lesions of the left cerebral hemisphere. *Brain*, 1960, **83**, 243–260.

Milner, B., Taylor, L., & Corkin, S. Tactual pattern recognition after different unilateral cortical excisions. Paper presented at the 38th Annual Meeting of the Eastern Psychological Association, Boston, 1967.

Morgagni, G. B. *The seats and causes of diseases investigated by anatomy*. Translated by B. Alexander, A. Millar & T. Cadell, London, 1769.

Oppenheim, H. Über einen bemerkenswerten Fall von Tumor cerebri. *Berliner Klinische Wochenschrift*, 1906, **13**, 1001–1004.

Pourfour du Petit, F. *Lettres d'un médecin des hôpitaux du roy à un autre mèdecin de ses amis*. Namur: Charles Gèrard Albert, 1710.

Reichardt, M. *Allegemeine und spezielle Psychiatrie: ein Lehrbuch für Studierende und Arzte*. (3rd ed.) Jena: Fischer, 1923.

Rieger, C. Über Apparate in dem Hirn. *Arbeiten aus der Psychiatrischen Klinik zu Würzburg*, 1909, **5**, 176–197.

Semmes, J. Hemispheric specialization: A possible clue to mechanism. *Neuropsychologia*, 1968, **6**, 11–26.

Semmes, J., Weinstein, S., Ghent, L., & Teuber, H. L. *Somatosensory changes after penetrating brain wounds in man*. Cambridge, Mass.: Harvard University Press, 1960.

Vaughan, H. G., Jr., & Costa, L. D. Performance of patients with lateralized cerebral lesions. *Journal of Nervous and Mental Disease*, 1962, **134**, 237–243.

Wyke, M. Postural arm drift associated with brain lesions in man. *Archives of Neurology*, 1966, **15**, 329–334.

6.

Tactile Perception of Direction in Normal Subjects*

Implications for hemispheric cerebral dominance

In previous studies[1,2] we reported that a substantial proportion of right-handed patients with disease of the right hemisphere show bilateral impairment in identifying the direction of linear tactile stimulation applied to the palms of the hands, but that patients with left hemisphere disease show impairment only in the right hand. We believed these results indicated that the right hemisphere plays a crucial role in subserving spatial perceptn in the tactile modality as well as in the visual and auditory modalities.

If this inference of function from symptom is correct, it should be possible to demonstrate a between-hands difference in the accuracy of tactile perception of direction in right-handed normal individuals. Since tactile information from the left hand is initially processed primarily in the right hemisphere and tactile information from the right hand is initially processed primarily in the left hemisphere, the special role of the right hemisphere in

processing spatial information should be reflected in a relative superiority of the left hand in tactile perception of direction. The performances of the control patients in our previous studies provided an opportunity to evaluate this prediction. The findings were negative; in neither study was a significant difference apparent in the accuracy of tactile perception of direction between the left and right hands of the control patients.

Two considerations led us to undertake a more intensive study of the question. First, the tactile perception tasks in these studies were fairly easy for the control patients, many of whom gave perfect or near-perfect performances. For example, in the study of Fontenot and Benton,[2] a majority of the control patients made two errors or fewer in 24 trials on each hand. Secondly, it seemed possible that the durations of the stimulus used in the earlier studies (three seconds in the first, two seconds in the second) were too long to disclose a between-hands difference. Tachistoscopic investigations have shown that the duration of exposure is a

* A. L. Benton, H. S. Levin, and N. R. Varney, *Neurology*, 1973, 23, 1248–1250.

crucial variable in eliciting lateral field differences in visual perception, with shorter
exposures favoring the disclosure of
between-field differences.[3,4] Accordingly,
in the present study the duration of tactile
stimulation was reduced to one second,
making the perceptual task more difficult
and at the same time increasing the
chances that lateral differences, if they
exist, would be brought to light.

METHOD

The subjects were 24 university students
(11 men, 13 women). All were strongly
right-handed by self-classification and all
reported preferential use of the right hand
in seven unimanual activities, including
writing, throwing a ball, and using a hammer. The range of ages in the group was
18 to 22 years.

Procedure

The instrument used to present the tactile
stimuli was the same one used in the
earlier studies, the electromechanical stimulator of Carmon and Dyson.[5] This
apparatus, which has been described in
detail elsewhere,[1,5–7] permits accurate
control of virtually all significant stimulus
variables, such as force, area of stimulation, duration of application, and direction of stimulation. The stimulus was a
linear array of three stainless steel rods,
each having a flat circular surface of 0.8
mm^2 and a weight of 20 g; the distance
between the rods was 15 mm. This stimulus was positioned 2 mm above the palm
and delivered in each of four different
directions, as shown in the illustration. (A
photograph of the mode of application of
the stimuli may be found in *Neurology*,
vol. 19, p. 528.) The duration of stimulation was one second and the intertrial
interval was 10 seconds.

The direction of stimulation was
guided by radial lines printed on a grid

stamped on the palms prior to testing.
Twenty-four linear stimuli, six in each
direction, were applied to the palm of
each hand. The ABBA order (i.e., 12 stimulations of left palm, 24 stimulations of
right palm, 12 stimulations of left palm)
was used with 12 subjects and the BAAB
order with the other 12.

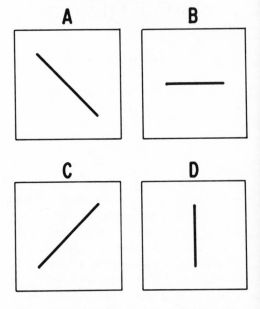

Fig. 4. Visual display card on which subject
identified direction of tactile stimulation.

A black curtain obstructed the subject's view of his hand. The visual display
(see Figure 4) was placed before him so
that he could easily point to it with his left
or right hand. The instructions to the subject were as follows: "I am going to touch
your hand with these metal rods in one of
the four directions shown on this card. I
want you to tell me in which direction you
feel the rods, either by pointing to the
direction on this card or by calling the letter printed above it, each time that I touch
you." One demonstration trial was given.
The 24 test trials were then presented to
each hand, and the subject's responses
were recorded. The score was the number

of correct choices in 24 trials for each hand.

RESULTS

The mean scores for the two hands are shown in Table 3. The accuracy of identification was significantly higher for the left hand than for the right. As the standard deviations indicate, there was considerable individual variation in the level of performance. The range of scores was 14 to 24 in the left hand and 9 to 24 in the right hand. No subject performed perfectly with both hands but four subjects made not more than one error on either or both hands, achieving total scores of 46 or 47. There was a fairly substantial positive correlation (rho = .74) between scores on the right and left hands, indicating the presence of a general capacity for the tactile perception of direction that is expressed in performance level on both hands.

The difference in accuracy of recognition in the two hands also was evaluated by comparison of the number of subjects who showed superior recognition in each hand. The data are presented in the table. A significantly higher number of subjects showed superior recognition in the left hand when the between-hands difference is defined either by a minimal, one point difference in score or by a difference in score of at least three points.

DISCUSSION

The finding of a left-hand superiority in the tactile recognition of direction in normal subjects confirms the validity of the inference, drawn from studies of patients with unilateral brain disease, that the right hemisphere is in some sense "dominant" for the appreciation of the spatial aspects of perception. This conclusion is reinforced by the outcome of an analogous investigation of lateral field differences in the visual perception of direction in normal subjects; a significant superiority of the left visual field in the identification of the direction of lines presented tachistoscopically to each half-field was found.[3] Thus, results in normal subjects provide evidence complementary to that yielded by studies of patients with brain disease in favor of the basic hypothesis.

Table 3. Tactile perception of direction in 24 normal subjects

Mean number of correct choices (24 trials with each hand)	
Right hand	18.96 (S.D. = 3.7)
Left hand	21.00 (S.D. = 2.8)
Difference	2.04 (t = 3.5; p < .002)

Within-subject differences, 1 or more points[a]	
Differences	*No. of subjects*
Superior accuracy in right hand	5
Superior accuracy in left hand	17
Equal accuracy in the two hands	2

Within-subject differences, 3 or more points[a]	
Differences	*No. of subjects*
Superior accuracy in right hand	
Superior accuracy in left hand	10
Equal accuracy in the two hands	14

[a] Wilcoxon Matched Pairs Signed-Ranks Test (p < .01).

SUMMARY

The accuracy of tactile perception of the direction of linear punctate stimulation of brief duration on the palms of the right and left hands of right-handed normal subjects was investigated. Perception of direction was significantly more accurate on the left hand than on the right hand. The findings support the results of studies of patients with unilateral brain disease that have shown that lesions of the right hemisphere may produce bilateral impairment in this perceptual performance. It is concluded that the right hemisphere plays a distinctively important role in mediating spatial recognition in the tactile modality as well as in the visual and auditory modalities.

REFERENCES

1. Carmon A, Benton AL: Tactile perception of direction and number in patients with unilateral cerebral disease. Neurology (Minneap) 19: 525–532, 1969

2. Fontenot DJ, Benton AL: Tactile perception of direction in relation to hemispheric locus of lesion. Neuropsychologia 9: 83–88, 1971

3. ———: Perception of direction in the right and left visual fields. Neuropsychologia 10: 447–452, 1972

4. Adams J: Visual perception of direction and number in right and left visual fields. Cortex 7: 227–235, 1971

5. Carmon A, Dyson JA: New instrumentation for research on tactile sensitivity and discrimination. Cortex 3: 406–418, 1967

6. Carmon, A: Stimulus contrast in tactile resolution. Perception & Psychophysics 3: 241–245, 1968

7. Carmon A, Benton AL: Parametric aspects of tactile resolution. Perception & Psychophysics 10: 331–334, 1971

7.

The Interplay of Experimental and Clinical Approaches in Brain Lesion Research*

INTRODUCTION

Our knowledge of the effects of brain lesions on behavior has been gained through two approaches. The first is the experimental method in which structural or functional alteration of the central nervous system is deliberately induced and its behavioral outcome noted. The second is the clinical method in which the behavioral consequences of the lesions produced by disease are observed.

If the two approaches are compared, the experimental method is seen to have significant advantages in that the investigator can exercise some control over the size and locus of the lesion he produces, the degree of control being dependent upon a number of factors such as the prevailing state of surgical technology and the depth of understanding of the structural characteristics of the brain and the anatomic relationships between its parts. Theoretically the experimental investi-

gator has an unlimited number of animals at his disposal so that he can proceed systematically to compare the effects of lesions of different locus and size. He can also exercise a considerable degree of control over the genetic characteristics and life history of his animals as well as over other variables, such as age, that interact with experimental interventions to determine the consequences of these interventions. The clinical investigator enjoys none of these advantages. He must take the lesions as he finds them and, while some may approximate experimental lesions in discreteness, the majority are associated with one or more confounding factors that may make it difficult to draw confident conclusions about the relationship of the lesion to the behavior of the patient. Nor can the clinical investigator exercise direct control over extralesional factors such as age, health status, and the life history, although to some degree he may be able to reduce variability in these respects by an appropriate selection of cases.

But not all the advantages are on the

* A. L. Benton in S. Finger (Ed.), *Recovery from Brain Damage: Research and Theory.* New York, Plenum Press, 1978, pp. 49–68.

side of the experimentalist. Detailed study of the behavioral aspects of the brain–behavior relationship is much more easily acomplished in human subjects. Animals must be trained to respond in the laboratory situation, human subjects need only to be asked to. It is a commonplace observation that animals often behave in an inexplicably stupid manner in the unnatural environment of the laboratory, quite unlike their appropriate real-life behavior. The human subject can report what he sees, the animal cannot. The cognitive capacities of the human subject are incomparably greater, offering opportunities for the analytic study of diverse aspects of mentation which are not possible with animals.

Thus, each approach has its reciprocal strengths and weaknesses and complement each other well in the total research effort on the effects of brain lesions on behavior. Historical study shows that, in line with this complementarity, there has usually been a constant interaction between the two methods in pursuing a particular line of inquiry. In this chapter I shall illustrate the interplay of the two approaches as they were brought to bear on specific questions about brain–behavior relationships and try to show how they coalesced to provide some answers to these questions. The early history of two topics that have been investigated through both experimental and clinical brain lesion research will be sketched. The first is the evolution of our knowledge of cortical localization of visual function. The second deals with the method of double sensory stimulation which has become a standard feature of the clinical neurological examination. As will be seen, in both instances relevant findings were first generated by experimental investigation on animals and these led to analogous and more refined study of human patients.

CORTICAL LOCALIZATION OF VISUAL FUNCTION

Ferrier, Munk, and the clinicians

A detailed description of the early history of this topic may be found in the first two chapters of Polyak's (1955) monumental volume on the vertebrate visual system. As he states, "As far back in the human past as there is a record, the supreme importance of vision and of its instrument, the eye, has been recognized." Up to 1800, for practical reasons, investigation was primarily directed to the eye and its diseases. Nevertheless, the role of the brain in visual-information processing was also fully appreciated. The fact that there were structural connections between the eyes and the brain, in the form of "nerves," "ducts," or "tubes," was established very early. However, up to the middle of the nineteenth century, knowledge of details was scanty and often inaccurate. The cerebral center for vision was almost invariably placed below the cerebral hemispheres—in the lateral ventricles (Galen), the brainstem (Willis), the pineal body (Descartes), and other sites.

One reason for this was technical in nature. The limitations inherent in gross anatomical study made it very difficult indeed to trace the visual pathways beyond the optic tract. But an even more important reason was of a conceptual nature. The dominating influence of Flourens' doctrine of the equipotentiality of the cerebral hemispheres made it seem pointless to look for a focal center for vision above the level of the thalamus.

However, Flourens' dogma was challenged by two contributions in the 1850s, one of an anatomical nature and the other consisting of experimental and clinical observations, and these laid the groundwork for the subsequent identification of a cortical center for vision. By means of careful dissection of fixed specimens, Gratiolet (1854) was able to demonstrate the optic radiations arising from the lateral geniculate nuclei and fanning out to the cortex of the occipital and parietal lobes. He described the radiations as "expansions of the optic nerve terminating in a specific region of the cortex of the hemispheres." A year later, Gratiolet's anatomical discovery was complemented by the observations of Panizza (1855), who established a rough correlation between lesions in the occipitoparietal area and visual impairment, both in human case material and in dogs subjected to experimental ablations. Panizza reported that bilateral destruction of this area resulted in complete blindness while unilateral damage caused blindness in the opposite eye. A clinicopathologic study by Chaillou (1863) of a patient with extensive destruction of the "posterior" lobes and concomitant visual impairment provided an additional bit of evidence in support of Panizza's correlation. Similarly, Meynert's (1869) description of the course of the optic radiations from the thalamic level to the occipital and temporal lobes partially substantiated the observations of Gratiolet.

A more intensive search for the site of the cortical center for vision, as well as for the other senses, followed upon the discovery of the motor area of the cortex by Fritsch and Hitzig (1870). Ferrier (1876, 1878, 1890) carried out a long series of studies involving both destruction and stimulation of different cortical areas in animals, primarily the monkey, and sought confirmation of his experimental findings in relevant clinical observations. He concluded that the angular gyrus was the site of the cortical visual center since its "unilateral destruction has the effect of causing temporary blindness of the opposite eye, while bilateral destruction causes total and permanent blindness in both eyes" (Ferrier, 1878, p. 122). Con-

fronted by a substantial amount of contradictory evidence from the studies of other investigators, he later modified his position and conceded that the visual center occupied the territory of *both* the angular gyrus and the occipital lobes. But he still insisted that "the angular gyrus is the special region of clear or central vision of the opposite eye, and perhaps to some extent also of the eye on the same side" (Ferrier, 1886, p. 288). And he maintained that the occipital lobes "can be injured, or cut off bodily, almost up to the parieto-occipital fissure, on one or both sides simultaneously, without the slightest appreciable impairment of vision" (Ferrier, 1886, p. 273).

What could have led Ferrier to these inaccurate inferences? Given his crude surgical techniques, the suggestion by Starr (1884) and Schäfer (1888) that Ferrier had destroyed fibers of the underlying optic radiations in his angular gyrus ablations is probably correct. His notion that the opposite eye was affected by unilateral destruction of the angular gyrus rested on the conception (still held at the time by some experimentalists and clinicians including Charcot) that those retinogeniculate fibers which did not decussate at the optic chiasm crossed over to the opposite hemisphere through the colliculi so that the whole retina of a single eye was represented in a single lateral cortical area.

Studies by a number of experimentalists and clinicians in the 1870s and 1880s generated unassailable evidence that the locus of the cortical center for vision was to be found in the occipital lobes. The preeminent experimentalist of the period was the Berlin physiologist Hermann Munk, a painstaking investigator, whose studies on the dog and the monkey were technically and methodologically superior to those of most of his contemporaries. He was able to keep some of his operated animals alive for years and to study them thoroughly. Thus, he had the opportunity to note restitution of function, when it occurred, as well as certain peculiarities in visual behavior that could not be observed in the acutely operated animal. In 1876 he initiated a series of studies designed to elucidate the cortical basis of sensory and motor functions, the results of which were reported in detail in 16 lengthy communications (Munk, 1890).

With respect to vision, Munk demonstrated beyond reasonable doubt that, at least in dogs and monkeys, complete destruction of both occipital lobes produced permanent loss of vision, a condition which he designated as "cortical blindness." He also showed that complete destruction of a single occipital lobe produced a contralateral hemianopia and not blindness in the opposite eye, as supposed by Ferrier and others. Thus, he established that in the animals which he had studied the cortical "center" for vision was located in the occipital lobes.

Munk's early reports encountered a skeptical reception from other animal experimentalists, particularly on the part of antilocalizationists such as Goltz and close rivals such as Ferrier. But clinicians, already prepared by case reports such as those of Levick (1866) and Pooley (1877), which raised the possibility of an association between hemianopia and occipital lobe disease, viewed his conclusions much more favorably. Only a year after the publication of Munk's first communication, Baumgarten (1878) described a patient with persistent left homonymous hemianopia and no other signs of brain disease in whom autopsy disclosed a large cyst in the right occipital lobe. He commented that, despite the clear association between the occipital lesion and the hemianopia, he would hesitate to infer a causal connection on the basis of a single case, if it were not for the observations of Munk, who

"has been able to produce a lateral hemianopia (corresponding to our case) in monkeys by unilateral extirpation of the cortex of the occipital lobe." A year later, a very similar case was reported by Curschmann (1879). His patient, with a left homonymous hemianopia persisting until death, showed no other signs of brain disease. A focus of softening in the right occipital lobe was found on autopsy, leading Curschmann to conclude that his case confirmed Munk's correlation and to remark with some pride that "in view of the absence of other focal brain symptoms, it has the status of an experiment in man."

Within a few years, Munk's occipital localization of vision was widely accepted, although some of his more specific ideas proved to be incorrect. Reviewing Munk's work through 1883, Starr (1884) concluded that "the large number of animals used, the uniform results of the experiments in all cases, the length of time during which the symptoms persisted, and the minute care displayed in the observations combine to establish the truth of the conclusions reached." Starr added that "it remains for the pathologist to determine whether these facts which are true in the case of monkeys, are true also in the case of man." He proceeded to do this by means of a review of the relevant literature.

In fact, analysis of the evidence bearing on the question had already been published. The first of these was by Exner (1881) in his monograph on cortical localization of function in man. In his review of the findings in 167 autopsied cases reported in the literature through 1879, Exner distinguished between "absolute" cortical fields, lesions of which almost always produced a particular defect, and "relative" cortical fields, lesions of which produced the defect with notable frequency but not invariably. Thus, he classified a major part of the precentral gyrus as an absolute cortical field for motor function in the contralateral limbs since lesions in that area produced impairment in close to 100 percent of the cases. A larger surrounding territory was designated as a relative cortical field since lesions there produced contralateral motor impairment in 40 to 90 percent of the cases.

Although Exner's series was a large one, in only 6 cases were visual disturbances mentioned. (In contrast, no less than 100 cases presented with motor impairment of an upper extremity.) He was not able to identify an absolute cortical field for vision in that he found no area in which lesions always produced visual disturbances. However, he did find that lesions in a number of loci on the lateral and medial surfaces of the occipital lobes did produce impairment with frequencies ranging from 33 to 75 percent and hence he classified the occipital lobes as a relative field for vision. The highest frequency (60 to 75 percent) was associated with lesions in the superior part of the first occipital gyrus, leading to his designation of this area as the most "intensive" part of the relative cortical field for vision. Conversely, he found that lesions in the territory of the angular gyrus were associated with visual defect in only about 12 percent of the cases.

Insofar as vision was concerned, the weakness of Exner's review lay in the fact that even the very few cases with visual disturbances in his series were poorly described and of a heterogeneous character. [Neither Baumgarten's (1878) case nor that of Curschmann (1879) was included in his series, although both were published before 1880.] His sparse data could show only that the occipital lobes appeared to be more important than other regions of the cerebral hemispheres in the mediation of visual function. The subsequent analyses of Marchand and Starr of the site of lesion in patients with hemianopic defects were far more informative and convincing.

Marchand (1882) reviewed 22 cases, 11 with a right hemianopic defect and 11 with a left hemianopic defect. Within each subgroup, autopsy study showed involvement of the opposite thalamus or optic tract in 5 cases, the lesions being for the most part tumors. In the remaining 6 cases in each subgroup, lesions in the opposite occipital lobe were invariably found, the majority of these being vascular in origin. Stressing the importance of small, circumscribed vascular lesions for the study of cerebral localization, Marchand described a patient with a complete left hemianopia following a stroke whom he studied in 1876. Autopsy disclosed only an area of necrosis in the right occipital lobe. The unsuspected absence of a lesion at the level of the thalamus or the optic tract was at the time quite puzzling and "only after Munk's discoveries did this case gain clarity and interest."

Starr's (1884) case material consisted of 32 cases presenting a right (15 cases) or left (17 cases) hemianopia, either in isolation or as part of an ensemble of deficits. With one exception, all the cases had come to autopsy, the pathology in the exceptional case having been described during the course of surgical intervention. Of the 32 cases, 5 involved unilateral lesions at the thalamic level, 2 of these being neoplastic lesions also extending into the occipital lobe. Thirteen cases of right hemianopia were found to have lesions in one or another part of the left occipital lobe. In 2 of these cases, the field defect had been the only permanent symptom. Similarly, a lesion of the right occipital lobe was found in 14 cases with a left hemianopia, as part of an ensemble of defects in 9, as the only symptom in 4, and as the only permanent symptom in 1 case.

Starr concluded that "anatomical research, physiological experiment, and pathological observation unite in assigning to the occipital lobes of the brain the function of sight. The right occipital lobe receives impressions from the right half of both eyes, and the left occipital lobe receives impressions from the left half of both eyes. The visual area of the brain lies in the occipital lobes."

Precise localization of the visual center

From his ablation studies, Munk reached the conclusion that, although complete removal of the occipital lobes was required to produce cortical blindness (and complete removal of one lobe to produce a contralateral hemianopia), their upper convex surface represented the center of clearest vision. He proposed the idea that this area was the site of termination of the pathways from the foveal region of the retina but did not undertake any anatomical studies to demonstrate the point. This was as far as Munk was able to go and, as will be seen, a certain amount of confusion was engendered by his contention that lesions of the same area were also responsible for the production of another type of visual defect which he called "mindblindness." Munk, in 1879, was also the first investigator to propose that there was a fixed relationship between elements of the retina and corresponding loci in the occipital lobe.

The evidence that the primary cortical center for vision was to be found in the calcarine region of the mesial surface of the occipital lobes came from clinicopathologic correlations in patients with discrete lesions in that area. The first case of this type, reported by Huguenin (1881; Haab, 1882), concerned an 8-year-old tubercular girl who developed a left homonymous hemianopia during the course of an illness of 5 months' duration.

She suffered from headache, convulsions, and general mental impairment, but showed no motor, auditory, somatosensory, or speech defects. Autopsy disclosed two discrete neoplastic lesions, a small one in the left prefrontal area and a slightly larger one on the mesial surface of the right occipital lobe. Since the small left prefrontal lesion could be safely dismissed as the cause of the hemianopia, it was evident that the mesial occipital tumor (Figure 5A) was the crucial lesion.

It was Haab (1882) who first raised the question of whether the mesial, rather than the convex, region of the occipital lobes might be the site of the cortical visual center. Commenting on the findings in Huguenin's case, he remarked: "It is of interest to see that in this case the tumor destroyed precisely the center of the cortical area in which the stripe of Vicq d'Azyr is found. Has this peculiarly structured cortex perhaps specific connections with the visual sense?" (Haab, 1882, p. 149). He went on to describe the findings in a second case which reinforced this possibility. It was that of a 61-year-old man with a left homonymous hemianopia in whom autopsy study again disclosed a lesion in the mesial area of the right occipital lobe. The visual field defect and a slight awkwardness in moving the right arm and leg were the only symptoms shown by this intelligent patient 5 months after a stroke. The hemianopia persisted until the patient's death 3 years later. The only lesion found on autopsy was an area of necrosis surrounding the calcarine fissure in the right occipital lobe (Figure 5B).

An even more precise localization of the cortical visual center in a specific area of the occipital lobe was indicated by the subsequent case report of Hun (1887), describing a 57-year-old patient with a left homonymous inferior quadrantanopia of about 2 years' duration. The only finding on autopsy, apart from slight dila-

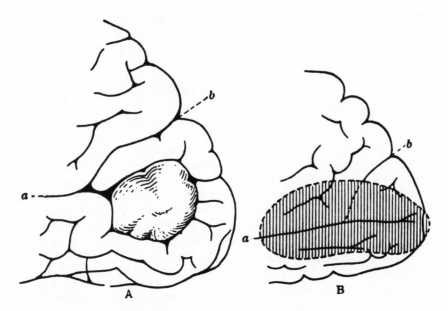

Fig. 5. (*A*) Site of lesion on the mesial surface of the right occipital lobe in the case of Huguenin (1881); (*B*) in the case of Haab (1882). Both patients showed a left homonymous hemianopia during life.

tation of the lateral ventricles, was a circumscribed atrophic area of cortex just above the calcarine fissure in the right occipital lobe, i.e., in the lower part of the cuneus.

In this case there is a lesion which destroys the lower half of the right cuneus, and there is one constant symptom which is present during the whole course of the disease: a blindness limited to the lower left quadrant of the field of vision of each eye. In the absence of any other cerebral lesion the destruction of the lower half of the right cuneus must be regarded as the cause of the blindness in the lower left quadrant of each field of vision. ... This case makes it probable that the fibres from the right upper quadrants of each retina terminate in the lower half of the right cuneus (Hun, 1887, pp. 144–145).

Hun's anatomic inference (or guess) that there was a topographic representation of the retinae onto the mesial surface of the occipital lobes was fully supported by subsequent investigators. Their work has been so well described by Brouwer (1936, pp. 459–482) and Polyak (1955, 179–203) that there is no point in reviewing it once again. It need only be pointed out that the leading investigators of the period, Wilbrand (1887, 1890; Wilbrand & Saenger, 1904, 1917) and Henschen (1890–1896), were primarily clinical researchers who correlated the perimetrically defined visual field defects shown by patients during life with autopsy findings. On the basis of an enormous case material, they were able to demonstrate that there was indeed a "cortical retina," as Henschen called it, on the mesial aspect of the occipital lobes, reflecting a point-to-point correspondence between the receptor surface and the cortical area.

Thus, clinicopathologic study of patients, rather than animal experimentation, provided the first indications of the locus and organization of the cortical visual center. The experimental demonstration that the calcarine region was the primary cortical end-station for vision was made by Minkowski (1911). He first showed that ablation of the cortical area on the convex surface that Munk had designated as the center for foveal vision produced no visual disturbances at all in the dog. He surmised that Munk's results were obtained because of inadvertent injury to the visual radiations which course directly under the cortex of the second and third occipital gyri, and in fact he showed by study of serial sections that, when an ablation presumably limited to the cortex did lead to visual defects, the radiations had been invariably injured. Minkowski went on to make complete and partial ablations of the striate area and found, in line with expectations, that complete bilateral destruction caused permanent blindness, complete unilateral ablation produced a contralateral hemianopia, and partial ablations of the superior and the inferior surface of the striate area produced an inferior and a superior hemianopia, respectively. Hence, he felt confident in concluding that the striate area constituted the cortical center for vision in the dog and that within this area there was a fixed correspondence between retinal loci and cortical loci.

Visual agnosia

If locus A_1 of the cerebral cortex of a dog is extirpated on both sides a peculiar disturbance in vision is noticeable 3–5 days after the injury, at a time when the inflammatory reaction has passed and no abnormality of hearing, smell, taste, movement, and sensation in the animal is present. The dog moves quite freely and easily indoors as well as in the garden without bumping against a single object. If obstacles are placed in his path, he regularly goes around them or, if a detour is not possible, he overcomes them adroitly, e.g., by crawling under a stool or carefully climbing over the man's foot or the animal's body which obstructs his path.

But now the sight of people whom he had always greeted joyfully leaves him cold, as does the company of other dogs with whom he used to play. He may be so hungry and thirsty that he is overactive; yet he no longer looks for food in the part of the room where he used to find it. And if the bowl of food and bucket of water are placed directly in his path, he repeatedly goes around them without paying attention to them. Food presented to him visually evokes no response as long as he does not smell it. A finger or fire brought close to the eye no longer makes him blink. The sight of a whip, which invariably used to drive him into a corner, no longer frightens him at all. He had been trained to present the ipsilateral paw when one waved a hand in front of an eye. Now one can wave one's hand indefinitely, the paw remains at rest until one says, "paw." And there are other observations of this nature. There can be no doubt about their interpretation. As a result of the extirpation, the dog has become mindblind, i.e., he has lost the visual ideas which he possessed, his memory images of previous visual perceptions, so that he does not know or recognize what he sees. However, the dog sees. Visual sensations reach consciousness and the stage of perception. They make it possible for ideas about the presence, form, and location of external objects to arise so that new visual ideas based on new memory images of the visual perceptions can be acquired.

Thus Munk (1878, pp. 162–163; 1890, pp. 21–22) described for the first time the condition to which he gave the name "mindblindness," and which later came to be designated as "visual agnosia" or "optic agnosia." Concomitantly, he offered an explanation for the condition. The animal had lost his "memory images" of previously perceived stimuli. Consequently, he could not relate current experience to past experience and hence he failed to grasp the "meaning" of a perceived stimulus.

But Munk found that mindblindness was only a temporary condition. Within a few weeks, the dog once again could recognize his master and other dogs and once again responded in a normal fashion to them. His explanation was that during the course of postoperative experience, new memory images were laid down in parts of the occipital cortex other than locus A_1. It will be recalled that Munk had specified that locus A_1 was the cortical center for foveal vision as well as the depository of memory images.

Munk's concept received a mixed reception. The fact that mindblindness appeared after a relatively superficial lesion in the very same area that subserved foveal vision and that it was a temporary condition made it seem probable that the animal's impaired behavior was due simply to loss of central vision. His notion that the mindblind dog was reduced to the status of a puppy without a store of visual memory images who could now deposit new images in another part of the occipital cortex seemed quite farfetched. Even his assumption that the mindblind dog's behavior was clearly deviant was questioned. Minkowski (1911), having removed locus A_1 from dogs without finding either a loss of central vision or signs of "mindblindness," remarked that he had often observed normal dogs to behave "unintelligently" in the face of visual stimuli, showing no response to the brandishing of a whip or sticking their paw in a piece of burning wood.

Consequently a substantial number of investigators, the earliest of whom was Mauthner (1881), interpreted mindblindness as the product of defective central vision perhaps coupled with postoperative mental blunting. For example, Siemerling (1890) studied a patient with mindblindness and was able to demonstrate a reduction in both visual acuity and color sensitivity which he concluded was responsible for the impairment in visual recognition.

But Munk's concept of mindblindness was accepted by other clinicians who observed a similar condition in some of their patients. Wilbrand (1887) and Lissauer (1890) described such patients who did not recognize objects or persons despite seemingly adequate visual acuity, and they related the condition to focal disease of the occipital lobes. Wilbrand agreed with Munk in attributing the defect to a loss of visual memory images but deviated from his thinking by postulating the existence of a discrete occipital cortical area, separate from the center for visual perception, which he designated the "visual memory field."

For his part, Lissauer (1890) not only presented a detailed description of the behavior of a patient with mindblindness but also offered a thoughtful discussion of the mechanisms that might be operating to produce the defect. The complete act of recognition involves two processes. The first is apperception, i.e., the conscious perception of an object, person, or event, implying the integration of the received sensory data into a unity or entity. The second process is the linking of the content of the perception with past experiences, implying associative activity and conferring meaning on the perception. Theoretically a patient might be rendered mindblind by a defect in one or the other mechanism. In practice, every patient suffering from mindblindness probably suffers from defects in both mechanisms because of the intimate interactive relationship between them. However, the severity of impairment in each might differ significantly. Thus, Lissauer felt that his patient exhibited a primarily associative type of mindblindness since a number of test performances indicated that he had excellent visual discriminative capacity.

One of the points made by Freud (1891) in his monograph on aphasia was the necessity for distinguishing between defects in naming objects and defects in recognizing them if clarity of thinking about the aphasic disorders was to be achieved. He therefore proposed that the term "agnosia" be employed to denote impairment in recognition within the context of adequate basic sensory capacity. His suggestion was generally adopted and "mindblindness" was discarded in favor of "visual agnosia" or "optic agnosia."

Up to this time, the structural characteristics of the occipital lobes and their connections with other hemispheric regions had received little attention. This gap was now filled by detailed anatomic study. Smith (1907) distinguished between morphologically differentiated striate and extrastriate occipital cortex, subdividing the latter into parastriate and peristriate areas. Brodmann (1909) similarly divided extrastriate cortex into an area 18 immediately surrounding striate cortex (area 17) and an outlying preoccipital area 19, a parcellation roughly corresponding to Smith's classification. At the same time, beginning with the work of Flechsig (1901), the connections of the occipital lobes with other cortical areas were investigated. Short association fibers connect area 17 with areas 18 and 19, from which arise longer association tracts leading to other parts of the cerebral hemispheres. These findings provided an anatomical framework for inferences about the lesional basis for disturbances in visual performance. Area 17 was the center for elementary visual experience. Elaboration of that experience into meaningful percepts required the functional integrity of areas 18 and 19, for these regions were the essential link between the primary visual center and the rest of the cortex. Thus, visual agnosia could be conceived as the outcome of lesions in area 18 and 19 which prevented the transmission and eventual integration of information arriving in area 17.

The concept of visual agnosia has had a checkered career since its introduction by Munk and the early studies of human subjects. On the one hand, the "reductionist" interpretation of Mauthner and Siemerling that the disorder is not a higher-level impairment in perceptual integration, association, or memory but only the expression of basic sensory deficit has been supported by some outstanding experimentalists and clinical investigators. The issue is, of course, whether or not the agnosic animal or patient does in fact have at his disposal the sensory information necessary for an accurate cognitive response. For example, Pavlov (1927, 1928) interpreted the mindblindness of Munk not as a higher-level psychological impairment but simply as loss of the capacity to make fine visual discriminations, and he suggested that the classical formula, "the dog sees but does not understand," should be reversed to read, "the dog understands but does not see sufficiently well" (Pavlov, 1927, p. 343). Similarly, Bay (1950, 1953, 1954) contended that visual agnosia in patients is explainable in terms of certain defects in visuosensory capacity, these defects typically occurring within the context of general mental impairment which itself hampers the process of drawing conclusions on the basis of inadequate visual information. He placed particular stress on alterations in rate of sensory adaption as the defect which may underlie the type of behavior called "visual agnosia." Critchley (1964) and Bender and Feldman (1965) also have advanced the view that visual agnosia is essentially the outcome of defective sensory capacity coupled with an overall decline in intellectual level. The "reductionists" have supported their position by citing the fact that practically every patient with visual agnosia is found to have *some* type of visual impairment, such as a field defect, inadequate visual scanning, or a disturbance in ocular fixation.

But the concept of visual agnosia as a "higher-level" disorder was fully accepted by other clinical investigators who described different subtypes of visual agnosia. The rather gross disability shown by Munk's dogs and Lissauer's patient was designated as "visual object-agnosia" while less pervasive disabilities involving one or another aspect of visual perception such as "visual form agnosia," "facial agnosia," and "visuospatial agnosia" were singled out for special study. Countering the argument that these disorders merely represent a partial impairment in basic sensory capacity, the "antireductionists" have pointed to the innumerable cases of severe visual defect that do not show the perceptual–integrative or associative disturbances characteristic of the agnosic patient.

THE METHOD OF DOUBLE SENSORY STIMULATION

Jacques Loeb

In 1884, the physiologist Jacques Loeb, who had worked with Goltz in Strasbourg, published a paper on the visual disturbances that follow experimental ablations of the brain in dogs. In it and two subsequent papers (Loeb, 1885, 1886), he described for the first time the responses of operated animals to double bilateral visual stimulation. Having noted that the most frequent immediate effect of unilateral destruction of one cerebral hemisphere is to produce a contralateral hemiamblyopia in which the animal is completely nonresponsive to visual stimulation on that side, he then described the course of recovery from the defect. In the first stage, the dog still does not perceive objects brought slowly into the affected field of vision but may respond to oscillat-

ing objects or to those that are rapidly introduced into the field. Further recovery of function then occurs.

The intensity of stimulus in the crossed visual half-field, which is necessary to elicit a reaction on the part of the dog, decreases steadily. After a time, if a single piece of meat is presented to the dog, he will react to it, even if it is not moved. In addition, when the meat is moved or thrown to the right, the dog follows it just as he would if it were moved or thrown to the left. It would appear from these tests that a visual disturbance is no longer present. However, if two pieces of meat are suddenly presented simultaneously to the dog, one in the right and the other in the left visual field, the animal who has been operated in the left hemisphere will without exception take the piece of meat to the left (Loeb, 1886, p. 294).

He then pointed out that such an impairment to double visual stimulation may be the only functional outcome of a less destructive cerebral lesion.

These findings record the course of a rather severe hemiamblyopia from the time of operation to the restitution of visual capacity; however, after superficial lesions and favorable conditions of operation and recovery, the initial disturbance is not as severe as here described. In the majority of cases, only the last described stage is present from the very beginning: the dog takes single pieces of meat under all conditions and favors that situated on the side of the lesion only upon simultaneous presentation of two pieces of meat (Loeb, 1886, pp. 275–276).

Seeking a physiological explanation of this pattern of responsiveness in which stimulation in the affected field is perceived when it is presented in isolation but not reacted to when presented in combination with concurrent stimulation in the healthy field, Loeb postulated that a unilateral hemispheric lesion produced impaired conduction in the involved neural pathways. As a consequence, the reactions mediated by these pathways are slower and weaker than those mediated by the neural connections of the intact hemisphere. In support of this interpretation, he cited the observation that if, under a condition of double stimulation, the intensity of the stimulus in the affected field is augmented to a sufficient degree, it would be perceived along with the stimulus to the healthy field.

Clinical application

Loeb demonstrated the behavior of his dogs to the clinical neurologist Hermann Oppenheim, who immediately applied the method of double sensory stimulation to patients with brain disease and found some who showed the predicted pattern of responsiveness (Oppenheim, 1885). Thus, two patients who perceived tactile stimulation on their affected side when it was presented in isolation failed to perceive it in combination with stimulation on the healthy side. Another patient showed failure to respond to tactile or visual stimuli when each was paired with corresponding stimulation on the healthy side. Still another patient showed failure to respond adequately to double simultaneous tactile or auditory stimulation. Confirming Loeb's observations on dogs, Oppenheim also reported that augmentation of the intensity of the stimulus on the affected side could lead to the normal perception of both stimuli on the part of a patient.

Finding that the procedure was of clinical value in an occasional case, Oppenheim adopted it as a diagnostic maneuver and described it in his famous textbook of neurology.

In certain cerebral diseases, which lead to unilateral sensory disturbances, I have often employed the following method of examination: two symmetrical locations on both sides of the body are simultaneously stimulated with touching by a brush or by pinpricks; under these conditions it happens that the patient invariably perceives only the stimulus which has been applied to the healthy side, while with single stimulation he feels every stimulus on the affected side. We shall designate this mode of examination as the method of double stimulation (Oppenheim, 1898, p. 51).

Subsequently the method of double sensory stimulation was utilized for investigative purposes in patients with suspected unilateral lesions by a few neurologists. Poppelreuter (1917) designated defective responsiveness to double visual stimulation as a "hemianopic weakness of attention." Thiébaut and Guillaumat (1945) called the deficit a "relative hemianopsia." The phenomenon was studied in detail by Bender and his coworkers (Bender & Teuber, 1946; Bender, Teuber, & Battersby, 1950; Bender, 1952; Bender & Feldman, 1952), who showed that it occurred in the different sensory modalities, gave it the name of "extinction," and described the diverse forms it may take. It was possible to show with human patients, who could give a verbal report of their experience, that partial extinction of response in the double stimulation paradigm may occur, i.e., the patient perceives the stimulus on the affected side or field but experiences it as weaker than when the stimulus is presented in isolation. Bender called this phenomenon "obscuration."

Utilizing a method of subjective magnitude estimation, Benton and Levin (1972) were able to produce the "obscuration" response in normal subjects by appropriate manipulation of the relative strength of competing tactile stimuli. Another type of deviant response, originally described by Jones (1907), was a tendency on the part of patients with unilateral lesions to report that both limbs had been touched when in fact stimulation had been applied only to the ipsilateral limb.

Eighty years after Loeb's pioneer studies, extinction to bilateral sensory stimulation was once again investigated experimentally in animals by Schwartz and Eidelberg (1968). Having been trained to respond differentially to electrical stimulation of the right, left, and both hands, monkeys were subjected to unilateral parietal and frontal ablations. Postoperatively a tendency to respond to double tactile stimulation as if single stimulation had been delivered to the hand ipsilateral to the side of lesion was observed. Daily fluctuations in the relative frequency of extinction responses, noted by Bender in patients, were also noted. Moreover, some animals showed the phenomenon of "synchiria" reported by Jones in patients, i.e., they responded to single stimulation of the limb ipsilateral to the side of the lesion as if double stimulation had been applied.

CONCLUDING COMMENTS

This sketch of the successive stages in the development of investigative work on two topics in the area of brain lesion research indicates how the experimental and clinical approaches interacted to advance understanding of the specific problem. As was mentioned earlier in the chapter, the initial observations were made on animals and these provided the impetus for analogous and more refined study of human subjects. In turn, the results of clinical study led to more detailed experimental investigation in animals. Thus, Munk's conclusion that the cortical mechanisms mediating visual function were located in the occipital lobes received a much more favorable reception from clinicians than from his fellow experimentalists, whose own preconceptions hindered acceptance.

In contrast, as Marchand and others pointed out, clinicians found Munk's results helpful in explaining previous observations, the significance of which had not been at all clear. Once Munk's experiments showed clinicians where to look for the cortical lesions producing visual impairment, they took full advantage of the experiments of nature that came their way and they were able to go far beyond the experimentalists of the period in establishing precise anatomical–behavioral correlations. Given this background of knowledge, Minkowski could once again investigate the problem in greater depth and provide experimental confirmation of the clinical correlations.

Is it the rule that the interplay of experimental and clinical research on a brain–behavior problem is like to be initiated by observations in animals? There is probably no such rule. The choice of a starting point in recounting the history of investigative work on a particular topic is largely determined by one's perception of whose work was particularly influential in determining the direction of subsequent research. With respect to vision, the experiments of Ferrier and Munk certainly meet this criterion and, hence, one regards them as pioneers. But their efforts were surely inspired by the discovery of the excitable motor cortex by Fritsch and Hitzig, who, on their part, cited earlier clinical observations relating discrete paralyses to focal brain lesions in support of the principle of cortical localization of motor function.

As early as 1874, Jackson advanced the concept that the posterior area of the right hemisphere subserved visual recognition and visual memory in human subjects. Subsequently, he published a case report in support of it (Jackson, 1876). Ferrier was quite familiar with Jackson's ideas along these lines and indeed referred to them as "hypotheses deserving consideration and further investigation" (Ferrier, 1878, p. 119). Thus, one could consider that Jackson was the "real" pioneer in pointing to a posterior representation of visual function or even Panizza (1855), whose early contribution seems to have been completely ignored at the time of its publication. Attention was called to it only after the publication of Munk's research (cf. Tamburini, 1880). And Panizza reported both experimental findings and clinical observations to make his point.

Thus, it seems rather fruitless to attempt to determine a starting point in an absolute sense and to ask whether this was represented by animal experimentation or clinical observation. The important fact is that, generally speaking, both the experimentalists and the clinicians kept themselves informed about developments in the others' field and took full advantage of these developments.

REFERENCES

Baumgarten, P., Hemiopie nach Erkrankung der occipitalen Hirnrinde. *Centralblatt für die Medicinischen Wissenschaften*, 1878, *16*, 369–371.

Bay, E. *Agnosie und Funktionswandel.* Berlin: Springer-Verlag, 1950.

Bay, E. Disturbances of visual perception and their examination. *Brain*, 1953, *76*, 515–550.

Bay, E. Optische Faktoren bei den räumlichen Orientierungsstörungen. *Deutsche Zeitschrift für Nervenheilkunde*, 1954, *171*, 454–459.

Bender, M. B. *Disorders in perception.* Springfield, Ill.: Charles C. Thomas, 1952.

Bender, M. B., & Feldman, D. S. Extinction of taste sensation on double simultaneous stimulation. *Neurology*, 1952, *2*, 195–202.

Bender, M. B., & Feldman, M. The so-called "visual agnosias." *Proceedings, VIII International Congress of Neurology*, 1965, 153–156.

Bender, M. B., & Teuber, H. L. Phenomena of fluctuation, extinction and completion in visual perception. *Archives of Neurology and Psychiatry*, 1946, *55*, 627–658.

Bender, M. B., Teuber, H. L., & Battersby, W. S. Discrimination of weights by men with penetrating lesions of parietal lobes. *Transactions of the American Neurological Association*, 1950, *75*, 252–255.

Benton, A. L., & Levin, H. S. An experimental study of "obscuration." *Neurology*, 1972, *22*, 1176–1181.

Brodmann, K. *Vergleichende Lokalisationslehre der Grosshirnrinde.* Leipzig: J. A. Barth, 1909.

Brouwer, B., Chiasma. Tractus opticus, Sehstrahlung und Sehrinde. In O. Bumke & O. Foerster (Eds.), *Handbuch der Neurologie*, Vol. 6, Berlin: Springer-Verlag, 1936.

Chaillou, F. H. Ramollissement multiple du cerveau. *Bulletin de la Société Anatomique de Paris*, 1863, *8*, (2nd Ser.), 70–73.

Critchley, M. The problem of visual agnosia. *Journal of the Neurological Sciences*, 1964, *1*, 274–290.

Curschmann, H. Die Lehre von der Hemianopsie und von den cerebralen Centren des Gesichtssinnes. *Centralblatt für Praktische Augenheilkunde*, 1879, *3*, 181–182.

Exner, S. *Untersuchungen über die Localisation der Functionen in der Grosshirnrinde des Menschen.* Wien: Wilhelm Braunmüller, 1881.

Ferrier, D. *The localisation of cerebral disease.* London: Smith, Elder and Co., 1878.

Ferrier, D. *The functions of the brain.* London: Smith, Elder and Co., 1876; 2nd Ed., 1886.

Ferrier, D. *The Croonian lectures on cerebral localisation.* London: Smith, Elder and Co., 1890.

Flechsig, P. Developmental (myelogenetic) localisation of the cerebral cortex in the human subject. *Lancet*, 1901, *2*, 1027–1029.

Freud, S. *Zur Auffassung der Aphasien.* Leipzig und Wien: Deuticke, 1891.

Fritsch, G., & Hitzig, E. Über die elektrische Erregbarkeit des Grosshirns. *Archiv für Anatomie, Physiologie und Wissenschaftliche Medizin* (Leipzig), 1870, 300–332.

Gratiolet, P. Note sur les expansions des racines cérébrales du nerf optique et sur leur terminaison dans une région determinée de l'écorce des hémisphères. *Comptes Rendus de l'Académie des Sciences*, Paris, 1854, 29, 274–278.

Haab, O. Über Cortex-Hemianopie. *Klinische Monatsblätter für Augenheilkunde*, 1882, 20, 141–153.

Henschen, S. E. *Klinische und anatomische Beiträge zur Pathologie des Gehirns*, Parts 1–3 Upsala: Almqvist & Wiksell, 1890–1896.

Huguenin, G. Über Hemiopie. *Korrespondenz-Blatt für Schweizer Aerzte*, 1881, 11, 43–44.

Hun, H. A clinical study of cerebral localization, illustrated by seven cases. *American Journal of the Medical Sciences*, 1887, 93, 140–168.

Jackson, J. H. On the nature of the duality of the brain. *Medical Press and Circular*, 1874 (reprinted in *Brain*, 1915, 38, 80–103.)

Jackson, J. H. Case of large cerebral tumour without optic neuritis and with left hemiplegia and imperception. *Royal London Ophthalmic Hospital Reports*, 1876, 8, 434–444.

Jones, E. The precise diagnostic value of allochiria. *Brain*, 1907, 30, 490–532.

Levick, Abscess of brain. *American Journal of the Medical Sciences*, 1866, 52, 413–414.

Lissauer, H. Ein Fall von Seelenblindheit nebst einem Beitrag zur Theorie derselben. *Archiv für Psychiatrie und Nervenkrankheiten*, 1890, 21, 222–270.

Loeb, J. Die Sehstörungen nach Verletzung der Grosshirnrinde. *Pflüger's Archiv für die Gesamte Physiologie*, 1884, 34, 67–172.

Loeb, J. Die elementaren Störungen einfacher Functionen nach oberflächlicher, umschriebener Verletzung des Grosshirns. *Pflüger's Archiv für die Gesamte Physiologie*, 1885, 37, 51–56.

Loeb, J. Beiträge zur Physiologie des Grosshirns. *Pflüger's Archiv für die Gesamte Physiologie*, 1886, 39, 265–346.

Marchand, F. Beitrag zur Kenntnis der homonymen bilateralen Hemianopsie und der Faserkreuzung im Chiasma opticum. *Graefe's Archiv für Ophthalmologie*, 1882, 28, 63–96.

Mauthner, L. *Gehirn und Auge*, Wiesbaden: Bergmann, 1881.

Meynert, T. Beiträge zur Kenntnis der centralen Projection der Sinnesoberflächen. *Sitzungsberichte der Kaiserlichen Akademie der Wissenschaften, Mathematisch-Naturwissenschaftliche Classe*, Wien, 1869, 60, 547–566.

Minkowski, M. Zur Physiologie der corticalen Sehsphäre. *Deutsche Zeitschrift für Nervenheilkunde*, 1911, 41, 109–118.

Munk, H. Weitere Mittheilungen zur Physiologie der Grosshirnrinde. *Archiv für Anatomie und Physiologie*, 1878, 2, 162–178.

Munk, H. Weiteres zur Physiologie der Sehsphäre der Grosshirnrinde. *Archiv für Anatomie und Physiologie*. 1879, 3, 581–592.

Munk, H. *Über die Functionen der Grosshirnrinde*. Berlin: August Hirschwald, 1890.

Oppenheim, H. Über eine durch eine klinisch bisher nicht verwerthete Untersuchungsmethode ermittelte Form der Sensibilitätsstörung bei einseitigen Erkrankungen des Grosshirns. *Neurologisches Zentralblatt*, 1885, 4, 529–533.

Oppenheim, H. *Lehrbuch der Nervenkrankheiten für Aerzte und Studirende*, II Aufl. Berlin: Karger, 1898.

Panizza, B. Osservazioni sul nervo ottico. *Giornale, Istituto Lombardo di Scienze e Lettere*, 1855, 7, 237–252.

Pavlov, I. P. *Conditioned reflexes*. London: Oxford University Press, 1927.

Pavlov, I. P. *Lectures on conditioned reflexes*. New York: International Publishers, 1928.

Polyak, S. *The vertebrate visual system*. Chicago: University of Chicago Press, 1955.

Pooley, T. R. Rechtseitige binoculare Hemiopie bedingt durch eine Gummigeschwulst im linken hinteren Gehirnlappen. *Archiv für Augen und Ohrenheilkunde*, 1877, 6, 27–29.

Poppelreuter, W. *Die psychischen Schädigungen durch Kopfschuss im Kriege 1914–1916: die Störungen der niederen und höheren Sehleistungen durch Verletzungen des Okzipitalhirns*. Leipzig: Voss, 1917.

Schäfer, E. A. Experiments on special sense localisation in the cortex cerebri of the monkey. *Brain*, 1888, 10, 36?–380.

Schwartz, A. S., & Eidelberg, E., "Extinction" to bilateral simultaneous stimulation in the monkey. *Neurology*, 1968, *18*, 61–68.

Siemerling, E. Ein Fall von sogenannter Seelenblindheit nebst anderweitigen cerebralen Symptomen. *Archiv für Psychiatrie und Nervenkrankheiten*, 1890, *21*, 284–299.

Smith, G. E. New studies on the folding of the visual cortex and the significance of the occipital sulci in the human brain. *Journal of Anatomy*, 1907, *41*, 198–207.

Starr, M. A. The visual area in the brain determined by a study of hemianopsia. *American Journal of the Medical Sciences*, 1884, *87*, 65–83.

Tamburini, A. Rivendicazione al Panizza della scoperta del centro visivo corticale. *Revista Sperimentale di Freniatria e Medicina Legale*, 1880, *6*, 153–154.

Thiébaut, F., & Guillaumat, L. Hémianopsie relative. *Revue Neurologique*, 1945, *77*, 129–130.

Wilbrand, H. *Die Seelenblindheit als Herderscheinung und ihre Beziehungen zur homonymen Hemianopsie*. Wiesbaden: J. F. Bergmann, 1887.

Wilbrand, H. *Die hemianopischen Gesichtsfeld-Formen und das optische Wahrnehmungzentrum*. Wiesbaden: J. F. Bergmann, 1890.

Wilbrand, H., & Saenger, A. *Die Neurologie des Auges*. Vol. 3, 1904, Vol. 7, 1917. Wiesbaden: J. F. Bergmann.

8.

Focal Brain Damage and the Concept of Localization of Function*

Cherchez dans l'homme et dans la bête
Quel siège a la raison, soit le cœur, soit la tête

HISTORICAL REVIEW

These lines from La Fontaine's fable, *Démocrite et les Abdéritains*, serve to remind us that "localization of function" is not only a very old concept but also one that was not necessarily related to the brain. Indeed no less an authority than Aristotle maintained that the heart was the seat of the psychic life while the brain served the function of cooling the body heat generated by the heart. These inferences apparently were derived from his observations that the brain was cold to the touch and that animals whose brains were touched did not seem to feel any sensation. As Clarke (4) points out, this cardiocentric theory of the seat of the mental life had many supporters during the Middle Ages and the Renaissance, including Andrea Cesalpino and William Harvey.

But, of course, the "cerebrocentric" theory of functional localization also had

its supporters, at least since the time of Alcmaeon of Croton, Democritus and the Hippocratic physicians (i.e., 400–500 B. C.), and the conflicting claims of the two schools generated the controversy as to whether the seat of mind was "in the heart or in the head." Clarke (4) describes how some medieval writers tried to resolve the controversy by suggesting that the heart and brain work together to support mental functions. Avicenna (980–1037), for example, stated that while the brain is the seat of sensation and thought, it is controlled by the heart. Alfredus Anglicus (fl. ca. 1215) wrote in a very similar vein: although the brain is the seat of intelligence, nevertheless, it is secondary to the heart, which is the source of its energy and which transmits emotional disturbances to it (4, 24).

Thus these early students postulated that mentation was mediated by a system rather than by a single organ.

Having been advanced by the early Greek physicians, the cerebrocentric theory evolved in the direction of increasing differentiation. This first took the

* In honor of Cornelio Fazio. A. L. Benton in C. Loeb (Ed.), *Studies in Cerebrovascular Disease.* Milan, Masson Italia Editore, 1981, pp. 47–56.

form of localization of different mental functions within the brain along its longitudinal axis, either in the brain substance itself or in the ventricles. Thus Nemesius (fl. ca. 400) placed sensation and perception in the anterior (lateral) ventricles, reasoning in the middle (third) ventricle and memory in the posterior (fourth) ventricle. Once formulated in an explicit way, this ventricular theory of cerebral localization in one or another version dominated medical thinking for over 1000 years and was seriously challenged only in the sixteenth and seventeenth centuries.

Localization of function in the substance of the brain displaced ventricular theory in the seventeenth century. At that time Thomas Willis (1621–1675) placed the seat of sensation in the corpus striatum. According to his schema, sensations were then transformed into meaningful percepts in the corpus callosum and these percepts were stored as memory images in the cerebral cortex. It is not exactly clear why "brain substance" theory supplanted ventricular theory at this particular juncture. Case reports describing patients with ventricular injury but without impairment of mental functions may have had an influence and the derisive attitude of Vesalius (who pointed out that even the ass, the most stupid of animals, possessed all four ventricles) also may have played a role in facilitating this shift in emphasis.

Other medical scientists proposed various localizations within the brain. Having observed that most parts of the brain could be absent or injured without producing mental impairment, La Peyronie (1678–1747) concluded that the corpus callosum was the seat of intelligence. On his part, Swedenborg (1688–1772) placed the higher mental faculties in the cells of the cerebral cortex and suggested that different cortical areas are concerned with different modalities of sensory experience. He also considered the basic ganglia to be centers of motor control (1).

Relatively broad concepts of cerebral localization, such as those of Willis and La Peyronie, were the rule in the eighteenth century. A quantum leap to another mode of thinking took place in the early decades of the nineteenth century when the anatomist and phrenologist, Franz Joseph Gall (1758–1828), expounded his ideas and made cerebral localization a central issue in neurophysiology and neuropsychology. Gall's basic postulate was that the human brain was not a single organ but an assemblage of organs, each of which formed the material substrate of a specific cognitive faculty or personality trait. He found no difficulty in identifying the locus in the brain of some thirty mental traits, most of which he took from the analyses of the Scottish school of psychology, as represented by Thomas Reid (1710–1796) and Dugald Stewart (1753–1828).

Gall's hypothesis that the brain is not a unitary equipotential organ, but instead consists of an aggregate of specialized areas, attracted both loyal supporters and vigorous opponents. The controversy was waged on several planes. Philosophical idealists and the religious establishment denied that specific parts of the brain could form the material substrate of mental faculties since this idea seriously weakened the concept of an abstract mind or of an immortal soul on which their philosophy or religious system rested. For essentially the same reasons, materialist philosophers and anticlerical groups embraced the idea.

However, the question was also addressed on an empirical scientific plane. Gall's major opponent, Pierre Flourens (1794–1867), was not a complete antilocalizationist. He divided the brain into four basic units, each of which served a distinctive function. The cerebellum controlled movement, the medulla was a vital center, the colliculi served as an organ of vision, and the cerebral hemispheres served as the organ of mentation, "of willing, judging, seeing, hearing, in a word, remembering." But Flourens was an anti-localizationist in respect of the functions of the hemispheres which, he insisted, acted as a unit with the different mental functions residing in all parts of the cerebral lobes. He reached this conclusion from ablation experiments on the pigeon and the chicken in which he observed that the degree of impairment of function was related to the mass of tissue ablated and not to its locus. He further noted that, when there was recovery of function, all the functions returned together. Apparently Flourens did not hesitate to apply these conclusions from his observations on birds to all organisms, including man, and he interpreted his findings as a refutation of Gall's theory. Karl Lashley (1890–1958) was in direct line of descent from Flourens. His conclusions, derived from ablation studies on the rat, were expressed in his "law of equipotentiality" (any specific area of the hemispheres is functionally equivalent to any other specific area) and his "law of mass action" (the severity of behavioral impairment following ablation of brain tissue is proportional to the amount of tissue removed).

In any case, clinical observation was more pertinent to the issue since Gall's conceptions dealt with localization of function in the human brain, not that of the pigeon or the rat. For centuries clinicians had suggested that the occurrence of discrete functional defects following injury to the brain, such as a monoplegia restricted to an arm or a leg or sensory loss in a limited area of the skin surface, argued for the validity of the concept of localization of cerebral function. On the other hand, it had also been noted repeatedly that a patient could sustain the loss

of an appreciable amount of hemispheric tissue, particularly in the frontal area, without showing evident functional deficit and this argued for mass action of the cerebral hemispheres. In more recent years the researches of Harold Wolff (1898–1962) and his collaborators on the relationship between objectively assessed degree of behavioral impairment and estimated amount of neuronal loss in both patients who had undergone surgical removals of cerebral tissue and those with degenerative brain disease also adduced evidence in support of Lashley's laws of equipotentiality and mass action (3, 16).

Apart from the question of the validity of his basic conceptions, the specific aspect of Gall's scheme which engaged the greatest scientific interest was his placement of the centers of speech and language in the frontal lobes. The spirited controversy over the validity of this localization began with Bouillaud's vigorous defense of it in 1825 and was resolved only when Broca demonstrated the association between motor aphasia and left frontal lobe disease and Wernicke and others established the crucial role of the posterior region of the left hemisphere in the mediation of language functions.

At the same time, beginning with the discovery by Fritsch and Hitzig in 1870 of the excitable motor cortex in the frontal lobes, experimental and clinical investigators were able to relate a variety of functions to different cortical areas, for example, vision to the occipital lobes, somesthesis to the peri-rolandic region, and so on. The experimentalists did this through ablation studies in which they noted the loss of function resulting from discrete removals of tissue. The clinicians accomplished it by relating the functional disturbances shown by patients during life to autopsy findings.

Thus by 1890 the view that the human brain is a functionally equipotential organ had been shown to be quite untenable. Nevertheless, there was still uncertainty concerning the degree to which sensory, perceptual, motor and cognitive capacities could be localized in the brain substance. This uncertainty applied with particular force to the question of the localization of strictly cognitive capacities, such as memory in its various forms, linguistic functions and reasoning ability.

TOWARDS A DEFINITION OF CEREBRAL LOCALIZATION

However, not all neurologists suffered from such doubts and extremely detailed systems of cerebral localization were developed by S. E. Henschen (15) (1847–1930), Karl Kleist (17) (1879–1960) and Oskar Vogt (26) (1870–1959). Henschen (14) (15), for example, undertook an exhaustive review of pertinent clinicopathologic reports in the literature and formulated a schema that postulated the existence of numerous independent cortical centers for almost every aspect of linguistic, mathematical, musical and perceptual activity. Thus he identified specific centers for word reading and number reading, for the understanding of word sounds and the understanding of word meanings, for different arithmetical operations, for rhythm, musical perception and musical praxis. On his part, Kleist (17) localized about 60 sensory, perceptual, linguistic and cognitive capacities in specific areas of the cerebral cortex. In line with his cytoarchitectonic orientation, Vogt (26) attempted to relate specific cognitive capacities to the status of specific cortical fields and layers and thus to provide a neurological basis for individual differences in talent.

Despite the fact that these systems of cerebral localization were proposed by highly respected investigators of great abi-

lity and unquestioned integrity, they were received with the utmost skepticism by neurologists. The very fact that the models were so detailed was itself cause for suspicion since clinical experience showed that there were exceptions to even the most widely accepted correlations, e.g., the association of motor aphasia with destruction of Broca's area or that of fluent receptive aphasia with destruction of Wernicke's area. There were also grounds for objection on a deeper level. These had to do with the basic assumptions underlying most of these localizational systems, simple as well as complex, which made specific parts of the brain the seat or center of specific behavioral capacities and which endowed the neurons comprising these sites or centers with truly extraordinary functional properties. For example, according to the classical doctrine of aphasia as formulated by Wernicke, Lichtheim and Bastian, Broca's area was the repository of memory-images (or representations) for the articulation of syllables; hence destruction of this "center" produced disturbances in speech articulation. Wernicke's area in the first temporal gyrus was the repository of memory-images (or representations) of the sounds of words; hence its destruction produced disturbed understanding of speech as well as a specific disturbance of speech expression related to this auditory amnesia. Mindblindness or visual object-agnosia was related by Wilbrand (29) to destruction of an "optic memory-field" (optisches Erinnerungsfeld), the individual cells of which contained representations of past visual experience. Similarly, Wernicke (27) ascribed tactile object agnosia or pure astereognosis to "a loss of the memory-images of the tactile sensations of concrete objects which are located in the postcentral gyrus." In short, specific mental capacities were subserved by specific parts of the brain.

As functional localization became a major topic of scientific inquiry, a few philosophers, physicians and physiologists perceived the difficulties inherent in these assumptions that equated particular aspects of mentation with particular parts of the brain. One of the first to do so was the philosopher, Friedrich Albert Lange (18) (1828–1875). In his history of materialism, he reviewed the early pre-Broca controversy about localization of function. As a positivist and humanist, he was sympathetic to the localizationist position. But then, using a homely example, he pointed out the fallacy involved in inferring the positive from the negative or, in physiological terms, inferring function from symptom. He wrote:

If someone shows me that a small lesion in a particular part of the brain of an otherwise healthy cat leads him to give up chasing mice, I will believe that one is on the right path for making psychological discoveries. However, I will not assume that the locus in which ideas of mouse-hunting have their seat has been found. If a clock strikes the hours incorrectly because a wheel is broken, it does not follow from this that the wheel struck the hours (18, p. 447).

A decade later, Hughlings Jackson (1855–1911) made the same point when he warned that "to locate the damage which destroys speech and to locate speech are two different things." Jackson's disciple, Henry Head (12) (1861–1940) dealt with the issue at greater length, pointing out that:

An act of speech is a march of events, where one changing condition passes insensibly into another. When speech is defective, this easy motion or transition is impeded; one state cannot flow into another because of some mechanical imperfection in the process. The power of finding words, the rhythmic modulation and balance of a phrase, the appreciation of meaning and intention, verbal or general, are thrown into disorder.

The processes which underlie an act of speech run through the nervous system like a prairie fire from bush to bush; remove all inflammable material at any one point and the fire stops. So, when a break occurs in the functional chain, orderly speech becomes impossible, because the basic physiological processes which subserve it have been disturbed. The site of such a breach of continuity is not a "centre for speech," but solely a place where it can be interrupted or changed (12, [Vol. 1,] p. 474).

In a similar fashion, Jacques Loeb (1859–1924) emphasized that the efforts of physiologists in the 1870s to localize mental functions in discrete cortical areas were, in principle, not different from the placement of mental functions in the ventricles or the earlier attempts of theologians to find the seat of the soul. He pointed out that the concept of "function" is only a short-hand term for a whole range of events and that "cerebral localization" consists essentially in describing how the course of these events is changed by induced changes in the nervous system. As he put it, the question of where intelligence is located in the brain cannot be answered. What can be answered is the question of the site in the brain of those lesions that produce disturbances in intelligence.

Jackson and Head were not antilocalizationist in the Flourens-Lashley sense. They certainly did not believe in the functional equipotentiality of all regions of the cerebral hemispheres. Indeed, Jackson was the first to present clinical evidence in favor of a specific association between disease of the posterior right hemisphere and disturbances in visual recognition and orientation. Despite his withering critique of the "diagram makers" with their neat models of interconnecting centers of speaking, writing, reading, and understanding, Head (12, Vol. 1, pp. 431–473) related different forms of aphasic disorder to focal lesions in different loci in the left hemisphere and, as Geschwind (6, 7) has pointed out, his localization was in essential accord with traditional practice. However, this does not imply, as Geschwind (6, 7) suggests, that Head's basic position with respect to localization was thereby vitiated. His quarrel with the "diagram makers" was not with their localizations of lesions but with their postulation of discrete centers which served as the seat of functions. "That lesions situated in different localities in one hemisphere can produce specific changes in the power to employ language is one of the most remarkable facts which emerge from the study of aphasia" (12, Vol. 1, p. 499). This explicit statement is sufficient to show that Head was concerned with the meaning of localization, not with elementary clinical findings.

No doubt the fact that clinical localization was so often successful fostered the confusion between "symptom" and "function." If nonfluent aphasic disorder was generally found to be associated with an anteriorly located lesion, a fluent aphasic disorder with a lesion in the posterior temporal region and acquired alexia with a lesion in the region of the angular gyrus, it was perhaps "natural" to conceive of these areas of being the seat or center of the disturbed functions. Lange, Jackson, Loeb, and Head perceived the fallacy in this reasoning and insisted that the brain and its mechanisms form a far more complex system than that envisaged by the diagram markers.

In essence, these critics argued that traditional models of brain function were too simplistic to do justice to the facts of cerebral organization. Jackson and later writers such as Arnold Pick (1851–1924), Constantin von Monakow (1853–1930) and Kurt Goldstein (1878–1965) further insisted that classical theory also oversimplified the facts on the behavioral side of the brain-behavior equation.

They pointed out that terms such as alexia, agraphia, word deafness, auditory agnosia, and visual agnosia lacked the specific denotative meaning that they were assumed to possess in studies which attempted to correlate lesions with symptoms. Instead, each term referred to a whole spectrum of behavioral disabilities on different levels and sometimes of a fundamentally different nature. Agraphia, for example, had such a variety of meanings from an operational standpoint that the designation of a patient as "agraphic" without further specification (as was the rule in clinical reports) was not truly informative. One did not know whether the term meant that the patient could not write spontaneously, to dictation or from copy, whether his disability was of a linguistic, praxic, or spatial nature, whether it was complete or partial, permanent or transitory.

Jackson urged the student to "put down what the patient does get at and avoid all such terms as 'amnesia, etc.' " (2, p. 33). On his part, Goldstein (8, 9, 10) emphasized the necessity for detailed qualitative analysis of a patient's performance on a given task if insight into the nature of his disability is to be achieved. Criticizing the simplistic tendency to record a performance as successful or not by marking it "plus" or "minus," he showed how a variety of factors, including some of affective nature, can determine the character and level of the patient's behavior.

There is no doubt that the point was well taken. Behavioral and linguistic study has demonstrated that even seemingly specific functions such as that of understanding ordinary conversational speech or reading simple text consists of multiple components, any of which may be disturbed as a consequence of brain disease and cause failure in performance. Hence, terms such as "impaired understanding of aural speech" or "alexia" (even when subdivided into "literal alexia" and "verbal alexia") are, like "agraphia," informative only in the global sense of indicating that something is wrong with the patient's understanding or reading. Luria, (21) distinguished between three levels of impairment in auditory comprehension among aphasic patients: acoustic or phonemic, in which the patient cannot discriminate speech sounds; amnesic, in which the meaning of words is not grasped; and semantic, in which propositions embodied in sentences are not understood. Goodglass, Gleason, and Hyde (11) employed a classification of the dimensions of speech comprehension which contained two of the components described by Luria (21) (word recognition and the understanding of propositions) but which also included the dimensions of memory for auditory sequences and the recognition of correct grammatical usage. They found that aphasic patients in different diagnostic categories showed different patterns of performance on the set of four tests. With respect to reading, Marshall and Newcombe (22) and other investigators (19) have distinguished between phonemic and semantic types of impairment in alexic patients.

PRESENT VIEWS

The implications of these developments in clinical behavioral analysis for the problem of cerebral localization are fairly clear. Since reading (or writing or the comprehension of oral speech) is an act that involves the simultaneous processing of a number of kinds of information on different levels and of a diverse nature, the neural system serving it must be quite extensive and complex. It must provide for the reception and transmission of these types of information and for their parallel processing. Consequently, there must be, not one, but a number of critical points or junctures in the system, injury to which will impair one or another of the components of reading. Since these components are not independent, e.g., phonemic impairment will retard word recognition and defective word recognition will retard phonemic analysis, the entire process of reading is likely to be disrupted by impairment of a single component.

The task of the localizer is to try to identify these critical junctures in the neural system. One possible approach is through the analysis of the characteristics of the patient's performance. Luria (21), for example, was able to correlate impairment in phonemic discrimination with wounds in the neighborhood of Wernicke's area and higher-level semantic dysfunction with involvement of parieto-occipital territory of the dominant hemisphere. Goodglass, Gleason, and Hyde (11) found that patients with Broca's aphasia (whose lesions were presumably located anteriorly) showed particularly severe impairment in memory for auditory sequences, while auditory word recognition remained relatively intact.

The agnostic disorders have always presented difficult problems of localization and they illustrate how complex the true state of affairs may be. Prosopagnosia provides an instructive example. Ever since the initial description of this peculiar disability by Quaglino in 1867, its close association with symptoms of disease of the right hemisphere, such as left visual field defect, spatial disorientation and constructional apraxia, has been quite evident (13).

A recent study by Whitely and Warrington (28) has presented radiological evidence to support the correlation between prosopagnosia and right hemisphere disease. However, the anatomical findings in the nine cases of prosopagnosia that have come to autopsy present a different picture. Bilateral lesions, most commonly in both occipital lobes but occasionally a rightsided occipital lesion in combination with a left hemisphere lesion in another area, have been found in every case (2, 20, 23, 25).

Thus, if the post-mortem findings are accepted at face value, bilateral disease would seem to be the necessary condition for the occurrence of prosopagnosia. Within this setting, a lesion situated in the region of the right lingual and fusiform gyri, i.e., at the occipito-temporal junction, appears to be a characteristic feature of the anatomic picture. This lesional localization in the basal occipital area is reflected in the remarkably high frequency of left upper quadrantic field defects in prosopagnosic patients, as Faust (5) and Meadows (23) have noted. The field defect per se, due to involvement of the underlying lower part of the optic radiations, probably has little functional significance in this context. The crucial lesion, according to Meadows (23), is damage to the inferior longitudinal fasciculus and tapetal fibers of the corpus callosum which interrupts the connections of occipital cortex with the middle temporal, inferior temporal and hippocampal gyri as well as those between the right and left occipito-temporal areas.

Thus, it appears in the case of prosopagnosia that there is a crucial lesion but it is crucial only in combination with disease in the opposite hemisphere. That is to say, the right inferior occipital lesion will derange a system that has been rendered vulnerable by a left lesion but it will not derange an intact system. It is not possible to say how many other behavioral disabilities follow this paradigm. The fact that prosopagnosia is a rare symptom suggests that this is not a very common combination of circumstances. The important point is that the symptom arises from derangement of a system which is its necessary and sufficient cause. The right occipital lesion is a necessary, but not a sufficient condition, for the appearance of the perceptual-mnesic disability. To generalize, symptoms must be viewed as expressions of disturbances in a system not as direct expressions of focal loss of neuronal tissue. Symptoms may change in time since the system is dynamic in nature and alters its mode of function in an attempt to meet the demands of organismic adaptation. When this attempt is successful, the symptoms disappear, as is likely to be the case with agnosia and apraxic disabilities which are so often transitory in nature.

What then is "cerebral localization?" It consists of the identification of the neuronal mechanisms within the brain that are responsible for the mediation of defined behavioral capacities. These mechanisms are never located in a single discrete neural aggregate but are always defined by dynamic sets of interrelationships among neuronal aggregates. Lesional localization consists of identifying those specific junctures within a system of interrelationships that derange the system with sufficient severity to impair its mediating functions. This functional impairment may be temporary if the system can reorganize itself to support the functions once again. Thus, the cerebral "localizer" must be prepared to encounter transitory defects as well as permanent ones and negative cases as well as positive ones. But the transitory defects and the negative cases should not be regarded as inexplicable exceptions to a simplistic rule but as valuable clues to the nature of neural mechanisms which he is seeking to elucidate.

REFERENCES

1. Akert, K., Hammond, H. P. (1962): *Eman-*

uel Swedenborg (1688–1772) and his contribution to neurology. Medical History
6:255–266.

2. Benton, A. L. (1979): *Visuoperceptive,
visuospatial and visuoconstructive disorders.*
In: Clinical neuropsychology, edited by K. M.
Heilman & E. Valenstein. New York, Oxford
University Press.

3. Chapman, L. F. Wolff, H. G. (1959):
*The cerebral hemispheres and the highest inte-
grative functions of man.* Arch. of Neurol. 1:
357–424.

4. Clarke, E. (1963): *Aristotelian concepts
of the form and function of the brain.* Bulletin
of the History of Medicine 37: 1–14.

5. Faust, C. (1955): *Die zerebralen Herdstörungen bei Hinterhauptsverletzungen und
ihre Beurteilung.* Stuttgart, Thieme.

6. Geschwind, N. (1964): *The paradoxical
position of Kurt Goldstein in the history of
aphasia.* Cortex 1: 214–224.

7. Geschwind, N. (1970): *The organization of language and the brain.* Science, 170:
940–944.

8. Goldstein, K. (1934): *Der Aufbau des
Organismus.* Den Haag, Nijhoff.

9. Goldstein, K. (1939): *The Organism.*
New York, American Book Co.

10. Goldstein, K. (1942): *After effects of
brain injury in war.* New York, Grune & Stratton.

11. Goodglass, H., Gleason, J. B., Hyde,
M. (1970): *Some dimensions of auditory
language comprehension in aphasia.* J. of
Speech and Hearing Research, 13: 595–606.

12. Head, H. (1926): *Aphasia and kindred
disorders of speech.* 2 vol. London, Cambridge
University Press.

13. Hécaen, H., Angelergues, R. (1962):
Agnosia for faces (prosopagnosia). Arch. of
Neurol. 7: 92–100.

14. Henschen, S. E. (1919): *Über Sprach-,
Musik- und Rechenmechanismen und ihre
Lokalisationen im Grosshirn.* Zeitsch. ges.
Neurol. und Psych., 52: 273–298.

15. Henschen, S. E. (1922): *Klinische und
Anatomische Beiträge zur Pathologie des
Gehirns, 5., 6., 7. Teil.* Stockholm, Nordisk
Bokhandeln.

16. Kiev, A., Chapman, L. F. Guthrie, T.
C., Wolff, H. G. (1962): *The highest integra-
tive functions and diffuse cerebral atrophy.*
Neurology, 12: 385–393.

17. Kleist, K. (1934): *Gehirnpathologie.*
Leipzig, Barth.

18. Lange, F. A. (1866): *Geschichte des
Materialismus.* Iserholm, J. Baedeker.

19. Lesser, R. (1978): *Linguistic investigations of aphasia.* London, E. Arnold.

20. Lhermitte, F., Chain, F., Escourolle,
R., Ducarne, B., Pillon, B. (1972): *Etude ana-
tomo-clinique d'un cas de prosopagnosie.* Rev.
Neurol. 126: 329–346.

21. Luria, A. R. (1970): *Traumatic aphasia.* The Hague, Mouton.

22. Marshall, J. C., Newcombe, F. (1973):
*Patterns of paralexia: A psycholinguistic
approach.* J. of Psycholinguistic Res. 2:
175–199.

23. Meadows, J. C. (1974): *The anatomical basis of prosopagnosia.* J. of Neurol.
Neurosurg. and Psych., 37: 489–501.

24. Pagel, W. (1958): *Medieval and renaissance contributions to knowledge of the brain
and its functions.* In: The brain and its functions, edited by F. N. L. Poynter, Oxford,
Blackwell.

25. Rondot, P., Tzavaras, A. (1969): *La
prosopagnosie après vingt années d'etudes cliniques et neuropsychologiques.* J. Psychol.
Normale et Pathol. 66: 133–166.

26. Vogt, O. (1951): *Die anatomische Ver-
tiefung der menschlichen Hirnolokalisation.*
Klin. Wochenschrift 29: 111–125.

27. Wernicke, C. (1895): *Zwei Fälle von
Rindenläsion.* Arbeiten der Psychiatrischen
Klinik in Breslau 2: 33–53.

28. Whitely, A. M., Warrington, E. K.
(1977): *Prosopagnosia: A clinical, psychological, and anatomical study of three patients.* J.
Neurol., Neurosurg. and Psych. 40: 395–403.

29. Wilbrand, H. (1887): *Die Seelenblindheit als Herderscheinung und ihre Beziehungen
zur Homonymen Hemianopsie.* Wiesbaden,
Bergmann.

9.

Hemispheric Dominance before Broca*

INTRODUCTION

A persisting question in the history of neuropsychology is why so many astute clinician–pathologists before 1860 failed to grasp the connection between aphasia and disease of the left hemisphere or, indeed, between aphasia and the occurrence of right hemiplegia. With the benefit of hindsight, one can see that the ingredients for establishing a correlation were already present in ancient medical writings. There is the statement in the Hippocratic corpus that associates temporary speechlessness following convulsions "either with paralysis of the tongue or of the arm and right side of the body" (5, p. 248). Coupled with this is the well-known Hippocratic observation that "an incised wound in one temple produces a spasm in the opposite side of the body" (5, p. 263). Some 500 years later Aretaeus of Cappadocia sought to explain this observation of contralateral motor

impairment following a head wound by postulating a crossing of the nerve tracts from the brain to the spinal cord (1, p. 306). It is not unreasonable to think that an integration of these statements would have suggested a specific association between speech disorder and left hemisphere disease.

A possible reason for the failure to make the correlation is that Aretaeus' remarkable conception was by no means universally accepted. Many physicians interpreted the occurrence of paralysis on the side contralateral to the side of injury as being the result of concussion, diffuse inflammation or a contrecoup effect. However, in the eighteenth century these factors were effectively eliminated as putative causes when Pourfour du Petit demonstrated the crossing of the descending nerve tracts at the level of the pyramids and Morgagni assembled an impressive mass of clinicopathologic case material to support the association between paralysis of one side of the body and disease of the opposite hemisphere.

No doubt a systematic survey of the early medical literature would disclose a

* Dedicated to the memory of Henry Hecaen. A. L. Benton, *Neuropsychologia*, 1984, 22, 807–811.

trend for "speechlessness," "aphonia," "alalia" and "speech amnesia" to be associated with paralysis of the right side of the body. But at the same time the unbiased compiler would have noted many cases that did not follow the rule, i.e. speechlessness without paralysis or with left-sided paralysis and left hemisphere disease without speech disorder. Thus he would have to conclude there was no obligatory association between aphasia and right-sided paralysis (or left hemisphere disease). Moreover, he would find that the early literature did not yield as rich a harvest as might have been anticipated. These reports were generally only a few lines in length and lacking in essential details. When speechlessness or disordered speech is mentioned, it is usually impossible to determine whether the impairment in expression was aphasic in nature or a reflection of neuromotor disability, stupor, confusion, dementia or psychosis.

Descriptions of aphasic patients that are sufficiently detailed to be informative first appeared in the late seventeenth century. At least nine such case reports were published before 1800—Schmidt (1673), Rommel (1683), Linné (1745), Dalin (1745), Gesner (1770, two cases), Spalding (1783), Herz (1791) and Crichton (1798) (Summaries and, in some instances, the complete texts of these reports can be found in the review by Benton and Joynt [3]). Of the nine patients, three had right-sided paralysis and a nonfluent aphasia. The other six patients had no paralysis and five of them had a fluent aphasic disorder. A reviewer of this series of cases might have noted that, when paralysis was present, it was always on the right side and never on the left. But evidently no student at that time was fortunate enough to be endowed with such serendipity. A possible distraction was the fact that medical interest in the eighteenth

century was largely focused on patients showing the more florid forms of fluent aphasia, as reflected in jargon aphasia and "wild" paraphasic utterances, and these patients generally did not show motor disability.

Three monumental treatises on clinical pathology, each of which dealt at some length with brain–behavior relationships, appeared in the eighteenth and early nineteenth centuries—Morgagni's *De sedibus et causis morborum per anatomen indigatis* (1761), Bouillaud's *Traité clinique et physiologique de l'encéphalite* (1825) and Andral's *Clinique médicale* (1829–1840). The present paper attempts an analysis of the basic data in each of these treatises with the aim of evaluating the strength of the latent evidence supporting a specific association between aphasic disorder and disease of the left hemisphere and discusses possible reasons for the failure to perceive the association. The singular story of the one man who did grasp the relationship but who elected at the time to withhold his discovery from the public will then be reviewed.

MORGAGNI

The first volume of Morgagni's great compilation includes numerous brief descriptions of speechlessness associated with apoplexy, head injury and fever, together with the findings at autopsy. He repeatedly emphasizes the connection between paralysis of one side of the body and the presence of disease in the opposite cerebral hemisphere. Many patients are described as speechless but more often than not the disability is noted within the context of stupor or a rapidly worsening condition resulting in death within hours. Consequently there are relatively few cases that are suitable for our analysis.

From an inspection of the 1769 English translation by Benjamin Alexander of

De sedibus, I identified ten cases of unilateral paralysis in patients who were not comatose, stuporous or dying in whom autopsy disclosed a purely or predominantly unilateral hemispheric lesion and in whom it was possible to ascertain whether or not speech was disordered. Five patients had a right-sided paralysis and four of them were impaired in speech. Five patients had a left-sided paralysis and one was impaired in speech.

BOUILLAUD

Beginning in 1825 and for a half-century thereafter, Jean-Baptiste Bouillaud was the great champion of Gall's localization of the centers of speech and language in the frontal lobes and he argued repeatedly, vigorously and, at times, rancorously that aphasic disorder resulted only from lesions in this territory. In his *Traité . . . de l'encéphalite* (1825), he presented 29 cases with and without aphasia and with and without lesions in the anterior, middle and posterior lobes. All of the aphasic patients had lesions that were in or close to the anterior lobes. Neither then nor subsequently could he find a valid example of aphasic disorder that was not a consequence of disease of the anterior lobes.

Inspection of Bouillaud's 29 cases shows that 25 had lesions confined to a single hemisphere, 11 in the left hemisphere and 14 in the right. Eight (73%) of the 11 left hemisphere cases were aphasic. Four (29%) of the right hemisphere cases were aphasic.

Perhaps one reason why Bouillaud did not perceive this trend toward a higher frequency of aphasic disorder in his left hemisphere patients is that not only was he obsessed with the frontal lobe localization of aphasic disorder but he also accepted Gall's dual localization of the centers of speech and language in both hemispheres. Thus whether a lesion was found to be in the left or right hemisphere was a matter of indifference to him.

ANDRAL

Gabriel Andral was one of the luminaries of French clinical pathology in the 1830s and 1840s. His *Clinique médicale* and *Précis d'anatomie pathologique* were widely used in France and known throughout the world in English, German and Italian translations. In Vol. 5 (*Maladies de l'encéphale*) of the *Clinique médicale* he addressed the question of the localization of speech disorder with special reference to the Gall–Bouillaud doctrine and presented his conclusions in the following succinct statement:

M. le professeur Bouillaud a publié, il y a déjà plusieurs années, un mémoire rempli de faits curieux desquels il a cru pouvoir déduire la conséquence que la formation de la parole a pour instrument l'extrémité antérieure de chaque hémisphère, attendu qu'il a trouvé cette partie lésée, toutes les fois que pendant la vie la parole elle-même avait été perdue. Voici, à cet égard, ce que nous ont appris nos recherches.

Sur trente-sept cas observés par nous ou par d'autres, relatifs à des hémorrhagies ou à d'autres lésions, dans lesquels l'altération résidait dans un des lobules anterieurs ou dans tous les deux, la parole a été abolie vingt-et-une fois, et conservé seize fois.

D'un autre côté, nous avons rassemblé quatorze cas où il y avait abolition de la parole, sans aucune altération dans les lobules antérieurs. De ces quatorze cas, sept étaient relatifs à des maladies des lobules moyens, et sept autres à des maladies des lobules postérieurs.

La perte de la parole n'est donc pas le résultat nécessaire de la lésion de lobules antérieurs, et, en outre, elle peut avoir lieu dans des cas où l'anatomie ne montre dans ces lobules aucune altération (2, p. 368).

It is quite evident from inspection of

the *Clinique médicale* (4th Edition, 1840) that not all 37 cases mentioned by Andral are described in the book. I was able to identify 11 cases of unilateral disease, 5 with lesions in the left hemisphere and 6 with lesions in the right hemisphere, where the status of the patient's speech during his illness is described. Of the 5 left hemisphere cases, 3 were aphasic. Of the 6 right hemisphere cases, none was aphasic.

A collaborator and admirer of P. C. A. Louis, who introduced the statistical approach into medical observation, Andral applied the latter's *méthode numérique* to his case material in evaluating Bouillaud's claims. Evidently it did not occur to him to extend its application to the question of a right-left hemisphere difference. The few lines he wrote on aphasia suggests that the topic was not of great interest to him and probably he was content with disproving the Gall-Bouillaud thesis. Bouillaud and Andral were polar opposites in temperament and in their approach to problems. Bouillaud was passionate, polemical and dogmatic; Andral was sober, analytic and wary of speculation. Moreover, the two men were opponents in other respects as well. Andral campaigned vigorously against the practice of blood-letting while Bouillaud was, as Garrison (8) describes him, "a furious bloodletter" who "favored pitilessly rapid bleeding, *coup sur coup.*"

In summary, the observations reported in each of the three treatises show a trend towards a specific association between speech disorder and left hemisphere disease. However, in no single instance is the trend statistically significant, as assessed by the Fisher Exact Probability Test (two-tailed), although it approaches significance ($p = .10$) in Bouillaud's sample. If it is permissible to combine the cases in the three samples and apply a chi-square test to the data, the resulting chi-square (10.3) indicates a

between-hemispheres difference which is significant at the .002 level.

Some of the possible reasons for the failure to perceive this difference have already been noted, such as the occurrence of exceptional cases, the presence of left hemisphere disease without speech disorder and the desparate conditions of so many patients. But perhaps the most important single reason is to be found in the circumstance that these men were very busy practitioners who at the same time actively pursued numerous and varied investigative interests. None of them was a specialist in the modern sense of the term, either in their medical practice or in their research. So far as can be seen, Morgagni had no interest in aphasia beyond noting on occasion that a patient was speechless and Andral had only a passing interest which quite clearly had been aroused by Bouillaud's claims.

Aphasia was a topic of major concern only to Bouillaud. Yet, when one considers his subsequent activity, it is understandable that, having embraced Gall's hypothesis of centers of speech in both frontal lobes, he proceeded to defend it vigorously without exploring the matter further. After 1825 he turned his attention to the fields of cardiology and rheumatology, to which he made a number of notable contributions, the most important of which was his demonstration of the association between rheumatic fever and endocarditis. Indeed, it was Bouillaud who introduced the terms "endocardium" and "endocarditis" into medicine (10).

Thus it is not unlikely that the major reason why the aphasia-left hemisphere association escaped the attention of Morgagni, Bouillaud and Andral is that their busy schedule and competing interests did not allow them the time to consider the data bearing on the association. It was left to a thoughtful country doctor with scholarly interests and the time to reflect on the meaning of his own observations and those of others to discover the correlation.

MARC DAX

In about 1836 this physician, who practiced in Sommières (about 25 km from Montpellier), wrote a paper purporting to show that aphasic disorder is exclusively associated with lesions of the left hemisphere. Marc Dax was born in 1770 and died in 1837. He was thus about 66 years old when he wrote his famous *mémoire*.

It is a remarkable document. Dax describes the successive observations that led him gradually to the conviction that aphasia was the product of left hemisphere disease. An aphasic patient with whom he had first become acquainted in 1800 had sustained a left parietal wound. At the time this meant to Dax only that Gall's frontal lobe doctrine could not be altogether correct. In 1809 he had an aphasic patient with an extensive tumor on the left side of the face who died some months later. He attached no special significance to the circumstance that the lesion was left-sided. However, when in 1811 he read that the naturalist Broussonet had become aphasic after a left hemisphere stroke, he reflected on the fact that the three cases with which he was familiar had left hemisphere lesions. From this time onward, Dax had a "prepared mind" and, when he encountered three additional cases of aphasia with presumptive left hemisphere disease over the period of 1812–1814, he formulated his hypothesis. He continued to collect cases over the ensuing 20 years, so that at the time of writing his paper he reported having a series of over 40 cases in whom the diagnosis of left hemisphere disease had been made, primarily on clinical grounds without pathological confirmation. It was on this empirical basis that he wrote:

De tout ci qui précède, je crois pouvoir conclure, non que toutes les maladies de l'hémisphère gauche doivent altérer la mémoire verbale, mais que, lorsque cette mémoire est altérée par une maladie du cerveau, il faut chercher la cause du désordre dans l'hémisphère gauche, et l'y chercher encore si les deux hémisphères sont malades ensemble.

Marc Dax's paper (7) was published in 1865 by his son, Gustav Dax (6), who stated that it had been read at a regional medical meeting in Montpellier in 1836. In fact there is no evidence that he did present the paper on that occasion (9). It is not mentioned in accounts of the meeting, nor could anyone be found who remembered having heard it. It seems almost certain that, if the paper had been presented, it would not have been totally neglected and would have had some repercussions.

The tone of Dax's paper is personally modest but firm in conviction. Its style indicates that it was meant to be a communication to his peers. He was quite aware of the importance of his discovery and he made one or two copies which he sent to professional friends. Why he did not make his discovery known at the time through publication or oral presentation is not clear. Perhaps he planned to publish after the collection of further data but death intervened. In any case, whether by intention or not, his manuscript became in effect a *paquet cacheté* that was brought to light only after Broca's discovery.

REFERENCES

1. Adams, F. *The Extant Works of Aretaeus, the Cappadocian.* Sydenham Society, London, 1856.
2. Andral, G. *Clinique médicale*, 4th Edn. Fortin, Masson, Paris, 1840.
3. Benton, A. L. & Joynt, R. J. Early descriptions of aphasia. *Arch. Neurol.* 3, 205–222, 1960.

4. Bouillaud, J. B. *Traité clinique et physiologique de l'encéphalite.* J. B. Bailliére, Paris, 1825.

5. Chadwick, J. & Mann, W. N. *The Medical Works of Hippocrates.* Blackwell Scientific Publications, London, 1950.

6. Dax, G. Notes sur le même sujet. *Gaz. hebd. Med. Chir.* (Paris). 2, 262, 1865.

7. Dax. M. Lésions de la moilité gauche de l'encéphale coincidant avec l'oubli des signes de la pensée. *Gaz. hebd. Med. Chir.* 2, 259–262, 1865.

8. Garrison, F. H. *An Introduction to the History of Medicine*, 4th Edn. W. B. Saunders, Philadelphia, PA., 1929.

9. Joynt, R. J. & Benton, A. L. The memoir of Marc Dax on aphasia. *Neurology* 14, 851–854, 1964.

10. Major, R. H. *A History of Medicine.* C. C. Thomas, Springfield, IL., 1954.

11. Morgagni, G. *The Seats and Causes of Diseases Investigated by Anatomy* (trans. by B. A. Alexander). A. Millar & T. Cadell, London, 1769.

III.
The Method of
Double Stimulation

10.

Jacques Loeb and the Method of Double Stimulation*

SENSORY EXTINCTION

The phenomenon of extinction of sensory responsiveness as a consequence of simultaneous double stimulation, which is observed in certain patients with cerebral disease, is currently a topic of considerable interest in both clinical neurology and physiological psychology. Extinction in the visual and tactual spheres has been extensively studied[1,7] and the deficit has been described as occurring in other modalities, such as proprioception,[4] taste,[2] and audition.

Visual extinction as a function of simultaneous double stimulation may be described in outline as follows: a single stimulus applied to either the right or left visual field is perceived by the patient. When, however, stimuli are applied to both fields, the patient reports seeing an object in only one of the fields. A favored method of testing for the deficit is to stimulate the suspected field, secure a report from the patient that he perceives the sti-

mulus, and, then, while continuing the initial stimulation, to apply a second stimulus to the healthy field, noting whether there is any change in responsiveness to the first stimulus.

The deficit occurs in varying degrees of severity. There may be complete cessation of responsiveness to the affected field with double stimulation ("extinction"). However, under this condition, the patient may still perceive the stimulus but report only that it has become somewhat dimmer or darker ("obscuration"). Sometimes the deficit cannot be elicited with standard testing procedures but becomes manifest if the patient is required to report or reproduce from memory what he has seen.[5] In other cases, significant augmentation of the strength of the stimulus in the affected visual field enables the patient to perceive both stimuli. Since the patient often behaves as if he were "neglecting" the stimulus in the affected field, the term, "hemianopic weakness of attention" was coined by Poppelreuter[17] as a name for this type of impairment. Thiébaut and Guillaumat[19] called the deficit "relative

* A. L. Benton, *Journal of the History of Medicine and Allied Sciences*, 1956, 11, 47–53.

hemianopsia." Finally, on the basis of the idea that the phenomenon may involve activity of assumed "suppressor systems" in the cortex, the designation of "sensory suppression" has been employed by some writers.[8,18]

Tactual extinction occurs in analogous fashion. A touch or pain stimulus applied, for example, to either shoulder, forearm, or palm is perceived by the patient, while double stimulation results in his reporting that he feels only the stimulus on one side.*

The clinical significance of the extinction phenomenon and the method of double stimulation lies in the fact that they disclose behavioral deficits which are not elicited by other methods of examination. In turn, these deficits point to dysfunction in the central nervous system and, in conjunction with other signs, are often of value in localizing the dysfunction. Thus, many of Bender's patients, who showed no visual field defects by routine perimetry, manifested behavioral impairment in the double stimulation test—impairment which disclosed the presence of central nervous system disease and which was helpful sometimes in the localization of the underlying lesions.

In addition, the phenomenon and the method possess broader psycho-physiological implications. As Bender and Teuber[3] have pointed out, it seems likely that the clinical findings represent a special case of a general principle of psychological functioning, viz., that in the interaction of simultaneously occurring stimuli or response tendencies, the stronger tendency will inhibit the weaker. In the intact subject, a marked difference in the strength of the

two stimuli is usually required to secure overt behavioral expression of the process. In the patient with nervous disease, the strength of the two response tendencies is differentially determined by intraorganismic factors so that the phenomenon may occur within the setting of double stimulation of objectively equal strength.

HERMANN OPPENHEIM

The method of simultaneous double stimulation was introduced into clinical neurology in 1885[14] by Oppenheim who wrote a paper on its possible clinical significance and subsequently made mention of it in the various editions of his well-known textbook of neurology.[15] Thus, Oppenheim is generally credited with being the discoverer of the method, at least insofar as its neuropathological application is concerned.†

In the second edition (1898) of the textbook, Oppenheim described the tactual stimulation procedure as follows:

In certain cerebral diseases, which lead to unilateral sensory disturbances, I have often employed the following method of examination: two symmetrical locations on both sides of the body are simultaneously stimulated with touching by a brush or by pin-pricks; under these conditions it happens that the patient invariably perceives only the stimulus which has been applied to the healthy side, while with single stimulation he feels every stimulus on the affected side. We shall designate this mode of examination as the method of double stimulation. (p. 51)

Following deliberate policy,‡ Oppen-

---

* These remarks actually cover only one form of extinction, that of the homologous crossed type. There are several other types (e.g., ipsilateral, nonhomologous crossed, interaction across sensory modalities) which are described in the monographs of Bender and Critchley. [1,7]

---

† One exception to this rule (the only exception of which the writer is aware) deserves mention. In a recent paper, Krueger, Price and Teuber,[9] citing Jacques Loeb's 1884 paper (vide infra), point out that he was the first to use the method of double stimulation in animal experimentation.

‡ See the preface to the first edition (1894).

heim did not include references to the literature in the earlier editions of his textbook, and there is no mention of previous work on the method of double stimulation, not even his own paper in the *Centralblatt*. However, beginning with the fifth edition (1908), he did add—with apparent reluctance—selected references.* In this edition, in the paragraph describing tactual extinction which is quoted above, reference is made to the *Centralblatt* paper. The seventh edition (1923) of the textbook, appearing after Oppenheim's death and revised by a number of his students, includes an additional reference with respect to the method of double stimulation: "At Oppenheim's suggestion, Medea (Atti della Soc. Milano, 1908) has studied this problem in detail."†

Thus, in the various editions of the famous textbook, there is no suggestion that Oppenheim might not have been the originator of the method of double stimulation and its application to problems of cerebral dysfunction. However, in his original paper in the *Centralblatt*, Oppenheim indicates clearly the direct source of the method. The paper begins as follows:

By means of superficial, circumscribed injury of the brain in dogs, Jacques Loeb elicited disturbances in function, the nature and interpretation of which he has reported in a brief communication in Volume XVII of Pflüger's Archiv. This author has had the kindness to demonstrate repeatedly the interesting phenomena in his experimental animals to me and thereby has stimulated me to make the investigations, the results of which I now briefly report.

Oppenheim then described four patients with focal lesions. Two of these showed tactual extinction on double stimulation, one showed both tactual and visual extinction and the fourth showed tactual and auditory extinction. He pointed out that the phenomenon never occurs in healthy subjects and, in fact, is found to be relatively infrequent in patients with cerebral disease. He also observed that augmentation of the strength of the stimulus to the affected side could lead to perception of both stimuli by the patient.

THE CONTRIBUTION OF JACQUES LOEB

Oppenheim's reference to "Volume XVII" of *Pflüger's Archiv* is evidently a typographical error. The paper which he almost certainly had in mind is in Volume 37 (1885) and bears the title, "Die elementaren Störungen einfacher Functionen nach oberflächlicher, umschriebener Verletzung des Grosshirns."‡ This paper was written on the basis of work which Loeb had done in the laboratory of Goltz in Strassburg.[16] In it he describes the method of simultaneous double stimulation with particular reference to the visual modality, reports his findings with the method on intact and operated dogs, and clearly indicates the neurophysiological significance of the extinction phenomenon, i.e., the implication of dysfunction in the contralateral half of the central nervous system. He begins the paper by stating two "laws of elementary disturbances of function."

* "The principal change which occurs in this new edition of my textbook is that, yielding to the pressures of friends of the work, I have decided, after much doubt and long hesitation, to cite references to the literature." (From the preface to the fifth edition.)

† The reference is to Medea.[13]

‡ In passing, it should be noted that in a comprehensive paper on visual and psychic disturbances following cerebral injury in the dog, which appeared a year earlier,[20] Loeb briefly described his findings with double stimulation. However, he reserved detailed discussion of its significance for the 1885 paper.

If we designate the side of the body and visual half-field which corresponds to the injured hemisphere as "same-sided" or the "side of operation" and the other as the "crossed" or "contralateral" side, the two laws of elementary disturbances of function read as follows:

I. If two stimuli, which are equal to each other in quality and intensity, are applied simultaneously to symmetrical parts of the retinae or skin, the stimulus applied to the crossed side is less effective than the one which is applied to the side of operation. However, by augmentation of the intensity of the stimulus to the contralateral side the same effectiveness can be achieved.

II. When a stimulus of a given quality and intensity is applied to the crossed side, the reaction has a longer latency and is slower than when the same stimulus is applied to the side of operation.

Three basic observations, which "can always and without exception be demonstrated, with constancy of a physical experiment," are then cited.

(1) If one suddenly and simultaneously presents pieces of meat in two symmetrical parts of the visual field of the hemi-amblyopic dog, the dog consistently takes the one situated on the side of the operation.—(2) If one lightly oscillates the meat situated on the contralateral side—a moving object is a stronger stimulus—, while the other piece of meat remains stationary, the animal will spring at the moving piece of meat. The rate of oscillatory movement which is necessary for this effect varies with different animals. Within certain limits, the more severe the hemi-amblyopia the higher the rate must be.—(3) If a piece of meat is presented alone in the crossed half-field to the dog, he regularly springs at it, even when it is not moved. Thus, while this stimulus, when it is presented alone, is adequate to elicit a reaction on the part of the dog, it remains always without effect if at the same time a second stimulus, of the same quality and intensity, is applied to the side of operation.

In a third paper,[12] which appeared a year later, Loeb again described the method of double stimulation as a means of disclosing half-field defects. He points out that the most serious immediate effect of this character after operative injury to a cerebral hemisphere is complete lack of responsiveness in the contralateral visual half-field, even to very strong stimulation. There is then gradual postoperative improvement so that after a few days oscillating objects or objects which are quickly introduced into the affected half-field are reacted to, while there is still no responsiveness to objects brought more slowly into the field. Progressive improvement continues beyond this intermediate stage.

The intensity of stimulus in the crossed visual half-field, which is necessary to elicit a reaction on the part of the dog, decreases steadily. After a time, if a single piece of meat is presented to the dog, he will react to it, even if it is not moved. In addition, when the meat is moved or thrown to the right, the dog follows it just as he would if it were moved or thrown to the left. It would appear from these tests that a visual disturbance is no longer present. However, if two pieces of meat are suddenly presented simultaneously to the dog, one in the right and the other in the left visual field, the animal who has been operated in the left hemisphere will without exception take the piece of meat to the left.

These findings record the course of a rather severe hemi-amblyopia from the time of operation to the restitution of visual capacity; however, after superficial lesions and favorable conditions of operation and recovery, the initial disturbance is not as severe as here described. In the majority of cases, only the last described stage is present from the very beginning: the dog takes single pieces of meat under all conditions and favors that situated on the side of the lesion only upon simultaneous presentation of two pieces of meat.

Specific observations on the animals' reactions to simultaneous double tactual stimulation are not recorded although references to it are made in the first "law" and in the statement that one-sided disturbances of sensibility, analogous to the visual disturbances, occur. Loeb's explanation of the extinction phenomenon was that injury to a hemisphere resulted in increased resistance to conductivity in the involved nervous pathways, with a consequent weakness and retardation in the behavioral reactions mediated by these pathways. He felt that his two "laws" had broad applicability to all central nervous system function, spinal as well as cerebral.

It seems evident that Loeb had a clear understanding of the significance of the method of simultaneous double stimulation. He described sensory extinction accurately and pointed out the importance of the factor of relative strength of stimulus in determining whether extinction would occur or not. He was obviously aware of the lateralizing neurophysiological implications of the phenomenon. One misses in his exposition any explicit indication that the extinction effect is a resultant of the interaction or "competition" of simultaneous stimuli, with the stronger stimulus in some way suppressing or inhibiting the effectiveness of the weaker one. However, this is equally true of Oppenheim's treatment, which is restricted to the practical clinical significance of the extinction phenomenon.

A year after the publication of Oppenheim's paper in the *Centralblatt*, Bruns, an assistant at Hitzig's clinic in Halle, published a confirmatory case report[6] of a patient who showed tactual extinction on double stimulation and credited Oppenheim with having "discovered a hitherto unrecognized type of sensory disturbance by means of a newly applied method of clinical examination." Loeb was not mentioned despite Oppenheim's frank acknowledgement of his work. This is perhaps understandable in view of the

purely clinical import of Bruns' brief paper. However, the failure to mention Loeb may also have been conditioned by the extremely acrimonious controversy on cerebral function between Goltz (and his able lieutenant, Loeb) and Hitzig (who was Bruns' chief), which was then going on.

In any event, Loeb's pioneer contribution was seemingly forgotten as the years passed and is only now once again being recognized.

REFERENCES

1. Bender, M. B. *Disorders in perception.* Springfield, Ill., Charles C. Thomas, 1952. 109 pp.

2. Bender, M. B. & Feldman, D. S. Extinction of taste sensation on double simultaneous stimulation. *Neurology*, 1952, 2, 195–202.

3. Bender, M. B. & Teuber, H. L. Phenomena of fluctuation, extinction and completion in visual perception. *Arch. Neurol. Psychiat.*, 1946, 55, 627–658.

4. Bender, M. B., Teuber, H. L., & Batterby, W. S. Discrimination of weights by men with penetrating lesions of parietal lobes. *Trans. Amer. neurol. Assoc.*, 1950, 75, 252–255.

5. Benton, A. L. *The revised visual retention test: clinical and experimental applications.* New York, Psychological Corporation, 1955, 68 pp.

6. Bruns, I., Ein Beitrag zur einseitigen Wahrnehmung doppelseitiger Reize bei Herden einer Grosshirnhemisphäre. *Neurol. Zbl.*, 1886, 5, 198–199.

7. Critchley, M. *The parietal lobes.* London, Edward Arnold & Co., 1953, 480 pp.

8. Furmanski, A. R. The phenomena of sensory suppression. *Arch. Neurol. Psychiat.*, 1950, 63, 205–217.

9. Krueger, E. G., Price, P. A., & Teuber, H. L. Tactile extinction in parietal lobe neoplasm. *J. Psychol.*, 1954, 38, 191–202.

10. Loeb, J. Die Sehstörungen nach Verletzung der Grosshirnrinde. *Pflüger's Arch.*, 1884, 34, 67–172.

11. Loeb, J. Die elementaren Störungen einfacher Functionen nach oberflächlicher, umschriebener Verletzung des Grosshirns. *Pflüger's Arch.*, 1885, *37*, 51–56.

12. Loeb, J. Beiträge zur Physiologie des Grosshirns. *Pflüger's Arch.*, 1886, *39*, 265–346.

13. Medea, E. Il metodo del doppio stimolo applicato alla ricerca di alcuni difetti visivi a tipo emianopsico in talune affezioni unilaterali del cervello. *Atti Soc. Milanese Med. Biol.*, 1908, *3* (4).

14. Oppenheim, H. Über eine durch eine klinisch bisher nicht verwerthete Untersuchungsmethode ermittelte Form der Sensibilitätsstörung bei einseitigen Erkrankungen des Grosshirns. *Neurol. Zbl.*, 1885, *4*, 529–533.

15. Oppenheim, H. *Lehrbuch der Nervenkrankheiten für Aerzie und Studierende.* Berlin, Karger, I Aufl., 1894; II Aufl., 1898; V. Aufl., 1908; VII Aufl., 1923.

16. Osterhout, W. J. V. Jacques Loeb. *J. Gen. Physiol.*, 1928, *8*, ix–lix.

17. Poppelreuter, W. Die psychischen Schädigungen durch Kopfschuss im Kriege 1914–16: die Störungen der niederen und höheren Sehleistungen durch Verletzungen des Okzipitalhirns. Leipzig, Voss, 1917.

18. Reider, N. Phenomena of sensory suppression. *Arch. Neurol. Psychiat.*, 1946, *55*, 583–590.

19. Thiébaut, F. & Guillaumat, L. Hémianopsie relative. *Rev. neurol.*, 1945, *77*, 129–130.

11.

An Experimental Study of "Obscuration"*

One of the observed effects of double sensory stimulation in patients with cerebral disease is diminution, rather than complete extinction, of the perception of the stimulus applied to the side of the body or visual half field opposite the side of lesion.[1,2] In such instances, the patient reports that the stimulus on the affected side looks darker or feels weaker than when it is presented alone. Since it was first noted in connection with double visual stimulation, the phenomenon has been called "obscuration." However, it applies equally to double tactile stimulation, where the patient may report a pinprick as duller or a pressure stimulus as weaker on one side than on the other. This partial form of extinction is often observed in the course of recovery of sensory function after stroke or trauma. Having manifested complete extinction on earlier occasions, the patient reports that he now feels or sees both stimuli with, however, a discernible difference in their

perceived intensities. This may be followed at a later date by the restitution of apparently normal responsiveness to double sensory stimulation.

Defective responsiveness to double stimulation in patients with cerebral disease is often conceived as being the exaggerated expression of a normal physiologic mechanism, wherein a stronger stimulus has the effect of inhibiting or suppressing the perception of a weaker one. The operation of such a mechanism is, of course, attested by numerous studies of sensory "masking" in human subjects, which have shown that the presentation of a more intense masking stimulus in close temporal association with a test stimulus will lead to an attenuation of the effect of the latter stimulus. The test stimulus is usually set at or near the threshold level, and the effect of concomitant presentation of the masking stimulus is assessed in terms of either a change in the frequency of detection of the test stimulus at threshold intensity[3-5] or a change in the threshold value itself.[6-10]

Two salient findings of these studies

* A. L. Benton and H. S. Levin, *Neurology*, 1972, 22, 1176–1181.

are pertinent to the problem of the mechanisms underlying the clinical phenomena of extinction and obscuration. The first is that contralateral masking (test stimulus and masking stimulus on opposite sides of the body or in opposite visual half fields) is markedly less effective than ipsilateral masking where the test and masking stimuli are positioned closely together.[5,9,11,12] The second is that test stimuli must be set at or near threshold value to demonstrate a contralateral masking effect. For example, Bird[4] was able to demonstrate the phenomenon of extinction of response to the weaker of two tactile pressure stimuli positioned on homologous sites of the two forearms in healthy subjects only when the intensity of the weaker stimulus was at a "minimal suprathreshold value," defined as the weakest intensity at which the subject detected the stimulus five times in succession. When the intensity of the test stimulus was raised slightly above that value, extinction was not produced.

These results stand somewhat in contrast to the clinical observation of the extinction phenomenon manifested by patients with cerebral disease. A stimulus applied to the side contralateral to that of the lesion in a patient with unilateral brain disease may be far above threshold intensity and, when presented in isolation, be readily perceived by him. Yet extinction of response to it can be relatively easily produced by concurrent stimulation of equal (or even lesser) intensity on the opposite side of the body. Thus there seems to be no necessity for the stimulus on the affected side to be at or near threshold level in order for extinction of perceptual response to occur within the context of double bilateral sensory stimulation. Nor can a raised threshold for single stimulation on the affected side be invoked to account for the phenomenon because, as Birch, Belmont and Karp[13]

have shown, patients with unilateral lesions still show extinction even when the relative intensities of the paired stimuli are adjusted to compensate for any differences in threshold sensitivity on the two sides.

This lack of concordance between the clinical findings in patients and the experimental results in healthy subjects poses difficulties for any theory that would explain extinction as the outcome of a normal physiologic mechanism wherein bilateral stimulation of unequal strength produces inhibition of response to the weaker of the two stimuli. The principle applies well enough when the weaker stimulus is at or near threshold intensity but, as has been indicated, healthy subjects are not likely to show extinction of perceptual response to the weaker stimulus if its intensity is clearly above threshold, while patients often will fail to perceive a relatively strong stimulus on the affected side in the context of competing stimulation on the unaffected side.

Experimental investigation of the phenomenon of obscuration offers a possible approach for gaining further understanding of the problem. The patient who reports a weakened perception of a suprathreshold stimulus applied to his affected side is clearly showing modified responsiveness as a function of simultaneous double sensory stimulation. The question the present investigation was concerned with was whether, using refined psychophysical methods and appropriate conditions of stimulation, it would be possible to demonstrate obscuration of perception of suprathreshold stimulation in healthy subjects who failed to show complete extinction of response to the weaker of two bilaterally applied tactile stimuli. The procedure was to train subjects to estimate the subjective magnitude of tactile stimuli (weights dropped on the skin surface) and, after this training, to secure their magnitude estimates under conditions of both single and double stimulation.

METHOD

The subjects were five male university students (age range 18 to 24 years), four of whom were strongly right-handed and one of whom was strongly left-handed as determined by their responses to a questionnaire assessing hand preference in various activities and by global self-rating of hand preference as being strong or moderate.[14] Each subject was given intensive training in the task of estimating the subjective magnitude of single tactile stimuli until he achieved stable estimates of the relative magnitudes of a series of stimuli varying along the dimension of intensity as defined by grams of pressure applied.

Apparatus

Punctate stimulation was delivered by a modified version of the electromechanical stimulator of Carmon and Dyson,[15] which drops probes on the skin surface and which permits precise control of force, duration, rate of application, and area of stimulation. The pressure delivered by each probe was determined by the weight within it above a tip which was 1.5 mm in diameter, as well as by the weight of the tip itself. The masking stimulus was a probe with a weight of 40 gm; the test stimuli were probes with weights of 1, 5, 10 and 20 gm. Upon impact of the probe on the skin, the tip of the probe retracted into the container. The duration of impact for all stimuli was 720 msec.

Experimental procedure

To familiarize the subject with the psychophysical procedure of subjective magnitude estimation, a line judgment task was given at the beginning of the first session. He was instructed to let the number 100 stand for the apparent length of a standard line (2 in.) and to assign numbers proportional to the apparent length of a series of subsequently presented lines. He was further informed that in making these estimates he could use any number, including fractions or decimals. Some examples were given to ensure that he understood the nature of the task. Estimates of magnitude were obtained for three series of presentations, each series consisting of a single presentation of each of five comparison lines (0.25, 1, 2, 4 and 6 in.). The standard 2 in. line was presented just before each series and identified as 100 by the experimenter. The lines were randomly ordered within each series.

The individual subjects assigned idiosyncratic values to the perceived lines. For example, on the third series of presentations, J. K. assigned values of 10, 60, 100, 250 and 400 to lines 0.25, 1, 2, 4 and 6, respectively, while D. A. assigned values of 20, 50, 100, 200 and 225 to the same lines. However, three series of training trials on this rather easy task were sufficient for each subject to achieve a correct rank ordering in respect to subjective magnitude in the sense that there was perfect correspondence between this ordering and the actual lengths of the lines.

Following the line judgment task, each subject was trained on the more difficult task of estimating the subjective magnitude of weights dropped on an area of the volar surface of the forearm which was 6 in. proximal to the wrist. Three subjects (including the left-handed subject) were trained and tested on the right arm and the other two subjects were trained and tested on the left arm. Instructions were identical to those used for the line judgment task. Each series of stimulations consisted of four weights (1, 5, 10, 20 gm) presented in random order. The standard weight (5 gm) was presented just before each series and identified by the examiner as 100. Training consisted of 48 series of stimulations, equally distributed among three training sessions. As a result of this training, each subject achieved stable estimates of the subjective magnitude of the weights as defined by a perfect correspondence between the rank order of his estimates and the rank order of the actual strengths of the weights for all of the last eight series of trials.

In the main experiment, the masking weight (40 gm) and each of the test stimuli (1 to 20 gm) were simultaneously delivered to homologous contralateral sites on the forearms, the test weights being applied to the arm which had been used in training. The task instructions were identical to those given for the training procedure, i.e., the subject was to assign a numerical value to the subjective magnitude of each test weight. He was informed that the procedure would differ from the previous procedure only in that, on occasion, a second weight would be simultaneously applied to his other arm. However, he was to attend only to the test weight and to report his estimates of its magnitude alone.

The session consisted of four trial blocks, each of which included four presentations of each of the four test weights. Within each trial block, two of the four presentations of a given test weight were accompanied by simultaneous application of the masking weight. Thus, each subject made 64 estimates (32 estimates for test weight trials alone and 32 estimates for test weight plus masking weight trials). The 16 stimulations within a trial block (four test weights presented twice alone and twice with the masking weight) were randomly distributed among four series to ensure that sensory adaptation and fatigue would not have a differential effect on the subject's sensitivity to the eight types of stimulation. Each series was immediately preceded by presentation of the standard weight (5 gm) which was identified as 100.

The subject was seated in front of the electromechanical stimulator with his arms resting on an adjustable platform connected to the stimulator. He extended his arms through the arm holders with the volar surfaces turned upward facing the stimulating probes. The probes were positioned 2 mm from the respective forearm surfaces. The subject was blindfolded during training and testing to eliminate any visual cues that might affect his judgment of the test stimulus. He was informed that movements of his arms would be detected by photocells and corrected by the experimenter. The duration of stimulation was 720 msec under all conditions. All trials involved the activation of both stimulator solenoids so that audible noises accompanying the operation of the stimulator would be constant for both types of trials. Each trial block was followed by a two minute rest period. The sessions lasted approximately 80 minutes. The interval between the last training session and the main testing session ranged from one to three days.

Supplementary study

This partial replication was done to assess the stability of the findings of the main experiment. It was identical in all respects to the main experiment except that the effects of simultaneous presentation of the contralateral masking weight were assessed only for the 5 and 10 gm weights. The five subjects (age range 17 to 25 years) were all right-handed. Having met the training criteria described above, they were given four blocks of trials, each of which consisted of two presentations of the four test weights alone and two presentations of the 5 and 10 gm weights in combination with the contralateral 40 gm weight. The 12 stimulations within a trial block were randomly distributed into three series of four stimulations, each series being preceded by the presentation of the standard 5 gm weight, which was identified by the examiner as 100. Thus, each subject made 48 magnitude estimates (32 estimates for test weight alone trials and 16 estimates for test weight plus masking weight trials).

RESULTS

Comparison of the subjective estimates of the magnitude of the test weights presented alone with the estimates of the magnitude of the same weights when presented in combination with the contralateral weight of greater strength provided unequivocal evidence of an overall obscuration effect. As part A of Table 4 shows, the mean magnitude estimate for the 32 test weights presented alone was 129.1, and the mean magnitude estimate for the same weights presented under a condition of simultaneous double stimulation was 106.5, the mean difference corresponding to a decline of 17.5 percent in perceived intensity from the single to the double stimulation condition. The distributions of the two sets of estimates were significantly different ($p < .001$), as determined by the Wilcoxon signed ranks test.

Part A of the table also discloses that the reduction in the perceived intensity of the test weights when they were applied in combination with the contralateral weight held for each of the four weights. However, the amount of reduction differed for the several weights, being fairly substantial and statistically significant for the 5 and 10 gm weights but smaller and nonsignificant for the 1 and 20 gm weights. Moreover, while each of the five subjects showed a decline in the perceived magnitude of the 5 and 10 gm test weights under

the condition of double stimulation, some subjects showed an augmentation of their estimates of the 1 or the 20 gm weight under this condition.

This discrepancy in the observed effects of double stimulation on the perceived magnitude of different test weights raised the question of whether the positive results for the 5 and 10 gm weights might have been a chance finding. The supplementary experiment, which was limited to a comparison of perceptual judgments of these weights under the two stimulation conditions, effectively disproved this possibility. As shown in part B of the table, the perceptual judgments of the magnitude of both the 5 and 10 gm weights declined significantly under the condition of double bilateral stimulation. This decline was consistent across subjects, i.e., each of the subjects reduced his magnitude estimates of each of the two weights when they were presented in combination with a heavier weight on the contralateral arm.

The correlation between the percentage reductions in estimates by the 10 subjects under the condition of double stimulation for the 5 gm and the 10 gm weight was calculated to determine whether there was any evidence for a general trait of susceptibility to masking in normal individuals. The obtained correlation coefficient (Spearman rank difference method) was .58, which approached significance ($p < .10$) for this small number of cases.

DISCUSSION

The purpose of this study was to determine whether a perceptual obscuration effect could be produced in healthy subjects under a condition of double sensory stimulation in which they do not show extinction of perceptual response to the weaker of the two stimuli. There were no

Table 4. Mean estimates of perceived magnitude of test weights presented alone and in combination with contralateral weight

	(A) Main experiment Weight (gm)					(B) Supplementary experiment Weight (gm)	
	1	5	10	20	All weights	5	10
Presented alone	27.8	109.2	157.3	222.2	129.1	106.3	164.3
Presented in combination	24.3	67.8	132.1	202.1	106.5	85.9	119.5
Difference	3.5	41.4	25.2	20.1	22.6	20.4	44.8
Significance of difference	NS	$p < .0001$	$p < .02$	NS	$p < .001$	$p < .01$	$p < .001$

firm grounds for predicting the direction of the results, and a number of outcomes were possible. It would not have been surprising if the perceived judgments of the magnitude of the test weights did not change from the single to the double stimulation condition. Conceivably the double stimulation condition could have had a facilitating effect and led to increased estimates of the intensity of the test weights. Finally, the obscuration effect that was the focus of interest, i.e., a decrease in the perceived magnitude of the test stimuli under double stimulation, might have occurred.

In fact, a stable, consistent and statistically significant obscuration effect of double sensory stimulation was observed for the two test weights (5 and 10 gm) that occupied a middle position in the series. For the extreme weights (1 and 20 gm), an overall obscuration effect was also present but it was slight, inconsistent across subjects and statistically nonsignificant. The possible reasons for this discrepancy in findings for the different weights may be considered. The fact that the mean subjective magnitude estimates made by two of the five subjects of the 1 gm weight when it was presented alone were quite small (2.5 and 11.3) effectively precluded a significant reduction in these estimates when the weight was presented in combination with the heavier contralateral weight. At the other end of the scale, the 20 gm weight was presented with a contralateral weight that was only twice as

heavy, and it may be that a greater difference in weight is required to produce the obscuration effect. It would be of interest to determine whether a still heavier contralateral weight of 50 or 60 gm would result in a reduction in the perceived intensity of a 20 gm test weight in normal subjects.

The major finding that, under certain conditions of double sensory stimulation, healthy subjects reduce their estimates of the subjective magnitude of tactile pressure stimuli, compared with their estimates when these stimuli are presented alone, may be interpreted as providing further support for the concept that the clinical phenomena of extinction and obscuration are exaggerated expressions of a normal physiologic mechanism. The indications of significant individual differences in susceptibility to this effect of double stimulation among healthy individuals accord with this view.

Since it requires intensive training of a subject, as well as his close attention and cooperation, the psychophysical method of subjective magnitude estimation can be applied to very few patients with cerebral disease. However, the design of the present study, in which stimuli of unequal strength are presented to opposite sides of the body, might prove useful in the assessment of patients with suspected unilateral cerebral disease who do not show extinction under a condition of double stimulation of equal strength. No healthy subject in this study showed anything approaching extinction of perception of the 5 gm weight when it was presented with a contralateral 40 gm weight. If a patient who showed no evidence of extinction under the conventional double stimulation condition should show extinction of perception of the 5 gm weight when it was presented with a contralateral 40 gm weight, presumptive evidence of abnormality in neural integrative function would be shown. The unilateral nature of this abnormality could then be assessed by reversing the direction of the stimulation so that the test weight is presented to the presumably healthy side and the heavy weight to the presumably affected side.

SUMMARY

Using a refined psychophysical method and appropriate conditions of stimulation, this study determined whether it would be possible to demonstrate "obscuration" of perception of suprathreshold tactile stimulation in healthy subjects who do not show extinction of perceptual response to the weaker of two bilaterally applied tactile stimuli. The procedure was to train subjects to estimate the subjective magnitude of weights dropped on the skin surface and, after this training, to secure their magnitude estimates of the same weights under conditions of both single and double stimulation. Comparison of these magnitude estimates under the two stimulation conditions provided unequivocal evidence of an obscuration effect, the estimates under the condition of double stimulation being significantly lower than those made under the single stimulation condition. There were also indications of individual differences in susceptibility to this effect of double stimulation. The results are interpreted as providing further support for the concept that the clinical phenomena of extinction and obscuration are exaggerated expressions of a normal physiologic mechanism. A modification of the procedure used in this investigation might be fruitfully applied in the study of patients with suspected cerebral disease who do not show extinction or obscuration of perception under the conventional condition of double sensory stimulation of equal intensity.

REFERENCES

1. Bender, M. B.: Disorders in Perception. Springfield, Ill., Charles C. Thomas, Publisher, 1952.

2. Critchley, M.: The Parietal Lobes. London, Arnold, 1953.

3. Halliday, A. M., Mingay, R.: Retroactive raising of a sensory threshold by a contralateral stimulus. Q. J. Exp. Psychol. 13:1, 1961.

4. Bird, J. W.: Parameters of double tactile stimulation. Cortex 1:257, 1964.

5. Abramsky, I., Carmon, A., Benton, A. L.: Masking of and by tactile pressure stimuli. Percept. Psychophysics 10:353, 1971.

6. Rosner, B. S.: Neural factors limiting cutaneous spatiotemporal discrimination. In Rosenblith W. A. (Editor): Sensory Communication. New York, MIT Press and Wiley & Sons, 1959.

7. Schmid, E.: Temporal aspects of cutaneous interaction with two-point electrical stimulation. J. Exp. Psychol. 61:400, 1961.

8. Uttal, W. R., Smith, P: Contralateral and heteromodal interaction effects in somatosensation: do they exist? Percept. Psychophysics 2:363, 1967.

9. Gilson, R. D.: Vibrotactile masking: some spatial and temporal aspects. Percept. Psychophysics 5:176, 1969.

10. Gold, C., Rosner, B. S.: Facilitatory spatial interaction with percutaneous electrical stimuli. Percept. Psychophysics 6:118, 1969.

11. Sherrick, C. E.: Effects of double simultaneous stimulation of the skin. Am. J. Psychol. 77:42, 1964.

12. Kietzman, M. L., Boyle, R. C., Lindsley, D. B.: Perceptual masking: peripheral vs.

central factors. Percept. Psychophysics 9:350, 1971.

13. Birch, H. G., Belmont, I., Karp, E.: The relation of single stimulus threshold to extinction in double simultaneous stimulation. Cortex 1:19, 1964.

14. Benton, A. L., Meyers, R., Polder, G. J.: Some aspects of handedness. Psychiat. Neurol. (Basel) 144:321, 1962.

15. Carmon, A., Dyson, J. A.: New instrumentation for research on tactile sensitivity and discrimination. Cortex 3:406, 1967.

IV.
Constructional Apraxia and Spatial Abilities

12.

Constructional Apraxia and the Minor Hemisphere*

Constructional apraxia has always held a special interest for neurologists and psychologists concerned with the "higher" functions of the nervous system. Undoubtedly a basic reason for their interest is that the questions which have been raised about the nature and neurological significance of this disorder apply with equal force to a topic of broader importance, namely, the issue of the distinctive functions of the minor hemisphere. Thus an understanding of the determinants and correlates of constructional apraxia is closely related to, and perhaps a prerequisite for, an understanding of hemispheric cerebral dominance in man.

THE PROBLEM OF DEFINITION

What is "constructional apraxia?" As is the case with so many of the behavioral deficits dealt with in clinical neuropsychology (e.g., "visual agnosia," "spatial dis-

orientation," "astereognosis"), a reasonably precise definition is not quite as easily formulated as one might assume. Kleist (1934), the originator of the concept, defined it in only the most general terms as a disturbance "in formative activities such as assembling, building and drawing, in which the spatial form of the product proves to be unsuccessful, without there being an apraxia of single movements." Thus constructional apraxia denotes an impairment in combinatory or organizing activity in which details must be clearly perceived and in which the relationships among the component parts of the entity must be apprehended if the desired synthesis of them is to be achieved. Obviously, this kind of ability can be assessed in a variety of ways and it is not surprising that many tasks have been used in the study of constructional apraxia. Among these are: block-arranging in the horizontal dimension; block-building in the vertical dimension; three-dimensional block-building; stick-arranging (as in the Goldstein-Scheerer test); construction of mosaic patterns from a

* A. L. Benton, *Confinia Neurologica*, 1967, 29, 1—16. By permission of S. Karger AG, Basel, Switzerland.

119

model (as in block-designs tests); copying designs, and free drawing. These constructional tasks may be extremely simple as in stick-arranging, block-building in the vertical dimension or copying single simple figures such as a square or a triangle. However, the level of difficulty can be augmented to practically any desired degree, e.g., by requiring three-dimensional construction instead of two-dimensional construction, by having the patient draw multiple figures with definite spatial and size relations among them or by having him make his construction not from an actual model but from a more or less abstract representation of it. Thus, in the block-designs task, it surely makes a difference whether the patient is required to copy an actual block model which shows the separation of the blocks or (as in the Kohs or WAIS block designs) a representation of it in reduced size which presents the global pattern but which does not show the separation of the blocks.

At this point, it is well to recall that tasks involving constructional praxis have long been utilized as tests of general intelligence. Block construction tasks, such as the building of a three-cube or a six-cube pyramid, and drawing tasks, such as the copying of a cross, square or triangle, occupy a prominent place in intelligence scales for preschool children. At higher levels, there are bead-stringing and formboard tests as well as tasks involving the drawing of more complex figures. The Block Designs test of Kohs (1923) was originally devised as a non-verbal test of general intelligence and not as a measure of a special ability. Kohs believed that his test assessed a broad and fundamental mental capacity which was not at all specifically associated with a "spatial relations" factor but rather one that could well be considered as the very core of intelligence. Defining intelligence as the capacity to analyze a situation, to discover

methods for solving it and, finally, to synthesize details into a consistent unity, he pointed out how the Block Designs test appeared to satisfy the requirements of a valid test of general intelligence.

In any case, the great variety of tasks which have been used to probe for the presence of constructional apraxia has made the concept rather fuzzy from an operational standpoint. As a consequence, when one reviews the extensive clinical literature on the deficit, one is often at a loss to know exactly what an author means by the term. Sometimes the task performances which define the concept for him are not even mentioned. Or defective copying of designs may be cited as evidence of constructional apraxia in one case while defective block construction may be cited as evidence of the deficit in the next case and one cannot help but wonder how the first patient performed on block construction (if in fact he was given the task) and how well the second copied designs (if in fact he was given that task). Sometimes imperfect performance on a rather difficult task such as the complex figure of Rey or constructing an elaborate three-dimensional structure is considered as evidence for a constructional deficit. Here one wonders what the performance level of the average person is and whether the performance of the brain-damaged patient actually may not be well within normal limits.

Thus, from an operational standpoint, constructional apraxia poses a definitional problem. An implicit assumption underlying investigative work in this area has been that we deal here with a unitary deficit which reveals itself in various ways, depending upon unspecified circumstances. Is this truly the case? Or is it possible that there is more than one discrete type of visuoconstructive disability?

The question has not been thoroughly explored but some relevant empirical evi-

Table 5. Concurrence of failure on 4 tests for constructional apraxia

Pair of tests	No. failing both	% failing both
Design copying and 3-dimensional block construction	7	41
Design copying and stick-construction	7	41
Design copying and block designs	5	29
3-dimensional block construction and stick-construction	9	53
3-dimensional block construction and block designs	9	53
Stick-construction and block designs	10	59

dence derived from recent studies in our laboratory can be cited. We have taken four representative constructional praxis tasks—copying visual designs (Benton, 1962), making stick-constructions from models (Fogel, 1962), building three-dimensional structures from models (Benton & Fogel, 1962) and the block-designs subtest of the WAIS (Wechsler, 1955)—and have given them to 100 brain-damaged patients and 100 control patients, the two groups being matched for mean age and educational level and variance in these characteristics. In passing, it may be noted that each task has a distinctive characteristic not shared by the other three. The copying test involves graphic activity; the other three do not. The stick-arranging test involves construction in two dimensions while the block construction test adds a third dimension. Finally, unlike the other three tests, block designs involve construction on the basis of a reduced and more or less schematic representation rather than from an actual model.

The 17 poorest performances on the part of the brain-damaged patients with respect to each test were identified; in the case of each test, this represented a performance level exceeded by 99–100% of the control patient group. The relationships among the 4 performances were then assessed by determining the degree of concurrence of failure for each pair of performances. The findings (Table 5) show that there is a general tendency for failure to occur on more than one task. On the basis of chance, one would expect three patients to fail both of a pair of tasks; the smallest number is five. This greater-than-chance concurrence is no doubt an expression of the inescapable common factor underlying practically all mental performances in human subjects. However, more importantly, one notes that the degree of communality between failure on the copying tests and the other three tasks is consistently lower than the degree of communality of failure among the other three tests themselves. Thus there is the suggestion that the copying test stands apart to some degree from the three assembling tests.

This impression is supported by the results of an overall correlational analysis which took into account the performances of the total group of 100 brain-damaged patients. Phi-coefficients for each of the pairs of test scores were computed (Table 6). Comparing the relative size of the phi-coefficients, it will be seen that the three coefficients between design copying and the three assembling tasks are consistently lower than are the coefficients among the three assembling tasks themselves.

These findings scarcely provide a definitive answer to the question of whether "constructional apraxia" is best conceived as a unitary type of impairment or simply as a collective name for a number of distinguishable deficits. They do show quite clearly that this *is* a real question. On the positive side, the results suggest that, given our present state of knowledge, it is probably useful to think in

Table 6. Correlations (phi-coefficients) among constructional performances of 100 brain-damaged patients

	3-dimensional block construction	Stick-construction	Block designs
Design copying	.24	.24	.28
3-dimensional block construction		.39	.32
Stick-construction			.39

terms of at least two types of constructional activity. Performance on assembling tasks, such as stick-arranging, block designs and three-dimensional block construction, appear to go together to form one type. On the other hand, the graphic performance of copying designs stands somewhat apart from the manual assembling performances and may be considered a second type of constructional activity. One implication of this conclusion is that provision should be made in investigative work or clinical evaluation for giving both a manual assembly test and a graphic test and the findings for each performance should be treated separately unless there is clear empirical justification for combining them.

Obviously, we do not have the final answer to the question of a possible typology of visuoconstructive performances. Fairly extensive analytic investigation will be required to provide it. It may well be a necessary precondition for the clarification of the vexed question of the role of the minor hemisphere in the mediation of visuoconstructive performances.

THE NATURE OF CONSTRUCTIONAL APRAXIA

Another question concerns the basic nature of the disability underlying defective visuoconstructive performances in brain-damaged patients. This is also in large part a definitional problem and one which must be thoroughly understood if a clear conception of the relationship between visuoconstructive disabilities and

hemispheric locus of lesion is to be achieved. Kleist had a quite definite idea about what he meant when he spoke of constructional apraxia. In his view, it was a particular type of visuoconstructive impairment which reflected an inability to translate an adequate visual perception into appropriate action, i.e., it represented a *perceptuomotor*, rather than a purely perceptual, deficit. He conceived of a rupture in the connection between visual and kinesthetic cerebral processes as being the essential basis for the disorder. At the same time, Kleist was fully aware that defective visuoconstructive performances could result from basic visuoperceptive impairment. But these did not belong to the specific category of constructional apraxia, which exemplified visuoconstructive impairment of an "executive" rather than a "perceptual" nature.

Following the publications of Kleist and of his pupil, Hans Strauss (1924), constructional apraxia was generally accepted as a distinctive category or type of behavioral deficit that might be shown by patients with cerebral disease. For the most part, however, subsequent workers tended to ignore the precise formulation of Kleist and instead employed the term "constructional apraxia" to cover all visuoconstructive disabilities. At the same time, they were inclined to see the performance deficit as being the motor expression of a more pervasive impairment in spatial thinking rather than as a defect which is shown only in constructional activity. This point of view was based on both theoretical and empirical considerations. Kleist, with his concept of a disconnection condition, represented the classical associationist approach which by then was rather out of fashion, having been supplanted by analyses in terms of perceptual and cognitive levels. Moreover, many students with a behavioristic orientation found it difficult to make a truly fundamental distinction between "perception" and "action" and were likely to see perception as being simply an implicit or covert form of action. At the same time, it was found empirically that as a rule patients with constructional apraxia did in fact show one or another form of impairment in visual perception or spatial orientation, e.g., in the discrimination of complex geometric figures, the recognition of hidden figures or fragmented figures, the identification of right and left body parts, or the recognition of individual fingers.

However, in recent years, the question of whether it is valid (or better expressed, whether it is *useful*) to make a distinction between perceptual and perceptuomotor disability has been raised once again. Duensing (1953) has postulated, on rather slim empirical grounds, that there are two types of visuoconstructive disability, an ideational-apractic and a spatio-agnosic type and has classified a number of the classic cases of constructional apraxia reported in the clinical literature into one or the other category. Bortner and Birch (1960, 1962), having shown that patients who perform defectively on the block designs task generally perform better on a discrimination task involving the same designs, interpret this result as evidence that perceptual and perceptuomotor abilities may show dissociated impairment in cases of cerebral disease. Other investigators (e.g., Ettlinger, Warrington & Zangwill, 1957; Costa & Vaughan, 1962) have sought to infer the existence of discrete types of visuoconstructive disability from analyses of the correlates of the disability as it presents in different groups of patients. Their tentative conclusion is that both an "executive" or "apractic" type of the disorder (as postulated by Kleist) and a "visuoperceptive" or "spatio-agnosic" type do exist. On the other hand, even more recent studies by Piercy and Smyth (1962) and Arrigoni and De Renzi (1964) have yielded findings that do not support the validity or clinical importance of such a distinction. There have also been attempts to infer the existence of discrete types of constructional apraxia from a study of qualitative features of performance.

Detailed analysis of these studies with a view toward assessing the weight of the evidence which each brings to bear on the problem of discrete types of visuoconstructive disorder cannot be attempted here and a summary statement must suffice. A fair conclusion, I think, is that neither the positive nor the negative reports present strong evidence for or against the thesis. I believe that the basic reason why investigation to date has failed to resolve this problem may be that it has not produced truly relevant information. This question of a possible typology of visuoconstructive disorders is a precise—one might almost say, delicate—question. It probably cannot be answered on the basis of findings obtained from the application of the usual tests for constructional apraxia. Nor is the answer likely to come from post hoc analyses of previously collected data which are in one's files. What is needed here is a series of true experiments that satisfy two requirements. The first requirement is that, prior to the study, the characteristics of the two postulated types of visuoconstructive disability must be precisely defined. Secondly, test methods and scoring systems specifically designed to assess these characteristics must be contrived. The application of these rationally developed techniques should answer the question of whether there are in fact distinguishable types of visuoconstructive disability. As has already been indicated, the answer to this question is a necessity before the role of the minor hemisphere in mediating visuoconstructive performances can be clarified.

CONSTRUCTIONAL APRAXIA AND THE MINOR HEMISPHERE

Turning to the question of the association between constructional apraxia and locus of cerebral lesion, one might first ask how frequently this group of deficits is shown by patients with brain disease in general. All studies agree that they are not uncommon deficits; in fact, they appear with relatively high frequency. For example, comparing our groups of brain-damaged and control patients and defining defective performance as a level exceeded by 95 per cent of control patients, we found that the incidence of deficit ranged from 25 per cent for design copying to 39 per cent for three-dimensional block construction. The analogous figures for some WAIS subtests, which were also given to these patients, may be cited to serve as a basis for interpretation. The Similarities, Comprehension, Arithmetic and Picture Arrangement subtests showed an incidence of defective performance ranging from 19 per cent (for Similarities) to 27 per cent (for Arithmetic). Thus it seems clear that these visuoconstructive disabilities represent a rather common type of impairment in brain-damaged patients (in contrast to, for example, ideational apraxia or facial agnosia).

When Kleist and Strauss first described constructional apraxia in the 1920s, they advanced the idea that the crucial lesion was in the posterior parietal area of the left hemisphere; it was here that the integration of visual and kinesthetic impulses necessary for successful constructional activity took place. This localization was generally accepted and the close association of constructional apraxia with other deficits referable to left hemisphere disease, such as finger agnosia, right-left disorientation and aphasic disturbances, was repeatedly noted. Nevertheless, as early as the 1930s, the observation had been made that visuoconstructive disability also may be shown by patients with lesions apparently confined to the right hemisphere with the implication that it could not be exclusively related to left hemisphere disease. In any case, the subsequent extensive studies of Zangwill and of Hécaen and their co-workers demonstrated an impressively high incidence of visuoconstructive disabilities in patients with right hemisphere lesions and this led to a rather remarkable shift of opinion regarding the relative importance of the two hemispheres in mediating visuoconstructive performances (cf. Paterson & Zangwill, 1944; McFie, Piercy & Zangwill, 1950; Hécaen, Ajuriaguerra & Massonet, 1951; Hécaen, Penfield, Bertrand and Malmo, 1956). In contrast to the earlier view, which regarded the deficit as a sign of disease of the dominant hemisphere, emphasis is now placed on the crucial role of lesions of the right hemisphere in producing the picture of constructional apraxia. From an empirical standpoint, there is rather general (although not universal) agreement today that patients with right hemisphere lesions show a higher incidence of deficit, and more severe deficit, than do those with disease of the left hemisphere (cf. Piercy, Hécaen & Ajuriaguerra, 1960; Benton, 1962; Benton & Fogel, 1962; Piercy & Smyth, 1962; Arrigoni & De Renzi, 1964; Warrington, James & Kinsbourne, 1966).

Although our own results, based on

strictly objective definitions of "deficit," provide general support for this belief, they also suggest that one may be dealing here with a rather complex state of affairs which changes character as a function of the type of task given to probe for the presence of constructional apraxia and the particular definition of "deficit" adopted. Our findings are presented in Table 7. As will be seen, the degree of bias in the direction of a higher frequency of deficit in patients with right hemisphere disease appears to be related to the specific task employed. When failure is defined as a performance level exceeded by 95 per cent of control patients, defective performance on copying designs and three-dimensional block construction is more than twice as frequent in the right hemisphere group as in the left hemisphere group. In contrast, there are only minimal differences between the two groups with respect to the relative frequency of defective performance on stick-arranging and block designs.

On the other hand, the picture changes somewhat when attention is restricted to the relative incidence of what might be called "severe" deficit, i.e., a performance level below the distribution of scores of the control patients. In the case of each test, the relative frequency of failure in the right hemisphere group increases. In this respect, our results support the belief that visuoconstructive defi-

cit tends to be more severe, as well as more frequent, in patients with right hemisphere disease. Finally, the picture shifts toward the opposite direction when attention is restricted to what may be called "moderate" deficit, i.e., the range of scores exceeded by 95–99 per cent of control patients but above that of the lowest 1% of that group. Here an attenuation of the difference between right and left hemisphere cases is seen. A clear predominance of failure in right hemisphere disease is shown only for three-dimension block-construction.

In summary, if these findings are generalizable (and this remains to be determined), they suggest that the degree of association between visuoconstructive deficit and hemispheric locus of lesion depends in part upon the type of constructional task selected by the investigator. A task such as three-dimensional block construction shows a larger difference between right and left hemisphere cases than does the somewhat more subtle block designs task. This finding provides incidental support for the view that block designs measure a more general cognitive ability which is likely to be impaired by cerebral damage independently of locus. The findings also suggest that the degree of association between visuoconstructive deficit and hemispheric locus of lesion is related to the defined severity of the deficit. Pronounced deficit is more likely to be

Table 7. Visuoconstructive deficits in patients with lesions of the right (N = 35) and left (N = 43) hemispheres

Test	Deficit[a]			"Severe" deficit[b]			"Moderate" deficit[c]		
	Right %	Left %	R/L ratio	Right %	Left %	R/L ratio	Right %	Left %	R/L ratio
Design copying	29	14	2.1	14.5	5	2.9	14.5	9	1.6
3-dimensional block construction	54	23	2.3	23	9	2.6	31	14	2.2
Stick-construction	34	26	1.3	14	7	2.0	20	19	1.1
Block designs	34	30	1.1	20	14	1.4	14	16	.9

[a] Performance level below that of 95–100 per cent of control patients (N = 100).
[b] Performance level below that of 100 per cent of control patients.
[c] Performance level below that of 95–99 per cent of control patients but above lowest 1 per cent.

shown by patients with right hemisphere disease while moderate deficit is found in patients with lesions of either hemisphere.

Given these reservations and qualifications, the empirical generalization that constructional apraxia is more frequent and more severe in patients with right hemisphere disease appears to have considerable validity. How is this empirical fact to be explained and what are its implications? Three major interpretations have been advanced and each needs to be considered.

One interpretation is that the observed difference between the two groups of patients is an artefact of case selection. It is pointed out that widespread disease of the left hemisphere is quite likely to produce severe aphasia and to make such a patient untestable. On the other hand, this limitation will rarely hold for right hemisphere disease in the right-handed patient. Moreover, since at a relatively early stage left hemisphere disease may produce significant disability (in the form of language disturbances and sensorimotor impairment of the preferred hand), it seems likely that on admission to a neurological service, the patients with left hemisphere disease will have more recent and less extensive lesions than those with right hemisphere damage. Both of these circumstances create a definite bias for testable patients with right hemisphere disease to have more extensive lesions than those with disease of the dominant hemisphere. As a consequence, comparison of unselected cases in the two hemispheric groups is essentially a comparison of a dominant hemisphere group with lesions of limited extension and a minor hemisphere group with lesions of unlimited extent. The higher frequency of visuoconstructive defect in the right hemisphere group is (or may well be) due to the fact that their lesions are larger than those of the patients with left hemisphere disease.

What shall we say about this point of view which disposes of the problem in such a summary way? First, it may be observed that the argument rests on the circumstantial considerations just mentioned and that no direct evidence has been adduced to support it. To be sure, the recent study of Arrigoni and De Renzi (1964), in which right and left hemisphere cases were compared not only in respect to constructional performance but also simple visual reaction time, is now being cited as evidence that right-left differences in constructional apraxia are determined by the factor of size of lesion (Warrington, James & Kinsbourne, 1966). Arrigoni and De Renzi observed a significantly higher frequency of constructional apraxia in their patients with right hemisphere disease but they also noted that the reaction times of these patients were longer than those of their patients with right hemisphere disease. Moreover, they found that the reaction times of apraxic patients were longer than those of non-apraxic patients, independently of hemispheric locus of lesion. When reduced groups of right and left hemisphere cases that were matched for reaction time were formed, the difference in respect to frequency of constructional apraxia was no longer significant. Interpreting retardation in reaction time as a measure of the extent, or at least the general disorganizing effects, of a lesion, they concluded that the differential occurrence of constructional apraxia in the two hemispheric groups was related to this factor of severity of brain-damage rather than to locus of lesion.

I cannot agree with this interpretation, for analysis of the actual findings of this valuable study shows that in fact the difference in relative frequency of constructional deficit between the two matched hemispheric groups was exactly as large as the difference between the original groups. Evidently, the failure of the difference between the matched groups to attain the magic .05 level of statistical significance was due simply to the smaller number of cases involved. Thus a convincing case for this "nihilistic" hypothesis (which admittedly does have the virtue of parsimony) has not been made. Its chief virtue at the present time is that is suggests an obvious methodological principle which should guide comparative investigations of the performances of patients with unilateral lesions.

A second major interpretation is that, although both hemispheres mediate constructional performances (and through the same mechanisms, whatever these may be), the contribution of the right hemisphere is more important from a quantitative standpoint. On first consideration, this may seem to be a mere restatement of the empirical facts rather than a real explanation. However, it does have an important implication which is amenable to empirical test, namely, that the performances of right and left hemisphere cases should be the same from a qualitative standpoint. More instances of deficit (and more severe deficit) will be found in patients with right hemisphere lesions but, except to the extent that qualitative characteristics of performance may be related to severity of deficit, the type of deficit shown by the two groups of patients will be identical. And this is perhaps the central issue in discussions of constructional apraxia today. For the third major interpretation (by far the most provocative) is that the minor hemisphere plays a special role in mediating visuoconstructive performances, a role which is analogous to that served by the dominant hemisphere in relation to language. In its most prominent form, this interpretation holds that the right hemisphere is "dominant" for at least certain aspects of visuo-

spatial cognition or (to avoid a possibly unjustified association with a single sensory modality) for certain aspects of spatial orientation. It is well known that a number of visuospatial deficits (e.g., neglect of the contralateral visual half-field, impairment in learning routes or locating places on a map, poor memory for spatial relations and dyspraxia for dressing) are shown with impressively higher frequency by patients with right hemisphere disease than by those with left hemisphere lesions. To this list may be added constructional disabilities, the ensemble of deficits being the expression of a basic disturbance in spatial thinking.

This profoundly important conception faces one major problem; at the same time, it has certain implications with respect to constructional apraxia. The problem is how to account for the relatively frequent occurrence of defective constructional performance in patients with lesions apparently confined to the left hemisphere. It has been met by drawing a distinction between the end-result (defective constructional performance) and the disability underlying the end-result. It is postulated that, while constructional defect in right hemisphere disease is one expression of a broad and multi-faceted visuospatial impairment, it is due to "executive" or "conceptual" defect in left hemisphere cases. If this is so, it is reasonable to expect that constructional deficit in right hemisphere disease will be correlated with other expressions of the postulated basic impairment while no such correlation would seem to be necessary in left hemisphere disease. Further, if there are distinctive determinants of defective performance in the two groups of cases, it would seem highly probable (although not absolutely necessary) that this circumstance would be expressed in distinctive features of performance, the behavior of the right hemisphere patient reflecting the spatial disorientation and that of the left hemisphere patients reflecting the executive or conceptual weakness.

It is apparent that this conception is related to the basic definitional questions discussed earlier in this paper. As pointed out, the results to date have not furnished a really satisfactory answer to the question of whether a valid and useful distinction between a visuospatial and a perceptuomotor type of deficit can be made. Correlational studies such as that of Costa and Vaughan (1962) suggest the possibility without, however, providing a convincing case for it. There is the further question of whether right and left hemisphere cases show qualitatively distinctive performances. This question can be considered independently of the issue of whether such differences as may be found are consonant with the notions of discrete visuospatial and executive types of underlying disability although, of course, the question derives much of its interest from this basic issue. Supposedly characteristic differences in the performances of the two hemispheric groups have been described. It is reported, for example, that it is typical of left hemisphere patients to draw better from a model than in response to verbal instructions, the difference perhaps being due to "conceptual" impairment (Piercy, Hécaen & Ajuriaguerra, 1960). However, the most recent study addressed to this question failed to confirm the dissociation (Warrington, James & Kinsbourne, 1966). The drawings of patients with right hemisphere disease have been described as complex and disorganized and including many strokes or elements (expressive of a "piece-meal" approach associated with loss of a visuospatial framework within which responses are organized) while the drawings of the left hemisphere cases are simple, primitive and impoverished. Rotational errors (reflecting disorientation in space) and neglect of the left side of a construction are likely to be shown by the patient with a right hemisphere lesion. Neither rotational errors nor a corresponding neglect of the right side of constructions are as likely to be shown by the patient with a left hemisphere lesion (Piercy, Hécaen & Ajuriaguerra, 1960). Some of these findings have been confirmed, others have not. The general picture is one of a few shreds and patches of empirical evidence which are far from satisfying and, at the same time, quite suggestive. The question is truly a tantalizing one. One *feels* that there is a real qualitative difference in the constructional performances of right and left hemisphere cases, the demonstration and definition of which are just beyond our grasp.

In summary, that there is a difference in the incidence of constructional defect in patients with right and left hemisphere lesions can scarcely be doubted. That this difference is an artefact of case selection is a possibility but a rather remote one. (In any case, the possibility can be eliminated by the institution of proper controls.) Thus it can be said that, in some sense, the right hemisphere plays a "dominant" role in the mediation of visuoconstructive activity in man. The statistics of the situation force us to concede that this "dominance" is relative, not absolute, since constructional apraxia in patients with disease apparently confined to the left hemisphere is not rare. A satisfying interpretation of the nature and determinants of this empirically established relative "dominance" of the right hemisphere has yet to be achieved. It may be that the abilities underlying constructional performances are (to use the expression of Piercy, Hécaen & Ajuriaguerra) "bilaterally but unequally represented," with the right hemisphere being somewhat more important from a quantitative standpoint.

Another possibility is that the two hemispheres play qualitatively distinctive roles in mediating constructional activity, with the right hemisphere being responsible for the visuospatial components of the activity. At the moment we are close to a stalemate in deciding among these and other interpretations. A basic reason for the stalemate is that to date the experimental designs and investigative methods of our studies have not been adequate to answer the questions posed.

SUMMARY

The concept of constructional apraxia has not been adequately defined from an operational standpoint. Intercorrelational analyses of various task performances utilized in clinical and investigative work to probe for the presence of the deficit suggest that at least two forms of impairment, a graphomotor form and an assembling form, can be identified. The nature of the disabilities underlying defective visuoconstructive performances is an unsettled question. Discrete types of "spatial-agnostic" and "executive-conceptual" disability have been postulated but the dichotomy still awaits empirical confirmation.

There is substantial evidence that patients with lesions of the right hemisphere show a higher incidence of constructional deficit, and more severe deficit, than do those with disease of the left hemisphere. However, detailed analysis suggests that the degree of association between defective performance and hemispheric locus of lesions depends in part upon the type of constructional task selected as a measure of performance and in part upon the particular definition of "deficit" adopted in classification.

A number of interpretations have been advanced to account for the observed association between constructional apraxia and disease of the right hemisphere. It is difficult to decide among these interpretations because the experimental design and investigative methods of studies to date have not been adequate to answer the crucial questions.

REFERENCES

Arrigoni, G. & De Renzi, E.: Constructional apraxia and hemispheric locus of lesion. Cortex *1*: 170–197 (1964).

Benton, A. L.: The visual retention test as a constructional praxis task. Confin. neurol. *22*: 141–155 (1962).

Benton, A. L. & Fogel, M. L.: Three-dimensional constructional praxis: a clinical test. Arch. Neurol., Chicago *7*: 347–354 (1962).

Bortner, M. & Birch, H. G.: Perceptual and perceptual-motor dissociation in brain-damaged patients. J. nerv. ment. Dis. *130*: 49–53 (1960).

Bortner, M. & Birch, H. G.: Perceptual and perceptual-motor dissociation in cerebral palsied children. J. nerv. ment. Dis. *134*: 103–108 (1962).

Costa, L. D. & Vaughan, H. G.: Performances of patients with lateralized cerebral lesions. I. Verbal and perceptual tests. J. nerv. ment. Dis. *134*: 162–168 (1962).

Duensing, F.: Raumagnostische und ideatorisch-apraktische Störung des gestaltenden Handelns. Dtsch. Z. Nervenheilk. *170*: 72–94 (1953).

Ettlinger, G.; Warrington, E. & Zangwill, O. L.: A further study of visual-spatial agnosia. Brain *80*: 335–361 (1957).

Fogel, M. L.: The Gerstmann syndrome and the parietal symptom-complex. Psychol. Rev. *12*: 85–99 (1962).

Hécaen, H.; Ajuriaguerra, J. de Massonet, J.: Les troubles visuoconstructifs par lésion pariéto-occipitale droite. Encépale *40*: 122–179 (1951).

Hécaen, H.; Penfield, W.; Bertrand, C. & Malmo, R.: The syndrome of apractognosia due to lesions of the minor cerebral hemisphere. Arch. Neurol., Chicago *75*: 400–434 (1956).

Kleist, K.: Gehirnpathologie (Barth, Leipzig 1934).

Kohs, S. C.: Intelligence Measurement (Macmillan, New York 1923).

McFie, J.; Piercy, M. F. & Zangwill, O. L.: Visual spatial agnosia associated with lesions of the right cerebral hemisphere. Brain 73: 167–190 (1950).

Paterson, A. & Zangwill, O. L.: Disorders of visual space perception associated with lesions of the right cerebral hemisphere. Brain 67: 331–358 (1944).

Piercy, M. F.; Hécaen, H. & Ajuriaguerra, J. de: Constructional apraxia associated with unilateral cerebral lesions. Brain 83: 225–242 (1960).

Piercy, M. F. & Smyth, V.: Right hemisphere dominance for certain non-verbal intellectual skills. Brain 85: 775–790 (1962).

Strauss, H.: Über konstruktive Apraxie. Mschr. Psychiat. 56: 65–124 (1924).

Warrington, E.; James, M. & Kinsbourne, M.: Drawing disability in relation to laterality of cerebral lesion. Brain 89: 53–82 (1966).

Wechsler, D.: Manual for the Wechsler Adult Intelligence Scale (Psychological Corporation, New York 1955).

13.

Visuoconstructive Disability in Patients with Cerebral Disease: Its Relationship to Side of Lesion and Aphasic Disorder*

INTRODUCTION

The relationship between visuoconstructive disorders (as reflected, for example, in failure on drawing and block assembling tasks) and side of lesion in patients with cerebral disease has long been an unresolved question. Kleist (1923, 1934), who defined "constructional apraxia" rather precisely as an executive disability due to faulty visual guidance of movement within a context of adequate visuoperceptive capacity per se, considered that the crucial lesion was situated in the posterior parietal area of the left hemisphere. It was presumably in this region that the integration of visual and proprioceptive information necessary for successful constructional performance took place. The association of constructional apraxia with other defects referable to disease of the left hemisphere (e.g., finger agnosia, right-left disorientation, aphasic disorder) supported Kleist's original localization (cf. Critchley, 1953; Benton, 1961). How-

ever, over the course of time it became quite evident that visuoconstructive disabilities could be shown by patients with lesions confined to the right hemisphere and indeed the indications were that such disabilities might be more frequent and more severe in these patients (cf. Piercy, Hécaen & Ajuriaguerra, 1960; Benton, 1962; Benton & Fogel, 1962; Piercy & Smyth, 1962; Arrigoni & De Renzi, 1964; Warrington, James & Kinsbourne, 1966).

Surveys of the relative frequency of visuoconstructive impairment in patients with unilateral cerebral disease generally show that defective performance is about twice as frequent in patients with right-sided lesions, the exact ratio apparently being dependent in part upon the type of task employed to assess constructional performance (Piercy & Smyth, 1962; Benton, 1967). On the other hand, the answer to the question of whether constructional disability is more severe (as well as more frequent) in patients with disease of the right hemisphere is not as clear. This is generally thought to be the case and at least one quantitative study (Benton,

* In honor of Hermann M. Burian. A. L. Benton, *Documenta Ophthalmologica*, 1973, 34, 67–76.

1967) has provided evidence to support the generalization. However, the recent study of Dee (1970), in which "constructional apraxics" with right or left hemisphere disease were compared with respect to severity of impairment in design copying and three-dimensional block building, failed to disclose the anticipated difference; gross failure (i.e., virtually complete inability to draw or build) was seen as frequently in the left-sided as in the right-sided cases.

It has proven to be difficult to formulate a satisfactory explanation for this rather modest bias toward a higher frequency of visuoconstructional defect in patients with right hemisphere disease. A straighforward concept of "hemispheric cerebral dominance" for visuoconstructive functions, analogous to that advanced for language functions, cannot be invoked for the two situations are not comparable. If one should investigate 100 right-handed clinically aphasic patients with unilateral cerebral lesions, one would find that 95 to 98 cases have disease of the left hemisphere. Moreover, in view of the possibility of error in classifying some patients as "right-handed" or in assuming that the disease process is strictly unilateral in nature, even this small number of cases of so-called "crossed aphasia" is probably an overestimate of the true frequency of right hemisphere "dominance" for language in right-handed persons. Given these circumstances, the characterization of the left hemisphere as "dominant" for language functions is quite justified. But the situation with respect to visuoconstructional performances is quite different. If one should investigate 100 right-handed patients with unilateral lesions who showed visuoconstructive defects, one would probably find that about 65 have disease of the right hemisphere. Given the relatively high frequency of 35 per cent of "exceptional" cases, there is

no need (or justification) for invoking the concept of hemispheric cerebral dominance.

Nevertheless, the fact remains that there *is* a bias toward a higher frequency of visuoconstructive defect in patients with disease of the right hemisphere and this empirical finding requires explanation. A number of interpretations of it have been advanced. The simplest is that the observed difference in frequency is merely an artefact of case selection. It is argued, on the one hand, that patients with right hemisphere disease are likely to have somewhat larger lesions on admission to hospital than those with left hemisphere disease and, on the other hand, that patients with severe receptive aphasia may be excluded from study because of their inability to understand what is required of them with respect to task performance. In either case, the net effect would be the formation of groups of patients with lesions of unequal size and different locus and it is this circumstance which may be responsible for the finding of a higher frequency of constructional deficit in the patients with right-sided lesions.

A second interpretation postulates that different mechanisms in each hemisphere combine to mediate constructional activity and that the integrity of both is required for successful performance. It is assumed, in harmony with the original formulation of Kleist, that a perceptuo-motor integrative mechanism located in the parieto-occipital area of the left hemisphere underlies the motor aspects of constructional activity. Consequently, a lesion in this area may disrupt the execution of performance even in the absence of visuoperceptive defects. In contrast, it is assumed that the right hemisphere mediates the spatial aspects of visual perception and these are an intrinsic component of constructional activity.

Hence impairment in visuospatial abilities resulting from right hemisphere disease will be reflected in defective constructional performance as well as in failure on recognition tasks requiring spatial thought. Thus constructional apraxia ensuing as a result of left hemisphere damage is viewed as being of a different character from the failure in constructional tasks observed in patients with disease of the right hemisphere. The former is an expression of a perceptuomotor or "executive" defect and corresponds to the "true" constructional apraxia of Kleist. The latter is only one of a number of behavioral expressions of impairment of higher-level perceptual ability.

A number of investigative approaches have been taken in an effort to validate this hypothesis. For example, it has been argued that, if defective constructional performance is the product of different mechanisms according to the side of lesion, this circumstance might well be reflected in qualitatively distinctive types of failure in the two groups of patients. On the whole, exploration of this possibility to date has yielded rather unimpressive results. A few qualitative performance features have been suggested as being characteristic of the performances of one or the other hemispheric group (e.g., spatial disorganization vs. simplification, differential performance in drawing from copy as compared to free drawing) but none has been convincingly demonstrated (cf. Benton, 1967; Warrington, 1969).

A more direct approach has been to determine the relationship between level of constructional performance and the status of perceptual abilities in patients with right and left hemisphere disease. If the theory of two discrete types of hemisphere-related disability is correct, defective constructional performance should be closely related to perceptual impairment

in patients with right hemisphere disease while a dissociation between the two categories of failure should be shown by at least some patients with disease of the left hemisphere. Investigating this question, Piercy & Smyth (1962) found that constructional apraxia was associated with poor visuoperceptive performance in patients with both right and left hemisphere disease and, further, that nonapraxic patients in each hemispheric group were superior in respect to visuoperceptive capacity to their non-apraxic counterparts. Similarly, Dee (1970) found that, irrespective of side of lesion, defective visuoconstructive performance (design copying, three-dimensional block building) was almost invariably associated with impairment in visual perception as assessed by multiple choice tests demanding complex form discrimination or spatial thinking. Thus it appears that this particular formulation of discrete types of hemisphere-related constructional apraxia in terms of the presence or absence of visuoperceptive impairment is not tenable.

The study which will be reported represents an attempt to clarify the question of the nature of the association between constructional apraxia and side of lesion by a comparison in which the role of aphasic disorder was examined somewhat more closely than has been done heretofore. The association between the status of language functions (as defined by scores on verbal tests or the presence of clinically evident aphasia) has been considered in some previous studies with rather inconclusive results (cf. Warrington, 1969). However, for the most part, these studies did not distinguish between motor and sensory aphasic disorder or assess the severity of defect. It was believed that an investigation of receptive and expressive language deficit, considered separately, might provide information which would have a bearing on the question of discrete hemispherically dependent types of visuoconstructive disability.

METHOD

Case material

The case material consisted of 48 right-handed patients from the neurological and neurosurgical services of the University of Iowa Hospitals, Iowa City, who showed evidence of cerebral disease which was apparently confined to one or the other hemisphere, the final diagnosis being based on clinical findings and the results of at least one ancillary procedure (angiography, radioactive brain scan, EEG). There were 34 patients with disease of the left hemisphere and 14 patients with disease of the right hemisphere in the sample. Of the 34 patients with left hemisphere disease, 26 showed expressive aphasia of either the fluent or non-fluent type. Receptive language capacity was assessed by a modified version of the Token Test (De Renzi & Vignolo, 1962) and, as described below, the aphasic patients were divided into groups with severe receptive language deficit (N = 9), moderate receptive language deficit (N = 9) and no receptive defect (N = 8).

Cerebrovascular disease was the most frequent diagnosis (28 cases) in the sample and neoplasm was the next most frequent (19 cases), the two categories accounting for all but 1 case, the exception being that of a patient with an atrophic focal lesion. The several groups were fairly comparable with respect to the relative number of cases with cerebrovascular or neoplastic disease in each, the proportion of cerebrovascular cases ranging from 50 per cent to 64 per cent. Intrahemispheric localization of lesions was not attempted.

In addition, a group of 30 control patients without history or evidence of cerebral disease was studied, their performances on the Token Test providing normative standards on which the judgment of receptive language capacity in the brain-diseased patients was based.

Tests

A 32-item version of the Token Test was utilized to assess receptive language capacity. The patient was given a credit of 2 points for each correctly executed command. If he failed an item, or asked to have the command repeated, it was given again and success on the second trial earned a credit of 1 point. The range of scores was 58–64 in the group of 30 control patients and 56–64 in the 14 patients (all non-aphasic) with right hemisphere disease. A score of 55 or less, representing a performance level exceeded by all the patients in the control and right hemisphere groups, was adopted as an index of receptive language disability. The severity of receptive language disability was classified as "moderate" if a patient's score was within the range of 46–55 points and as "severe" if it was 45 points or lower.

Constructional praxis was assessed by a standardized test requiring the building of three-dimensional structures with blocks (Benton, 1968). This is a fairly easy task for normal subjects, the great majority of control patients making errorless performances and 99 per cent of them making less than four errors. An error score of four or more was therefore considered to indicate a defective performance.

RESULTS

Of the 34 patients with left hemisphere disease, 8 showed no expressive or recep-

Table 8. Frequency of visuoconstructive defect in the several groups of patients

Classification	N	Frequency of failure[a]		
Left hemisphere disease				
A. Aphasic with severe receptive defect	9	66.7%		
			50%	
B. Aphasic with moderate receptive defect	9	33.3%		
				32.4%
C. Expressive aphasia only	8	12.5%		
			12.5%	
D. Not aphasic	8	12.5%		
Right hemisphere disease				
E. Not aphasic	14	35.7%		

[a] Performance level exceeded by 99 per cent of control patients.

tive language deficits and were classified as non-aphasic. Eight patients showed expressive language deficits but their Token Test performances were within normal limits (score of 56 or higher) and they were classified as "Expressive Aphasia Only." Of the remaining 18 aphasic patients, 9 showed moderate receptive impairment (scores ranging from 46–55) and 9 showed quite severe receptive defects, their Token Test scores ranging from 4–31. It is of some interest that the scores of the patients with receptive defects formed two clearly different distributions with the highest scores in the "severe" group being decidedly below the lowest score in the "moderate" group. At the same time, it may be noted that only one patient in the "severe" group showed virtually complete failure (score = 4) on the Token Test. The next poorest patient, who earned a score of 9 points, showed understanding of at least some simple commands. Thus, although this group was characterized by quite severe receptive impairment, the patients in it did show a modest degree of language understanding.

The constructional performances of the several groups of patients are shown in Table 8. Thirty-six per cent of the patients with right hemisphere disease showed defective three-dimensional block building, a figure which is comparable to

previous findings (Benton, 1968). In the total group of 34 patients with left hemisphere disease, 11 (32 per cent) performed defectively. However, a striking difference between the patients with and without receptive language defect is quite evident. While only 12.5 per cent of the patients without receptive deficit (including those with expressive aphasia) showed constructional impairment, 50 per cent of those with receptive defects were impaired. The highest frequency of impairment (decidedly higher than that shown by the patients with disease of the right hemisphere) was found in the group of aphasic patients with severe receptive defect.

DISCUSSION

The major findings of the study are: (1) the relatively high frequency of defective constructional performance in non-aphasic patients with disease of the right hemisphere; (2) the very low frequency of defective performance in non-aphasic patients with disease of the left hemisphere; (3) the equally low frequency of defective performance in those aphasic patients with left hemisphere disease who show only expressive defects without concomitant receptive difficulties; (4) the relatively high frequency of defective constructional performance in aphasic patients with receptive language impairment.

Thus it seems evident that, in patients with disease of the left hemisphere, visuoconstructive defect is associated with the presence of receptive language impairment. In this respect, the findings are quite similar to those of a recent study (Sauguet, Benton & Hécaen, 1971) in which it was found that body schema disturbances (e.g., defective finger recognition) were likely to be manifested only by patients with receptive language difficulties. Evidently both types of performance deficit are "language dependent" in patients with left hemisphere lesions in the sense that receptive aphasic defect appears to be a necessary condition for their appearance.

The implications of the findings for the questions raised earlier may now be considered. Is the generally observed trend toward a somewhat higher frequency of constructional deficit in patients with right hemisphere disease an artefact of case selection? Our results suggest that this may well be the case. If circumstances are such as to lead to the formation of a group of patients with left hemisphere disease which includes only a few cases with sensory aphasia, or none at all, the performance level of this group on constructional tasks is likely to be close to the normal level and, at the same time, clearly superior to that of patients with right hemisphere disease. On the other hand, if the left-sided group includes a substantial proportion of patients with receptive language impairment, its overall performance is likely to be comparable to that of the right-sided group. And, indeed, if a left-sided group composed exclusively of patients with sensory aphasia were formed, its performance level will probably be found to be inferior to that of an "unselected" group of patients with disease of the right hemisphere. There is, then, reason to believe that the findings of

at least some comparative studies of visuoconstructive disability in relation to side of lesion may be due to sampling bias.

At the same time, the results also support the concept of discrete types of visuoconstructive impairment in relation to side of lesion but not, however, in the form in which the concept is usually advanced. The findings of the study of Dee (1970) were quite clear in their implications that constructional difficulties are closely associated with perceptual impairment irrespective of side of lesion and hence a dichotomy of "visuoperceptive" versus "executive" types of deficit as related to side of lesion does not seem to be tenable. We did not give visuoperceptive tasks to our patients but, judging from Dee's results as well as those of Piercy & Smyth (1962), there is every reason to assume that the apraxic patients in all the subgroups would have shown concomitant perceptual impairment.

The striking feature of the results is the close association of failure in performance with sensory aphasia in the left-sided cases. There was, of course, no such association in the patients with right hemisphere disease and, in this sense, one can think of two types of visuoconstructive disability, the one being language-related and the other not. Not every patient with sensory aphasia showed constructional impairment; even some of those with quite severe receptive language deficit performed adequately on the block building test. One cannot therefore ascribe the constructional failure solely to the language deficit even though the latter appears to be a necessary precondition. Evidently an additional factor enters into the picture and our task would seem to be to try to identify the nature of this factor. These patients were also given tests assessing the traditional forms of apraxia, i.e., the capacity to execute symbolic movements and demonstrate the use of objects, and failure on these tasks was also found to be closely associated with the presence of sensory aphasia (Dee, Benton & Van Allen, 1970). The finding supports the view that, in patients with left hemisphere disease, constructional apraxia is an expression of a more general apraxic disorder while in patients with right hemisphere lesions it presents as a distinctive deficit.

Other possibilities that deserve to be explored in an effort to explain the findings are the relationship between visual field defect and visuoconstructive disability in the two hemispheric groups as well as the influence of size and locus of lesion on performance level. It is possible, for example, that the sensory aphasics with constructional apraxia are those whose lesions extend into the parieto-occipital region while those without constructional disability have disease confined to the temporal lobe.

In any case, this strikingly close association of visuoconstructive disability with sensory aphasia in patients with disease of the left hemisphere suggests that there are different determinants of failure in visuoconstructive tasks according to side of lesion. In this sense, it seems justified to speak of discrete "types" of constructional apraxia. The definition of these "types" in terms of underlying mechanisms remains to be formulated.

REFERENCES

Arrigoni, G. & E. De Renzi. Constructional apraxia and hemispheric locus of lesion. *Cortex*. 1: *170–197* (1964).

Benton, A. L. The fiction of the "Gerstmann syndrome." *J. Neurol. Neurosurg. Psychiat.* 24: *176–181* (1961).

———. The Visual Retention Test as a constructional praxis task. *Conf. Neurol.* 22: *141–155* (1962).

———. Constructional apraxia and the minor hemisphere. *Conf. Neurol.* 29: *1–16* (1967).

———. La praxie constructive tri-dimensionnelle. *Rev. Psychol. Appl.* 18: *63–80* (1968).

———. & M. L. Fogel. Three-dimensional constructional praxis: a clinical test. *Arch. Neurol.* 7: *347–354* (1962).

Critchley, M. The Parietal Lobes. Edward Arnold, London (1953).

Dee, H. L. Visuoconstructive and visuoperceptive deficit in patients with unilateral cerebral lesions. *Neuropsychologia.* 8: *305–314* (1970).

———, A. L. Benton & M. W. Van Allen. Apraxia in relation to hemispheric locus of lesion and aphasia. *Trans. Amer. Neurol. Assn.* 95: *147–150* (1980).

De Renzi, E. & L. A. Vignolo. The Token Test: a sensitive test to detect receptive disturbances in aphasics. *Brain.* 85: *665–678* (1962).

Kleist, K. Kriegsverletzungen des Gehirns in ihrer Bedeutung für die Hirnlokalisation und Hirnpathologie. In: Handbuch der ärztlichen Erfahrung im Weltkriege 1914/1918. Bd. IV, Geistes- und Nervenkrankheiten. (O. von Schjerning, Ed.) Barth, Leipzig (1923).

———. Gehirnpathologie. Barth, Leipzig (1934).

Piercy, M. F., H. Hécaen & J. De Ajuriaguerra. Constructional apraxia associated with unilateral cerebral lesions. *Brain.* 83: *225–242* (1960).

———, & V. Smyth. Right hemisphere dominance for certain non-verbal intellectual skills. *Brain.* 85: *775–790* (1962).

Sauguet, J., A. L. Benton & H. Hécaen. Disturbances of the body schema in relation to language impairment and hemispheric locus of lesion. *J. Neurol. Neurosurg. Psychiat.* 34: *496–501* (1971).

Warrington, E. K. Constructional apraxia. In: Handbook of Clinical Neurology, Volume 4. (P. J. Vinken & G. W. Bruyn, Eds.) North-Holland Publishing Co., Amsterdam (1969).

———, M. James & M. Kinsbourne. Drawing disability in relation to laterality of cerebral lesion. *Brain.* 89: *53–82* (1966).

14.

Spatial Thinking in Neurological Patients: Historical Aspects*

This chapter sketches the development of knowledge and ideas about diverse defects of spatial thinking in patients with brain disease. It covers the period beginning with the inception of these ideas somewhat over 100 years ago to the 1960s. The review is necessarily selective and incomplete since the literature on the topic is enormous. However, it should provide a historical background for discussion of the current status of the field.

HUGHLINGS JACKSON

The idea that a lesion in the brain could produce a specific defect in thinking, orientation, or action with respect to space arose within the context of the broader concept of agnosia. The origins of the latter concept can be traced in the evolving thought of Hughlings Jackson. As early as 1864, Jackson raised the question of whether perception, particularly

* A. L. Benton in M. Potegal (Ed.), *Spatial abilities: developmental and physiological foundations.* New York, Academic Press, 1982, pp. 253–275. Copyright 1982, Academic Press.

visual perception, might not have its seat in the right cerebral hemisphere. Ten years later, in his famous paper on the nature of the duality of the brain, he discussed the possibility in greater detail, expressing the opinion that the posterior part of the right hemisphere served the function of visual recognition and memory (Jackson, 1874). As he phrased it, "the hinder part of the brain on the right side is the chief seat of the revival of images in the *recognition* of object, places, etc. [p. 101]." As an example of a defect in this capacity caused by disease, he cited the case of a patient who exhibited what is now called disorientation for place. Although she was in the London Hospital, she asserted that she was in a place in Holborn where she had worked for some years. But Jackson admitted that the evidence for locating "perception" in the right hemisphere was not strong, remarking that "as will be seen, my facts are very few [p. 103]."

Two years later, Jackson's ideas took more definite form when he described a patient who proved to have a tumor in the posterior right hemisphere and whose "first symptoms were those of what I call imperception. She often did not know objects, persons and places." The first indication that something was amiss with this 59-year-old woman was when she lost her way going from her home to a nearby park, a route she had been taking for 30 years. Over the course of the next few weeks, she showed odd lapses of behavior. For example, she made mistakes in dressing herself, a type of disability that later was given the name of "dressing dyspraxia." After admission to the hospital, she was not able to identify the different nurses attending her. Collectively these deficits in recognition, orientation, and action constituted what Jackson called *imperception*, "a defect as special as aphasia." However, his term was not adopted by other clinicans who later described the same constellation of deficits under tbe rubric of *mindblindness* or *visual agnosia*.

The next major contribution to this topic came from the physiological laboratory. Having shown that extensive destruction of the occipital lobes produced blindness in dogs and monkeys, Hermann Munk (1878) then described the effects of a more limited lesion in the same area. The animal (in this case, the dog) obviously could see since he ambulated freely and avoided obstacles. Yet he seemed to have lost the capacity to grasp the meaning of many visual stimuli that he appeared to perceive clearly. For example, he showed no signs of special recognition of his master, nor did he react appropriately to a threatening gesture or to the sight of a piece of meat. Munk called this disturbance in visual behavior *mindblindness* and he ascribed it to a loss of visual memory images that prevented the animal from relating current visual experience to past experience.

Munk's idea of a higher order disturbance in which visual associational or

memory processes are impaired against a background of intact visuosensory capacity received a skeptical reception from his fellow physiologists, who were inclined to interpret mindblindness as an expression of defects in visual discrimination. Some clinicians also doubted the reality of mindblindness, feeling that the condition was essentially a reflection of defective visual acuity, and their position was supported by Munk's own contention that mindblindness resulted from a lesion in the same areas as served foveal vision. However, other clinical observers readily accepted the concept since they were convinced that they had seen patients with the same impairment Munk had described in dogs. Case reports, such as those by Wilbrand (1887) and Lissauer (1890), established that mindblindness or visual object agnosia did exist in human subjects. The primary deficit shown by these patients was an inability to recognize objects or persons despite apparently adequate visual acuity. In addition, some showed spatial disorientation, as reflected in losing one's way along familiar routes both indoors and outdoors, not being able to describe the location of familiar streets and buildings or to describe the disposition of the furniture in one's living room or bedroom. Since not all patients with visual object agnosia showed these spatial disabilities, the designation of *visuospatial agnosia* was given to them to indicate their essential independence from disorders of object recognition.

BADAL AND SPATIAL THINKING

Another trend in clinical investigation emphasized impairment in spatial thinking independently of sensory modality. The pioneer study of this type was that of a Bordeaux ophthalmologist, Jules Badal (1888), who entitled his paper "Contribution to the Study of Psychic Blindness,

Alexia, Agraphia, Inferior Hemianopsia, Disorder of the Sense of Space" (cf. Benton, 1969; Benton & Meyers, 1956). His patient showed a large number of diverse deficits but her chief complaint was spatial disorientation. She could not find her way in her apartment or in the immediate neighborhood and she would not leave home without a guide. She could not answer simple questions about the spatial relations of the main streets of Bordeaux although she had long been thoroughly familiar with them. Like Jackson's patient, she showed dyspraxia for dressing. "She could not dress herself alone without putting on her clothes in reverse, taking the left sleeve for the right. It took her an infinite time to determine the order in which the different articles of clothing should be put on." She showed faulty visual guidance of hand movements in reaching (cf. Damasio & Benton, 1979). "She also had great difficulty in finding objects which she needed, even when they were in front of her. She would reach for it and her hand would constantly pass over it as if influenced by a false projection due to paralysis of the eye muscles. However, there was no diplopia, no strabismus and the eye movements were executed in a normal manner [p. 101]." Her central visual acuity was excellent. If her attention could be directed to them—for she had great difficulty in maintaining and shifting ocular fixation—she could name the smallest letters on the eye chart and she showed no difficulty in recognizing or naming the smallest objects.

But, as suggested by the title of his paper, Badal's main point was that the patient suffered from an impairment in spatial perception that transcended the visual modality. Although her auditory acuity appeared to be intact, she made errors in identifying the direction of the source of sounds. Impairment of spatial perception in the somesthetic modalities

was manifested in defective body schema performances. She showed gross finger agnosia, not being able to state which of her fingers had been touched, and she could no longer distinguish between the right and left sides of her body. These errors in localization were made whether her eyes were open or closed.

Similar cases with visual disorientation and difficulty in making spatial judgements but with intact visual acuity and visual object recognition were described by Foerster (1890), Dunn (1895), Peters (1896), Meyer (1900), and Lenz (1905). Discussing the fact that one of his patients showed a serious disability in reading, Meyer pointed out that this type of reading failure, which reflected a disturbance in spatial orientation, was not to be confused with true alexia which was of a linguistic character.

In 1909 Balint described a patient with a rather distinctive assemblage of deficits associated with inaccurate visual judgments. The most prominent features of the syndrome, which Balint described as "psychic paralysis of gaze, optic ataxia, and spatial disturbance of attention [p. 51]" and which is now called *Balint's syndrome*, were maintenance of ocular fixation on a point in the visual field with seeming inability to shift fixation, inattention to objects and events in other parts of the visual field, and misreaching for objects. These impairments in oculomotor and visuomotor function were accompanied by a number of perceptual deficits, such as difficulty in estimating distances, in reading long polysyllabic words (although simpler words could be read), and in identifying figures such as a hexagon or an octagon although simpler figures such as a triangle or square were readily identified. Attention was generally fixated on a point in the right visual field with consequent neglect of stimuli in the left field. There were many expressions of impairment in the execution of visually guided movements. Besides misreaching for objects, the patient was unable to draw or copy or to use a knife accurately in cutting. But he could recognize objects and read single letters.

An interesting development of this early period is seen in Rieger's (1909) hypothesis that the brain contains two distinct but interacting apparatuses, one serving verbal–conceptual functions and the other spatial–practical functions. His ideas were developed further by Reichardt (1918) who described visuospatial and visuoconstructional defects in association with lesions of the right hemisphere and contrasted them with the linguistic impairments associated with left-hemisphere disease.

Thus, by 1910, a fairly large number of specific deficits in performance, indicative of impairment of spatial thinking, had been described. As Table 9 shows, these deficits could be perceptual, amnesic, or praxic in nature. Thinking about their neurological basis followed two lines. The dominant point of view was that these disabilities were the product of bilateral disease involving the occipital and posterior parietal and temporal areas, and this position received substantial support from autopsy study. Thus, the brain of Foerster's (1890) patient showed bilateral softening confined to the occipital and parietal lobes (Sachs, 1895) and the brain of one of Meyer's (1900) patients showed bilateral occipital lobe disease. Autopsy study of Balint's (1909) patient showed bilateral atrophy of the occipital, parietal, and temporal lobes with the most marked changes evident in the posterior parietal and temporal areas. The prevailing view was that this extensive destruction of visual association cortex resulted in a loss of visual memory images.

A second line of thought emphasized

Table 9. Performance deficits described in the literature as of 1910

1. Inability to follow routes
2. Defective topographic or geographic memory
3. Difficulty in judging distance
4. Difficulty in reading
5. Inattention in left visual field
6. Misreaching for objects
7. Dyspraxia for dressing
8. Difficulty in locating objects
9. Disturbances in ocular fixation

the role of the right hemisphere in the mediation of spatial thinking. As has been seen, Jackson considered the posterior part of the right hemisphere to be a center for visual recognition and memory, including spatial memory. In the 1890s, a Philadelphia physician, T. D. Dunn (1895), specifically localized spatial orientation in the right hemisphere. Having described a patient who could not remember the spatial relations of familiar streets or even of the rooms in his house but who could still recognize objects, faces, and simple words, he postulated the existence of a "geographic center" in the right hemisphere for what he called "the sense of location." Since his patient did not have visual object agnosia or facial agnosia, Dunn denied that it was necessary to invoke a generalized loss of visual memory images as the underlying disability, the patient having only loss of "optical images of locality."

Further support for a specific association between spatial disorientation and disease of the right hemisphere came from the observations of Peters (1896) and Lenz (1905), each of whom called attention to the relatively high frequency of spatial disorientation in patients with left homonymous hemianopia. However, in contrast to Dunn, both authors were extremely cautious in making inferences from their observations. Peters declined to draw a conclusion and Lenz only raised the question of whether "the right occipital lobe is perhaps more strongly related to orientation than the left."

THE CONTRIBUTION OF WALTHER POPPELREUTER

Study of patients with traumatic head wounds during and directly after World War I added further knowledge about the visuospatial defects associated with brain injury. The most comprehensive and detailed investigation was that of Poppelreuter (1917), who was the first to apply experimental–psychological methods such as tachistoscopy and the instrumental measurement of depth perception in the evaluation of these patients. As a consequence, he was able to show that defective depth perception was extraordinarily frequent in patients with occipital wounds. About one-third of them (with or without visual-field defects) proved to have some degree of impairment when acuity of depth perception was quantitatively assessed. Poppelreuter further pointed out that most of these patients did not complain of having difficulties in depth perception in everyday life.

He also studied accuracy in reaching for objects and found that misreaching could occur with different degrees of severity, that it might be present in the whole visual field or only in the periphery, and that patients with intact fields, as well as hemianopics, showed the defect. He emphasized the motor or behavioral aspects of misreaching and believed that the traditional explanation of it in terms of a disturbed "sense of locality" was incorrect. Rather it was a disturbance of coordination between sensory and motor processes, that is, an apraxia and not a disturbance in perception. Visuosensory capacity and distance judgment can be completely intact in a patient who misreaches. Thus, misreaching or defective

visual guidance of hand movements reflects "not an alteration in the content of perception but a disturbance of the mechanism of localization."

Poppelreuter studied the exploration of visual space in his patients by means of his "field of search" test in which 57 diverse visual stimuli (numbers, letters, geometric figures) were presented in an irregular array and the subject was required to point to stimuli named or shown by the examiner. Relying on quantitative measures of performance, Poppelreuter was able to demonstrate that visual exploration was significantly prolonged in many patients, particularly those with occipital or bilateral wounds. Hemianopic defect per se did not appear to have an important influence on performance. Decades later Teuber, Battersby, and Bender (1949; Teuber, 1964) utilized this procedure to investigate the exploration of visual space in both adults and children with brain damage and found prolongation in searching time not only in those with parieto-occipital lesions but also in those with frontal damage. In some patients with unilateral injury the deficit was particularly severe in the contralateral visual field.

Misreaching for objects or inaccurate pointing to them was only one form of what Poppelreuter called *visual apraxia*. Other forms of the disability were awkwardness in manipulating objects (e.g., cutting with scissors), defective visually guided locomotion (e.g., rail-walking), and visuoconstructional defects such as poor copying of designs, failure in block designs tasks, and inaccurate construction of block models. In discussing these performances he noted once again that visual-field defects were not closely related to them and he emphasized that these visuomotor deficits were independent of both disturbances in form perception, as disclosed by tachistoscopic or "mixed figures" tests, and impairment in distance judgment.

KARL KLEIST AND CONSTRUCTIONAL APRAXIA

One of Poppelreuter's more important contributions was his emphasis on visuoconstructive disabilities as a distinctive type of disturbance that could be shown by patients with brain disease. This theme was then taken up by Karl Kleist (1922/1934), who earlier had made similar observations (Kleist, 1912) and who now coined the term *constructional apraxia* for the disability he defined as a disturbance "in formative activities such as assembling, building, and drawing, in which the spatial form of the product proves to be unsuccessful, without there being an apraxia of single movements."

As a neurologist, Kleist was particularly interested in the site of the lesions that led to constructional apraxia. He agreed with Poppelreuter that, at least in its pure form, constructional apraxia represented a failure in integration between perceptual and motor processes rather than a perceptual defect per se. Thus it was, in modern terminology, a "disconnection symptom" (Geschwind, 1965). At the same time, Kleist was aware that impaired visuoperceptual capacity could also be expressed in defective visuoconstructive performances and he conceded that it was often difficult to decide whether an observed visuoconstructive disability was a "true" constructional apraxia or the direct reflection of visuoperceptive impairment. In any case, what *he* meant by *constructional apraxia* was the disconnection symptom, not the motoric expression of a perceptual deficit. Indeed, that is why he called it an *apraxia*, that is, a disturbance in purposeful motor activity within a setting on intact sensory and motor capacity. With respect to the

neurological basis for the disability, Kleist placed the crucial lesion in the parieto-occipital territory of the left or dominant hemisphere, the functional effect of such a lesion being to disconnect the visual association area (Areas 18, 19, 39) from anterior motor and premotor regions and hence to prevent visual information from reaching executive motor centers.

Kleist's description and particularly that of his student Hans Strauss (1924) established constructional apraxia as a form of motoric visuospatial disorder associated with brain disease. However, his insistence that it was purely a praxic or "executive" disability was for the most part ignored and sometimes actively challenged. For example, Kroll (1929), Kroll and Stollbun (1933), Lange (1936), and Schlesinger (1928) pointed out that disturbances in spatial orientation and visual perception were almost always part of the clinical picture of "constructional apraxia." Consequently, the term was generally applied to any visuoconstructional failure, whether or not it occurred within a setting of perceptual and orientational disability.

On the neurological side, Kleist's localization of the crucial lesion underlying constructional apraxia was also challenged by subsequent clinical study which indicated that in fact the deficit was more frequently shown by patients with right-hemisphere disease than by those with left-hemisphere damage (Benton, 1962; Benton & Fogel, 1962; Dide, 1938; Hécaen, Ajuriaguerra, & Massonet, 1951; Lange, 1936; McFie, Piercy, & Zangwill, 1950; Paterson & Zangwill, 1944; Piercy, Hécaen, & Ajuriaguerra, 1960; Piercy & Smyth, 1962). As has been mentioned, this point had already been made by Reichardt (1918), who contrasted visuospatial and visuoconstructive defects associated with right-hemisphere disease with the linguistic defects produced by lesions of the left hemisphere. Kleist took account of Reichardt's observations but questioned their validity on the grounds that his cases may have had left-hemisphere lesions that were not evident on macroscopic examination and also that some of his patients may have been left-handed.

Despite the accumulating evidence in its favor, the idea that there is a close association between constructional apraxia and disease of the right hemisphere was not readily accepted by neurologists. Admittedly, the early contributions to the topic, consisting of single case studies or global clinical impressions, could easily be discounted. Only after the more systematic studies of Zangwill, Hécaen, and their co-workers (1944–1951) were published was it necessary to consider the reported correlation seriously. However, even when the correlation was accepted, its neuropsychological meaning was not clear. It was not possible to consider the right hemisphere to be "dominant" for visuoconstructive or visuospatial activity in the same sense that the left hemisphere was considered to be dominant for language functions, for the two situations were not at all comparable. Aphasic disorder resulting from disease of the nondominant right hemisphere in a right-handed patient (i.e., so-called crossed aphasia), was recognized as a highly unusual phenomenon, occurring in not more than 1 or 2% of cases (Russell & Espir, 1961; Zangwill, 1960). But, of course, constructional apraxia resulting from disease of the left hemisphere in right-handed patients was not at all unusual. It was only a matter of a bias toward a somewhat higher frequency in patients with lesions of the right hemisphere (Benton, 1962; Benton & Fogel, 1962).

This empirical finding that, although it is more frequent and more severe in patients with right-hemisphere disease, constructional apraxia is also shown by a substantial proportion of patients with disease of the left hemisphere posed a problem of interpretation. One proffered explanation more or less reflected the observed facts. It hypothesized a partial "dominance" of the right hemisphere for visuoconstructive functions in the form of their "bilateral but unequal representation" in the two cerebral hemispheres (Piercy & Smyth, 1962). Another explanation, first advanced by Duensing (1953), held that there are two distinctive types of visuoconstructive disability, of fundamentally different character. One type, equivalent to the "true" constructional apraxia of Kleist, is of an executive or motor nature and is related to the disruption of mechanisms in the left hemisphere. The other type results from a basic impairment in visuospatial thinking and is related to disruption of mechanisms in the right hemisphere.

Piercy and Smyth (1962) undertook to evaluate the cogency of the two competing explanations by investigating the relationship between constructional performance and the status of visuoperceptive ability in patients with right- and left-hemisphere disease. A number of tests requiring the copying of designs and the construction of block and matchstick models were employed to assess constructional ability and Raven's Progressive Matrices provided the measure of visuoperceptive capacity. It was reasoned that if the hypothesis of two distinctive types of visuoconstructive disability in relation to side of lesion is correct, then a close association between defective constructional performance and visuoperceptual impairment should be seen in patients with right-hemisphere lesions but not in those with disease of the left hemisphere, at least some of whom should show constructional apraxia within a context of intact visuoperceptive capacity. The results were unequivocal. Constructional performances and score on the Raven test were very closely associated in both hemispheric groups. The two groups differed only in respect to level of performance, the patients with right-hemisphere damage showing more severe impairment on both the constructional and perceptual tasks. Piercy and Smyth concluded that the theory of two distinctive types of visuoconstructive disability could not be supported and that the concept of "bilateral but unequal representation" in the two hemispheres was the more likely possibility.

However, a study the same year by Costa and Vaughan (1962) generated different results. Giving the WAIS block designs and the Raven matrices to patients with unilateral lesions, they found a close correlation ($r = .83$) between the two performances in those with right-hemisphere disease but only a minimal positive association ($r = .33$) in those with left-hemisphere disease. Although the authors did not draw a specific conclusion, their findings were consonant with the existence of discrete visuoperceptual and executive types of constructional impairment.

Qualitative analysis of the constructional performances provided another approach to the question of whether there existed distinctive types of disabilities that were differentially related to side of lesion. It was argued that impaired visuospatial functions should be reflected in productions characterized by distortion of the spatial relations among the elements of the construction. Construction from a model should be as defective as construction to verbal command because of the pervasive visuoperceptual disability. In contrast, executive or psychomotor impairment with attendant awkwardness in manipulation of the pencil or blocks should be reflected in constructions that

are coherent and spatially correct but simplified and lacking in elaboration. Constructions from a model should be superior to those from verbal command since the model could facilitate slavish copying and the making of corrections when indicated. Fragmentary evidence in favor of this distinction was adduced by a number of investigators, among them Hécaen et al. (1951), Duensing (1953), McFie and Zangwill (1960), Piercy et al. (1960), and Arrigoni and De Renzi (1964). However, the detailed comparative study by Warrington, James, and Kinsbourne (1966) of drawing performance in relation to side of lesion failed to confirm most of the hypothesized qualitative differences in the productions.

Thus, by the 1960s there were a number of unresolved questions about constructional apraxia, the primary ones being whether it represented one or more than one disability and what was the exact nature of its relationship to side of lesion in patients with unilateral brain disease. In addition, the question of whether or not constructional apraxia was merely a reflection of general mental impairment was raised (Benton, 1967, 1969).

TYPES OF IMPAIRMENT

The casualties of World War I provided an abundance of case material for detailed study and this led to the development of classifications of types of visual disorientation. Gordon Holmes (1918; Holmes & Horrax, 1919) divided into two categories the disorders of visual orientation and attention that he observed: (1) disturbances in localization, orientation and distance perception, as reflected in misreaching for objects, inability to learn routes, and difficulty in reading connected text; (2) oculomotor defects, such as the inability to shift fixation on verbal command and absence of the blink reflex.

On his part, Kleist (1922/1934) distinguished between disturbances of visuospatial *perception* (as reflected in defective bisection of lines, pointing to objects, or distance judgments and visuospatial *agnosia* or *amnesia* (as reflected in the forgetting of geographic and topographic relationships). The neurological significance of the distinction was that the perceptual disorders were related to lesions in the calcarine region and its immediate vicinity (Areas 17 and 18). These lesions might be unilateral (producing, for example, mislocalization in one visual half-field) or bilateral (producing, for example, defective depth perception). In contrast, the agnosic or amnesic disorders were related to lesions of the outlying Area 19 primarily involving the left hemisphere.

Russell Brain (1941) made still another distinction between defective localization of stimuli within grasping distance (as in misreaching for objects) and defective localization of stimuli beyond arm's reach (as in poor distance judgments). Some of his patients showed impairment in one form of localization and not in the other, dissociations that he attributed to differences in the site of the causative lesions. He suggested that lesions involving the connections between visual cortex and the hand and arm area of the parietal somatosensory cortex produced mislocalizations within arm's reach whereas those affecting the connections between the visual cortex and the leg area resulted in impaired localization of more distant stimuli within "walking distance," as he phrased it. Later Birkmayer (1951) made a similar distinction.

Brain also offered a classification of forms of visual disorientation. The first form was defective localization of objects in space and this could be subdivided into three types, depending on whether it resulted from impaired visual acuity,

hemianopia, or impairment of cerebral integrative processes. This last type was true agnosia for spatial relationships and could be exhibited in either one half-field, as Riddoch (1935) had shown, or in the entire field. Patients with visuospatial agnosia, particularly if it is present throughout the visual field, "cannot find their own way round objects when they run into them, set out in the wrong direction to get to others which they clearly see, and have difficulty in finding their way about and learning the topography of a room [p. 268]."

A second type of disorientation was loss of stereoscopic vision, an uncommon disorder previously described by Riddoch (1917) and Holmes and Horrax (1919). Another rare disorder was visual allesthesia, that is, the referral of visual stimuli to the opposite half-field, comparable to the more extensively described tactile allesthesia in which stimuli applied to one side of the body are referred to the opposite side (cf. Benton, 1959). Brain had not seen such a case and mentioned it only for the sake of completeness in listing.

A more important type of disorientation was neglect or unawareness of the left half of visual space shown by patients with extensive lesions of the parieto-occipital territory of the right hemisphere. Comparable to the neglect of the left side of the body seen in patients with right parietal lesions, this unawareness of the left half of space produces an inability to follow routes because of a tendency to avoid making turns to the left when indicated.

Finally, Brain listed loss of topographical memory as an independent form of visual disorientation, pointing out that a patient may have serious visuospatial problems on the perceptual level and yet be able to describe routes and spatial interrelationships accurately. Although most of the cases of this type described in the literature had proven to have bilateral disease, Brain expressed the opinion that the crucial lesion was in the left occipital area.

DISTURBANCES OF THE BODY SCHEMA

As has been noted, Badal included his patient's inability to discriminate the left and right sides of her body and to identify her fingers as expressions of a "disorder of the sense of space." Many clinical investigators followed his example in viewing these and other disturbances of the body schema as reflecting a basic impairment in spatial thinking. After Gerstmann (1924, 1927) described finger agnosia as "a circumscribed disturbance of orientation towards one's body," Lange (1930, 1933) and Stengel (1944) suggested that this rather peculiar deficit as well as the other elements of the Gerstmann syndrome (right-left disorientation, agraphia, acalculia) should be considered as part of a more comprehensive syndrome of spatial disorientation involving external space and constructional praxis as well as the body schema.

There were, however, competing explanations. Head (1926) interpreted impairment in right-left discrimination to be a specific expression of the same disturbance in "symbolic formulation and expression" that defined aphasia. Consequently, he included tests of right-left orientation in his battery for the assessment of aphasic patients. Moreover, these "hand, eye and ear" tests, as he called them, included nonverbal imitation tasks as well as tasks requiring naming or understanding the names of body parts. Supporting Head's interpretation, Benton (1959) cited the extraordinarily high frequency with which aphasic patients showed disturbed left-right awareness and finger recognition as evidence that the occurrence of these deficits in patients with unilateral brain disease reflects a disturbance of language or symbolic thinking.

Ajuriaguerra and Hécaen (1949) and Benton (1959) pointed out that disorientation with respect to external space did not necessarily imply disorientation toward one's own body and, conversely, that disturbances in the body schema did not necessarily imply the occurrence of conventional visual disorientation as described by Poppelreuter and Kleist. However, the frequent concurrence of the two types of orientational disability, particularly in the form of neglect of the left half of space *and* of one's body, was noted by Pineás (1931), Brain (1941), Critchley (1953), and other observers. Brain believed that visuospatial orientation and body awareness were intimately related and that the posterior parietal region connecting the visual cortex with the somatosensory area in the postcentral gyrus provided an anatomical basis for this association.

AUDITORY-SPATIAL DISCRIMINATION

Apart from single case reports, such as those of Badal (1888), Penfield and Evans (1934), Ross and Fountain (1948), and Wortis and Pfeffer (1948), the spatial aspects of audition in patients with brain disease were not investigated until the 1950s when Sanchez-Longo and Forster (1958; Sanchez-Longo, Forster, & Auth, 1957) reported their studies of auditory localization. In the first study the performance of 5 patients with unilateral temporal lobe lesions were compared to a group of control patients with the finding that 4 of the 5 patients were grossly inaccurate, their mean error of localization being larger than the poorest of the 20 control subjects. Moreover, in analogy with visual localization, every patient showed a larger error of localization in the auditory field contralateral to the side of lesion. The results were confirmed in a second study of a larger number of patients. In addition, a group of patients with lesions not involving the temporal lobe were assessed with the finding that their overall performance level was within the normal range. The observation that patients with unilateral temporal lobe injury often show particularly severe impairment in localization in the contralateral field was consonant with the earlier case reports of Penfield and Evans (1934) and Wortis and Pfeffer (1948).

However, Walsh (1957), presenting click stimuli through earphones and manipulating time and intensity differences between the clicks as cues to localization of the apparent direction of the source of sound, reported that patients with temporal lobe lesions performed quite adequately. A second study, in which sounds were transmitted through air to assess "real" rather than "apparent" localization, produced the same results. The three patients with temporal lobe lesions were able to localize the source of the sound. Walsh's treatment of his data was rather impressionistic (in contrast to the quantitative analyses of Sanchez-Longo and Forster) and it is not clear that patients performed on a normal level of accuracy. In any case, his results were in accord with those earlier reported by Ross and Fountain (1948).

The study of Shankweiler (1961) introduced some new elements into an already rather confused picture. Two of his basic findings were negative. There was no evidence for particularly severe impairment of localization in the contralateral auditory field in patients with unilateral lesions nor did those with temporal lobe disease show more severe defects than those with parieto-occipital or frontal lesions. However, he did find that the patients with right-hemisphere lesions were poorer in performance than those with left-hemisphere lesions, significantly on one auditory localization task (pointing to the source of a sound) and nonsignificantly on a second task (discrimination of angular differences). Pointing out that auditory localization takes place in a visually organized space, Shankweiler considered that the observed between-hemispheres difference in accuracy of localization was not unexpected in view of the established association between visuospatial deficits and disease of the right hemisphere. Another finding, which perhaps explains some of the discordant results of previous studies, was that for both control subjects and patients the correlation between performances on the two auditory localization tasks (pointing versus verbal judgment) was not significant.

Teuber (1962), employing dichotic clicks with manipulation of time and intensity differences to assess auditory localization, reported results that were in accord with those of Shankweiler. Patients with right-hemisphere lesions performed more poorly than those with left-hemisphere disease. In addition, performance level tended to be specific to the task. A patient might perform adequately on the intensity difference task but not on the time difference task or vice versa. Teuber concluded that "brain injury can impair binaural localization based on time and intensity differences, but the effects are dissociable, suggesting at least partial separation of neural mechanisms underlying these two forms of localization [p. 154]."

TACTILE-SPATIAL PERFORMANCES

The concept that the tactile and kinesthetic senses have a spatial component as well as methods for measuring that component arose from the inspired work of Ernst Heinrich Weber (see Ross & Murray, 1978), two of whose studies have recently appeared in English translation (Weber, 1978). He devised the tactile compass to measure the accuracy of discrimination of two points on the skin and later developed the procedure of having a subject indicate a point on the skin that had been touched in order to measure the accuracy of tactile localization. The two-point threshold is primarily a measure of tactile acuity, analogous to visual acuity. Nevertheless, that there is a spatial component in the task of discriminating two points on the skin surface is indicated by the significant correlation between this performance and the error of tactile localization (Boring, 1930). However, it was generally agreed that the task of localizing a stimulated point on the skin was the more direct measure of the "sense of space."

Beginning in the 1870s, two-point discrimination and single-point localization were intensively studied both in patients with lesions of the central nervous system and in those with peripheral nerve injuries. It was readily established that impaired performance could occur as a consequence of disease of the somatosensory system at any level from the peripheral nerve to the cerebral cortex. Thereafter attention was focused on a number of questions. One of these was whether these tactile "spatial" deficits could occur independently of more basic defects in tactile sensitivity or were merely expressions of these defects. A second question concerned the neurological basis of impaired tactile-spatial performances.

With regard to the question of the relationships of tactile-spatial defects to impaired sensitivity, there was a gradual accumulation of evidence that defective two-point discrimination and point localization could be shown in the absence of defects in tactile sensitivity and, conversely, that patients with severely impaired tactile sensitivity (i.e., raised thresholds to pressure, pain, and temperature) could show intact localizing capacity. In 1901 Otfrid Foerster reviewed the pertinent literature and described the findings in a large sample of his own patients to establish these facts. However, at the same time he pointed to the close association between defects in tactile localization and disturbances in kinesthetic sensitivity, as reflected in raised thresholds for the detection of passive movements of the fingers, hands and arms.

Recalling the longstanding controversy between proponents of nativist and empiricist theories of the genesis of space perception, Foerster adduced clinical evidence to support the proposition that the apprehension of spatial characteristics and relations is not an inherent attribute of sensory experience but instead gradually develops as associations between different sensory experiences are formed. Thus, the tactile sense of space is the resultant of the establishment of connections between tactile, visual, and kinesthetic experience. If kinesthetic experience is impoverished, as in cases of congenital paralysis, or is impaired as a consequence of acquired disease of the nervous system, then tactile experience is deprived of its spatial component and this is reflected in defective performance on spatial tasks such as point localization.

At the same time, other somatosensory tests of a spatial character were developed and applied for clinical and investigative purposes. Position sense, that is, a patient's awareness of the position in which his arm, finger, or toe has been placed, was assessed by his verbal report or his imitation of the position. Recognition of the direction of lines drawn on the skin surface was another procedure used to assess the spatial aspects of tactile perception. A more complicated maneuver was to draw numerals or letters on the forearm, palm, or finger tips and determine whether or not the patient could identify them. His failure to do so was labeled *agraphesthesia*.

Over the decades there was much discussion about the meaning of failing performance on these spatial tasks. Broadly speaking, there were two schools of thought on the subject. One group saw these deficits as expressions of a primary disorder of spatial thinking in which the patient is unable to organize sensory information into a coherent spatial framework. Head (1920), for example, ascribed inaccurate point localization and position sense to the impairment of spatially organized "schemata" relating to the body surface and to posture. The other group insisted that failing performance was merely the result of more basic disorders in sensitivity such as raised or unstable sensory thresholds, disturbances in sensory processes over time, and fatigability, so that in fact the patient did not receive the sensory information required to localize accurately or discriminate between two stimulated points. The controversy is still not resolved.

However, all neurologists agreed that failure on these somatosensory spatial tasks was a sensitive indicator of the presence of brain disease and, specifically, of disease of the parietal lobes. The detailed investigation of sensory disturbances from cerebral lesions carried out by Head and Holmes (1911; Head, 1920; Holmes, 1927) showed this clearly and later work only confirmed their findings. The study of Shy and Haase (1957), in which 25 patients with verified focal lesions in the parietal lobe were given a battery of 12 sensory tests, found that four of the five most frequently encountered defects were of a spatial character, namely, impaired

position sense, inaccurate point localization, raised thresholds for two-point discrimination and inability to identify numerals drawn on the skin. The one non-spatial deficit in this set of five was a raised threshold for the perception of passive movement which, as Foerster (1901) had shown decades earlier, was closely correlated with tactile-spatial defects. In contrast, sensory thresholds for pressure, pain, and temperature were altered in relatively few patients and all of these showed one or more spatial deficits. Shy and Haase suggested that somatosensory deficits could be arranged in a hierarchical order in relation to overall severity of impairment, as shown in Table 10. They conceded, however, that there were cases whose pattern of deficits did not conform to the schema.

With respect to the neurological basis of these somatosensory deficits, clinical investigators such as Foerster (1901) and Head (1920) demonstrated that impairment could be produced by lesions at any level of the nervous system. Head and Sherren (1905), for example, found that defective two-point discrimination was closely associated with impaired sensitivity to tactile pressure in patients with peripheral nerve injuries and indeed was a remarkably persisting deficit that might be present after all other sensory capacities had returned to normal. Head and Thompson (1906) found that defective two-point discrimination was a frequent consequence of spinal cord disease but in this instance it could appear independently of any important disturbances of tactile sensitivity. Nevertheless, Head believed that lesions below the level of the cortex were more likely to result in basic sensory impairment (i.e., raised or unstable thresholds to light, pressure, pain, and temperature) than were cortical lesions, which primarily impaired the discriminative aspects of sensory experience.

Clinical study during the last two

Arthur Benton   Somesthesis & Cerebral Dominance

(Tactile, proprioceptive)   Somatosensory
                Somesthesis ?
- contralateral control sens, movement - but exceptions to the
generalization :

   1st to report : 1906   Oppenheim   - L. Parietal tumour
                                → impaired tactile sensitivity
                                   (astereognosis) R & L hands

    O - postulated L. Hem. dominant for higher level
         tactile cognitive performances <u>bilaterally</u>
         (as for language, praxis)

1914   Goldstein - similar case
1922   Foix   -   "
1925 - other 3a neurologists - a Left Handed patient - astereognosis

extra lemniscal system - ipsilateral input - may contribute to smallness of differences found in normals (compared to br. damaged)

2) 2 Pt Discrim   (Pa(ms)
3) Point Localization   (Pa(ms)
4) Threshold for Passive Movement (Mid Ring)

→ many cases bilateral impairment from unilateral lesions

Ss 1) Pressure — ipsilateral impairment
     2) 2 Pt — only contralateral

1. Bilateral sensory defect with unilateral lesions not rare,
2. The occurrence of bilateral impt. much more
   frequent in patients with L Hem disease

Semmes checked out: aph vs aphas.   contr-no-moro

R Hem - play activating impt role in mediating spatial attn
  - but underlying neurological mechanisms completely unknown
  - there is a mechanism in RHem : supra sensory for
                                    ; mediating spatial attn

maybe - because had to make 2 judgement
  ; made a simpler task
  → same results

RHem patients: 60% bilateral impairment

                                                RH
                                    ipsi   /
                                    contra   / LH

RHem disease - often bilateral impairment in
  ; judgement of direction , tactile realm

H: L Hand superior; perception of tactile stim   1.35 sec
  - looked at data ; no difference - but task too easy → 1 sec.   2.2 sec.
  then → difference ; college students
  ; small diff in fav. of L. Hand   17/2 y

 1 or 7 pts
 Normal   24   - R Hand   24   - Equal
 65

* using 30% criterion ;

Benton: Spatial Performances in Tactile Realm
would patient with R Hem disease show bil. impairment
< Hem disease '' contralateral

Corkin
- showed - <u>true</u> with complex task
- compared R & L Frontal Frontal-Temp) Temporal
(was a "Fr. lobe" perf.)
→ R Hem patients - worse deficits than L Hem

Hypothese - (any lesion - specific & general effect)

Z
(if unilesion → contralateral)
near ipsilateral

Benton: study : 2 or 3 probes dropped on palm
- showed [boxes] ① slope ② number
etc.

Ho - since #'s involved , L Hem lesion → bilateral impairment

Judgement of #('s) →

R Hem

L Hem

TPS   Contra

Judgement of Direction

R Hem

L Hem

← Judgement of Direction

Ipsi   Contra

# of errors would confirm lesion

IPSI   Contra

R Hem - bilaterally impaired on Judgement of direction

= quel
R Hand
☺5y

Hécaen - infl. of familial handedness
study: 6 groups R(R) R(LS) R(LP) NR(R) NR(LS) NR(LP)
Same task   74%

results:

degree of
L Hand
sup

47%   67%
         43%   48% R Handed
                  20% NR(R)
R   S   P

Famil Handedness Classification

study: feeling → stm. → identify an array
→ L Hand superiority; slightly stronger in men but
parametrically ✓ LH 14/24 sup.
            48% sup.   Both - 17/24
- majority didn't follow trend
due to kids; simplified — LH small diff sup.
- boys sim. / girls - less diff.

7/4/13 yr. gave to kids; simplified — LH small diff sup.
- boys sim. / girls - less diff.

LH
RH
7 yr   13 yr
   10 yr

A.D. press - 1 hr. - confirmed >R LHem

Corkin et al - couldn't confirm asymmetry
    but did confirm bilaterally

Wyke - Postural ArmDrift study →
some patients, Left Hem lesion showed bilateral weaving
          L Hem lesion

amt of
weaving
or Drift

R Hem lesion
Normals

LH   RH

Common(?)
- about same bilateral det either Hem
But - contralateral debris more freq. R Hem
Thus - L Hem disease showed relatively higher freq of
    ipsilateral defect

- simple sensory functions — bilateral innervation
- can more complex functions ⟷ gnosic defects
but - appeared even the elementary sens. funct → bilateral
      deficit
- most of these patient's ⁞
concluded — each side of body represented on both
      sides

        - anatomical evidence — ipsilateral proj. from
          each ear.

Head — never reported this, but was using patient's own control to
      test sensation on both side : can → considering
      same value as "normal" on side ipsilateral to lesion
      and "abnormal" on contralateral side (in different
      patients)
      - his analysis probably missed case

- most of these patient's — R Hand lesions
concluded — each side of body represented on both

(massive
  L Hans
  untestable)

1960 — Semmes, Weinstein, Ghent, Teuber (penetrating br. wounds)
      - large sample; controls
      - 4 performances :1) thresh. for light pressure (palms at hands)

Table 10. Levels of severity of defect in parietal lobe disease[a]

Level	Deficits
I	Impaired position sense
II	I plus slowed perception of passive movement (normal threshold)
III	II plus raised threshold for passive movement and defective point localization
IV	III plus raised two-point threshold and agraphesthesia
V	IV plus astereognosis, defective roughness discrimination and temperature sense
VI	V plus raised threshold for pressure and pain

[a] Adapted from Shy & Haase, 1957.

decades of the nineteenth century established that the cortical mechanisms mediating somatosensory responses were primarily located in the parietal lobe. However, the precentral gyrus, which today is usually designated as a motor area, was often included in the somatosensory region, the combined precentral and postcentral gyri constituting a sensorimotor region. Moreover, it was found that lesions in the posterior part of the parietal lobe, as well as in the postcentral gyrus, could produce various forms of impairment. Thus, Head (1920) concluded that "loss of sensation of the cortical type may be produced by a lesion of the pre- and post-central convolutions, the anterior part of the superior parietal lobule, and the angular gyri. These portions of the hemisphere contain the sensory centres [p. 759]." However, it was not possible to relate different forms of impairment to lesions in specific loci within this extended somatosensory cortical region.

It was understood that, in consonance with the facts of contralateral innervation, unilateral parietal disease would produce tactile impairment on the opposite side of the body. However, beginning in 1906 and extending through the 1930s, a number of clinicians reported instances of bilateral impairment in patients with apparently unilateral lesions. The earliest papers described bilateral defects in tactile object identification in association with unilateral lesions but later studies, such as those of Bychowsky and Eidinow (1934) and Koerner (1938), reported bilateral disturbances of sensitivity to pressure, pain, and vibration. Little attention was paid to these scattered papers until the publication of the large-scale study of Semmes, Weinstein, Ghent, and Teuber (1960) who demonstrated that bilateral impairment in pressure sensitivity, two-point discrimination, point localization, and the detection of passive movement was not a rare finding in patients with unilateral lesions. Subsequent studies generally confirmed their finding. A second observation that these bilateral defects were encountered with particularly high frequency in patients with left-hemisphere disease was not consistently supported. Subsequently, Carmon and Benton (1969) found bilateral impairment in the perception of the direction of punctate stimuli applied to the skin in patients with right-hemisphere disease but not in those with left-hemisphere lesions. They interpreted their findings as indicating that the right hemisphere plays a particularly important role in the mediation of behavior requiring the appreciation of spatial relations in the tactile as well as the visual modality. The significance of a supramodal spatial factor in the mediation of tactile form discrimination was emphasized in studies by Semmes (1965), De Renzi and Scotti (1969), and Dee and Benton (1970) which found a close relationship between defect on the tactile task and corresponding defect in visuospatial performances.

CONCLUDING COMMENTS

Disorders in spatial thinking associated with disease of the nervous system were recognized by clinicians as early as the 1880s. These disorders were typically studied within a single sensory modality. Vision was investigated in great detail and types of visuospatial disorder were formulated by Kleist, Brain, and other neurologists. The occurrence of specific disorders, which were often defined in terms of level (e.g., sensory, integrative, mnesic), was then related to the locus and extent of the causative lesion. Spatial deficits in the somatosensory modality, such as inaccurate tactile localization and impaired position sense, were also investigated, mainly in relation to their value in diagnosis but also as a vehicle for studying integrative processes in the central nervous system. In contrast, the spatial aspects of audition received relatively little attention. The concept that brain disease can produce a generalized impairment in spatial thinking that affects performance in all sensory modalities was advanced. Over the decades there was a slow accumulation of evidence pointing to the paramount importance of the right hemisphere in mediating spatial performances.

The exact nature of the interrelations among the diverse performance deficits that are regarded as indicative of "spatial disorientation" remains to be determined. Clinical observation attests that patients may show dissociated deficits, that is, failure on one spatial task but not the other. For example, although perceptuomotor spatial disability, as reflected in failing visuoconstructional performance, is usually associated with visuoperceptual spatial disability, as reflected in failing performance on discrimination tasks, some patients show one type of deficit but not the other (Costa & Vaughan, 1962; Dee, 1970). There is also evidence that the neuropathological bases for distinctive types of disabilities may differ. Defective three-dimensional block construction, a perceptuomotor spatial disability, is shown by a substantial proportion of aphasic patients with left-hemisphere disease but impaired appreciation of the direction of lines, a visuoperceptual-spatial disability, is not characteristic of these patients (Benton, 1973; Benton, Hannay & Varney, 1975; Benton, Varney & Hamsher, 1978). Moreover, despite theorizing about the dependence of orientation in external space on the integrity of the body schema, clinical observation discloses numerous instances of dissociated impairment, as documented in the section on disturbances of the body schema in our discussion.

The intriguing concept of a supramodal spatial disability deserves further exploration. An association of visuospatial (and visuoconstructive) performance deficits with tactile-spatial deficits has been described by a number of investigators (Corkin, 1965; Dee & Benton, 1970; De Renzi & Scotti, 1969; Milner, 1965). It seems likely that the basis for the relationship is that in sighted persons all spatial performances—visual, auditory, somesthetic—take place within a visually organized spatial matrix. However, the observed occurrence of dissociated visual and tactile spatial deficits raises the question of whether the determining factors may not be neuropathological rather than behavioral in nature.

REFERENCES

Ajuriaguerra, J. de, & Hécaen, H. *Le cortex cérébral*. Paris: Masson et Cie, 1949.

Arrigoni, G., & De Renzi, E. Constructional apraxia and hemispheric locus of lesion. *Cortex*, 1964, *1*, 170–197.

Badal, J. Contribution à l'étude des cécités psychiques: Alexie, agraphie, hémianopsie inférieure, trouble du sens de l'espace. *Archives d'Ophtalmologie*, 1888, *8*, 97–117.

Balint, R. Seelenlähmung des Schauens, optische Ataxie, räumliche Störung der Aufmerksamkeit. *Monatsschrift für Psychiatrie und Neurologie*, 1909, *25*, 51–81.

Benton, A. L. *Right-left discrimination and finger localization: Development and pathology.* New York: Hoeber-Harper, 1959.

Benton, A. L. The visual retention test as a constructional praxis task. *Confinia Neurologica*, 1962, *22*, 141–155.

Benton, A. L. Constructional apraxia and the minor hemisphere. *Confinia Neurologica*, 1967, *29*, 1–16.

Benton, A. L. Disorders of spatial orientation. In P. L. Vinken & G. W. Bruyn (Eds.), *Handbook of clinical neurology* (Vol. 3, Ch. 13), Amsterdam: North-Holland, 1969.

Benton, A. L. Visuoconstructive disability in patients with cerebral disease: Its relationship to side of lesion and aphasic disorder. *Documenta Opthalmologica*, 1973, *34*, 67–76.

Benton, A. L., & Fogel, M. L. Threedimensional constructional praxis. *Archives of Neurology*, 1962, *7*, 347–354.

Benton, A. L., Hannay, H. J., & Varney, N. R. Visual perception of line direction in patients with unilateral brain disease. *Neurology*, 1975, *25*, 907–910.

Benton, A. L., & Meyers, R. An early description of the Gerstmann syndrome. *Neurology*, 1956, *6*, 838–842.

Benton, A. L., Varney, N. R., & Hamsher, K. Visuospatial judgment: A clinical test. *Archives of Neurology*, 1978, *35*, 364–367.

Birkmayer, W. *Hirnverletzungen Mechanismus, Spätkomplikationen, Funktionswandel*, Wien: Springer-Verlag, 1951.

Boring, B. G. The two-point limen and the error of localization. *American Journal of Psychology*, 1930, *42*, 446–449.

Brain, W. R. Visual disorientation with special reference to lesions of the right cerebral hemisphere. *Brain*, 1941, *64*, 244–272.

Bychowsky, G., & Eidinow, M. Doppelsei-

tige Sensibilitätstörungen bei einseitigen Gehirnherden. *Nervenarzt.*, 1934, *7*, 498–506.

Carmon, A., & Benton, A. L. Tactile perception of direction and number in patients with unilateral cerebral disease. *Neurology*, 1969, *19*, 525–532.

Corkin, S. Tactually-guided maze learning in man: Effects of unilateral cortical excisions and bilateral hippocampal lesions. *Neuropsychologia*, 1965, *3*, 339–351.

Costa, L. D., & Vaughan, H. G. Performances of patients with lateralized cerebral lesions: Verbal and perceptual tests. *Journal of Nervous and Mental Disease*, 1962, *134*, 162–168.

Critchley, M. *The parietal lobes*. London: Edward Arnold, 1953.

Damasio, A. R. & Benton, A. L. Impairment of hand movements under visual guidance. *Neurology*, 1979, *29*, 170–178.

Dee, H. L. Visuoconstructive and visuoperceptive deficit in patients with unilateral cerebral lesions. *Neuropsychologia*, 1970, *8*, 305–314.

Dee, H. L. & Benton, A. L. A cross-modal investigation of spatial performances in patients with unilateral cerebral disease. *Cortex*, 1970, *6*, 261–272.

De Renzi, E., & Scotti, G. The influence of spatial disorders in impairing tactual discrimination of shapes. *Cortex*, 1969, *5*, 53–62.

Dide, M. Les désorientations temporospatials et la préponderance de l'hémisphere droit dans les agnoso-akinésies proprioceptives. *Encéphale*, 1938, *33*, 276–294.

Duensing, F. Raumagnostische und ideatorisch-apraktische Störung des gestaltenden Handelns. *Deutsche Zeitschrift für Nervenheilkunde*, 1953, *170*, 72–94.

Dunn, T. D. Double hemiplegia with double hemianopsia and loss of geographic centre. *Transactions, College of Physicians of Philadelphia*, 1895, *17*, 45–56.

Foerster, O. Untersuchungen über das Localisationsvermögen bei Sensibilitätsstörungen: Ein Beitrag zur Psychophysiologie der Raumvorstellung. *Monatsschrift für Psychiatrie und Neurologie*, 1901, *9*, 31–42.

Foerster, R. Über Rindenblindheit. *Graefes Archiv für Ophthalmologie*. 1890, *36*, 94–108.

Gerstmann, J. Fingeragnosie: Eine umschriebene Störung der Orientierung am eigenen Körper. *Wiener Klinische Wochenschrift*, 1924, *37*, 1010–1012.

Gerstmann, J. Fingeragnosie und isolierte Agraphie: ein neues Syndrom. *Zeitschrift für die gesamte Neurologie und Psychiatrie*, 1927, *108*, 152–177.

Geschwind, N. Disconnexion syndromes in animals and man. *Brain*, 1965, *88*, 237–294; 585–644.

Head, H. *Studies in neurology*. London: Oxford University Press, 1920.

Head, H. *Aphasia and kindred disorders of speech*. Cambridge: The University Press. 1926.

Head, H., & Holmes, G. Sensory disturbances from cerebral lesions. *Brain*. 1911, *34*, 102–254.

Head, H., & Sherren, J. The consequences of injury to the peripheral nerves in man. *Brain*, 1905, *28*, 116–338.

Head, H., & Thompson, T. The grouping of afferent impulses within the spinal cord. *Brain*, 1906, *29*, 537–741.

Hécaen, H., Ajuriaguerra, J. de, & Massonet, J. Les troubles visuoconstructifs par lésion pariéto-occipitale droite. *Encéphale*, 1951, *40*, 122–179.

Holmes, G. Disturbances of visual orientation. *British Journal of Ophthalmology*, 1918, *2*, 449–468; 506–516.

Holmes, G. Disorders of sensation produced by cortical lesions. *Brain*, 1927, *50*, 413–427.

Holmes, G., & Horrax, G. Disturbances of spatial orientation and visual inattention, with loss of stereoscopic vision. *Archives of Neurology and Psychiatry*, 1919, *1*, 385–407.

Jackson, J. H. Clinical remarks on defects of expression (by words, writing, signs, etc.) in diseases of the nervous system. *Lancet*, 1864, *1*, 604–605.

Jackson, J. H. On the nature of the duality of the brain. *Medical Press and Circular*, 1874, *17*, 19. (Reprinted in *Brain*, 1915, *38*, 80–103.)

Jackson, J. H. Case of large cerebral tumour without optic neuritis and with left hemiplegia and imperception. *Royal London Ophthalmic Hospital Reports*, 1876, *8*, 434–444.

Kleist, K. Der Gang und der gegenwärtige Stand der Apraxieforschung. *Ergebnisse der Neurologie und Psychiatrie*, 1912, *1*, 342–452.

Kleist, K. Kriegsverletzungen des Gehirns in ihrer Bedeutung für die Hirnlokalisation und Hirnpathologie. In O. von Schjerning (Ed.), *Handbuch der Ärztlichen Erfahrung im Weltkriege*, Bd. 4. Leipzig: Barth, 1922/1934.

Koerner, S. C. Die Beeinflussbarkeit der Sensibilität an symmetrischen Hautgebieten bei einseitiger Hirnschädigung und bei Gesunden. *Deutsche Zeitschrift für Nervenheilkunde*, 1938, *145*, 116–130.

Kroll, M. *Die neurologischen Symptomenkomplexe*. Berlin: Springer, 1929.

Kroll, M., & Stollbun, D. Was ist konstruktive Apraxie? *Zeitschrift für die gesamte Neurologie und Psychiatrie*, 1933, *148*, 142–158.

Lange, J. Fingeragnosie und Agraphie. *Monatsschrift für Psychiatrie und Neurologie*. 1930, *76*, 129–188.

Lange, J. Probleme der Fingeragnosie. *Zeitschrift für die gesamte Neurologie und Psychiatrie*, 1933, *147*, 594–620.

Lange, J. Agnosien und Apraxien. In O. Bumke & O. Foerster (Eds.), *Handbuch der Neurologie*. Bd. 6. Berlin: Springer-Verlag, 1936.

Lenz, G. *Beiträge zur Hemianopsie*. Stuttgart, 1905.

Lissauer, H. Ein Fall von Seelenblindheit nebst einem Beitrag zur Theorie derselben. *Archiv für Psychiatrie und Nervenkrankheiten*, 1890, *21*, 222–270.

McFie, J., Piercy, M. F., & Zangwill, O. L. Visual–spatial agnosia associated with lesions of the right cerebral hemisphere. *Brain*, 1950, *73*, 167–190.

McFie, J., & Zangwill, O. Visual–constructive disabilities associated with lesions of the left cerebral hemisphere. *Brain*, 1960, *83*, 243–260.

Meyer, O. Ein- und doppelseitige homonyme Hemianopsie mit Orientierungstörungen. *Monatsschrift für Psychiatrie und Neurologie*. 1900, *8*, 440–456.

Milner, B. Visually guided maze learning

in man: Effects of bilateral hippocampal, bilateral frontal, and unilateral cerebral lesions. *Neuropsychologia*, 1965, *3*, 317–338.

Munk, H. Weitere Mittheilungen zur Physiologie der Grosshirnrinde. *Archiv für Anatomie und Physiologie*. 1878, 2, 162–178.

Paterson, A., & Zangwill, O. L. Disorders of visual space perception associated with lesions of the right cerebral hemisphere. *Brain*, 1944, *67*, 331–358.

Penfield, W., & Evans, J. P. Functional defects produced by cerebral lobectomies. *Research Publications, Association for Research in Nervous and Mental Disease*, 1934, *13*, 352–377.

Peters, A. Über die Beziehungen zwischen Orientierungsstörungen und ein- und doppelseitiger Hemianopsie. *Archiv für Augenheilkunde*, 1896, *32*, 175–187.

Piercy, M. F., Hécaen, H., & Ajuriaguerra, J. de. Constructional apraxia associated with unilateral cerebral lesions—left and right sided cases compared. *Brain*, 1960, *83*, 225–242.

Piercy, M. F. & Smyth, V. Right hemisphere dominance for certain nonverbal intellectual skills. *Brain*, 1962, *85*, 775–790.

Pineas, H. Ein Fall von räumliche Orientierungsstörung mit Dyschirie. *Zeitschrift für die gesamte Neurologie und Psychiatrie*. 1931, *133*, 180–195.

Poppelreuter, W. *Die psychischen Schädigungen durch Kopfschuss im Kriege 1914–1916 Die Störungen der niederen und höheren Sehleistungen durch Verletzungen des Okzipitalhirns*. Leipzig Voss, 1917.

Reichardt, M. *Allgemeine und spezielle Psychiatrie: ein Lehrbuch fuer Studierende und Ärzte*. II Aufl. Jena, Germany: G. Fischer, 1918.

Riddoch, G. Dissociation of visual perceptions due to occipital injuries, with special reference to appreciation of movement. *Brain*, 1917, *40*, 15–57.

Riddoch, G. Visual disorientation in homonymous half-fields. *Brain*, 1935, *58*, 376–382.

Rieger, C. Über Apparate in dem Hirn. *Arbeiten aus der Psychiatrischen Klinik Würzburg*, 1909, *5*, 176–197.

Ross, H. E., & Murray, D. J. Introduction.

In E. H. Weber. *The sense of touch*. London: Academic Press, 1978.

Ross, S. J., & Fountain, G. Phenomenon of cutaneous sensory extinction. *Archives of Neurology and Psychiatry*, 1948, *59*, 107–113.

Russell, W. R., & Espir, M. L. E. *Traumatic aphasia*, London: Oxford University Press, 1961.

Sachs, H. Das Gehirn des Foerster'schen Rindenblinden. *Arbeiten aus der Psychiatrischen und Nervenklinik Breslau*, 1895, 2, 55–122.

Sanchez-Longo, L. P., & Forster, F. M. Clinical significance of impairment of sound localization. *Neurology*, 1958, *8*, 119–125.

Sanchez-Longo, L. P., Forster, F., & Auth, T. L. A clinical test for sound localization and its applications. *Neurology*, 1957, *7*, 655–663.

Schlesinger, B. Zur Auffassung der optischen und konstruktiven Apraxic. *Zeitschrift für die gesamte Neurologie und Psychiatrie*, 1928, *117*, 649–697.

Semmes, J. A non-tactual factor in stereognosis. *Neuropsychologia*, 1965, *3*, 295–315.

Semmes, J., Weinstein, S., Ghent, L., & Teuber, H. L. *Somatosensory changes after penetrating brain wounds in man*. Cambridge: Harvard University Press. 1960.

Shankweiler, D. Performance of brain-damaged patients on two tests of sound localization. *Journal of Comparative and Physiological Psychology*, 1961, *54*, 375–381.

Shy, G. M., & Haase, G. R. Sensorische Störungen bei Scheitellappenläsionen. *Deutsche Zeitschrift für Nervenheilkunde*, 1957, *176*, 519–542.

Stengel, E. Loss of spatial orientation, constructional apraxia and Gerstmann's syndrome. *Journal of Mental Science*, 1944, *90*, 753–760.

Strauss, H. Über konstruktive Apraxie. *Monatsschrift für Psychiatrie und Neurologie*. 1924, *63*, 739–748.

Teuber, H. L. Effects of brain wounds implicating right or left hemisphere in man: Hemisphere differences and hemisphere interaction in vision, audition and somesthesis. In V. B. Mountcastle (Ed.), *Interhemispheric relations and cerebral dominance*. Baltimore: Johns Hopkins Press, 1962.

Teuber, H. L. The riddle of frontal lobe function in man. In J. M. Warren & K. Akert (Eds.), *The frontal granular cortex and behavior*. New York: McGraw-Hill, 1964.

Teuber, H. L. Battersby, W., & Bender, M. B. Changes in visual searching performance following cerebral lesions. *American Journal of Physiology*, 1949, *159*, 592.

Walsh, E. G. An investigation of sound localization in patients with neurological abnormalities. *Brain*, 1957, *80*, 222–250.

Warrington, E. K., James, M., & Kinsbourne, M. Drawing disability in relation to laterality of cerebral lesion. *Brain*, 1966, *89*, 53–82.

Weber, E. H. *The sense of touch*: *De tactu*, translated by H. E. Ross: *Der Tastsinn* translated by D. J. Murray. London: Academic Press, 1978.

Wilbrand, H. *Die Seelenblindheit als Herderscheinung und ihre Beziehungen zur homonymen Hemianopsie*, Wiesbaden: J. F. Bergmann, 1887.

Wortis, S. B., & Pfeffer, A. Z. Unilateral auditory–spatial agnosia. *Journal of Nervous and Mental Disease*, 1948, *108*, 181–186.

Zangwill, O. L. *Cerebral dominance and its relation to psychological function*. Edinburgh: Oliver & Boyd, 1960.

V.
Reaction Time and Brain Disease

15.

Reaction Time in Unilateral Cerebral Disease*

Non-psychotic patients with cerebral disease show slower and more variable simple and choice reaction times than control patients who are comparable in age and educational level [1, 2]. These and similar findings have been interpreted as indicating that a fundamental cerebral function in man is to provide the necessary neural arrangements for the performance of simple high-speed tasks and that injury to any part of the brain will result in impairment in such performance [2, 3].

The purpose of the present study was to determine whether lesions localized within a single cerebral hemisphere would show differential effects on reaction time. In consonance with the idea that overall cerebral integrity is a necessary precondition for normal reaction time, it was predicted that patients with unilateral lesions would show retardation in simple reactions involving the side which is ipsilateral, as well as contralateral, to the side of the lesion. However, the possibility of a

supplementary focal cerebral effect was also investigated by comparing reaction times on the ipsilateral and contralateral sides in patients with unilateral cerebral lesions.

The following hypotheses were set up for test:

1. Patients with lesions of the right hemisphere would be slower than control patients in a simple reaction involving the right hand.

2. Patients with lesions of the right hemisphere would be faster than patients with lesions of the left hemisphere in a simple reaction involving the right hand.

3. In a choice reaction task, control patients would not show a difference in speed of reaction between the right hand and the left hand.

4. In a choice reaction task, patients with lesions of the right hemisphere would be faster in reactions involving the right hand than in those involving the left hand.

5. In a choice reaction task, patients with lesions of the left hemisphere would

* A. L. Benton and R. J. Joynt, *Confinia Neurologica*, 1959, 19, 247–256. By permission of S. Karger AG, Basel, Switzerland.

be slower in ractions involving the right hand than in those involving the left hand.

6. In a choice reaction task, the pattern of right hand-left hand performance in patients with lesions of the right hemisphere would differ from the pattern in patients with lesions of the left hemisphere.

METHOD

Subjects

Two groups of 20 patients each, one with lesions apparently restricted to the right cerebral hemisphere, the other with lesions apparently restricted to the left cerebral hemisphere, were formed on the basis of random selection. A variety of criteria (operation, autopsy, angiography, pneumoencephalography, clinical findings) had been utilized by the attending neurologists in making the judgment of unilateral cerebral disease in the patients, who were on the neurological and neurosurgical services of the University Hospital and Veterans Administration Hospital, Iowa City. The most frequent diagnosis were neoplasm and cerebrovascular disease. In the right hemisphere group, the lesion was localized in the frontal lobe in 6 cases, in a post-rolandic area in 8 cases, and involved both frontal and post-rolandic areas in 6 cases. In the left hemisphere group, the lesion was localized in the frontal lobe in 6 case, in a post-rolandic area in 7 cases, and involved both frontal and post-rolandic areas in 7 cases.

Although some patients had shown motor deficits at some time during the course of their illness, *at the time of testing, all had normal use of the upper extremities and sufficient vision to see both test lights at once, as judged by the usual clinical criteria (e.g., strength of grip, alternating motion rate).*

In addition, a control group of 20 patients on the neurological, neurosurgical, and medical services, who showed no evidence or history of cerebral disease, head trauma or epilepsy, was formed on the basis of random selection. Spinal cord disease was the most frequent diagnosis in this group.

No patient who was acutely ill, whose behavior raised the question of psychosis, who had a history of hospitalization for a psychiatric disorder or whose history suggested a mental defect state dating back to childhood was included in the groups. The mean age of the right hemisphere group (19 men, 1 woman) was 33.8 years ($SD = 11.1$) and mean educational level was 10.4 years ($SD = 2.5$). The mean age of the left hemisphere group (12 men, 8 women) was 39.9 years ($SD = 12.4$) and mean educational level was 10.1 years ($SD = 3.3$). The mean age of the control group (14 men, 6 women) was 36.7 years ($SD = 14.3$) and mean educational level was 10.1 years ($SD = 2.1$). As estimated by t and F tests, there were no significant differences among the groups with respect to mean age or education level or variance in these characteristics.

Procedure

The reaction time apparatus which was employed provided for the presentation of a light stimulus which was preceded by a buzz of 2 sec. duration, the latter stimulus serving as a "ready" signal. Two lights, that were mounted seven in. apart on the right and left sides of an upright panel which faced the patient, were connected respectively to microswitches attached to the right and left sides of the base of the apparatus.

In the simple reaction time task, the patient, having seated himself comfortably at the table, was instructed to rest the index finger of his right hand lightly on the right microswitch and to press the switch as soon as the right light appeared. The function of the buzz as a "ready" signal was explained to him. Five practice trials were given to acquaint the patient with the task. Thirty test trials then followed.

In the choice reaction time task, the patient was instructed to rest the index fingers of his right and left hands on the right and left microswitches and to press the appropriate switch when the right or left light appeared. As in the simple reaction time task, the light stimulus was preceded by a warning signal (buzz) of 2 sec. duration. The patient was warned not to press both keys at the same time. Lights on the investigator's side of the apparatus indicated the key which was pressed so that double pressing could be noted. Five practice trials were followed by 30 experimental trials, consisting of 15 stimulations on the right side and 15 stimulations on the left side presented in pre-determined random order.

The simple reaction time task was given first and was followed, after a rest period of 2–3 min., by the choice reaction time task. The reaction times were shown in .01 sec. units by an electrically driven clock which was activated by the onset of the light stimulus and stopped by the depression of the corresponding microswitch.

The times in .01 sec. for the 30 simple reactions, the 15 right hand choice trials and the 15 left hand choice trials were separately summed and averaged to the nearest .001 sec. for each patient. Because of skewness of some of the distributions of these mean scores, they were transformed to speed scores by taking the reciprocal of each patient's mean score in .01 sec. units and multiplying it by 1000. This transformation resulted in distributions of speed scores which were essen-

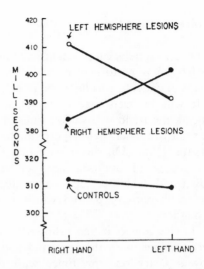

Fig. 6. Choice reaction times for right and left hands in control and brain-damaged patients.

tially normal and which were thus appropriate for statistical analysis.

RESULTS

Simple reaction time (right hand)

Mean simple reaction time in the control patients was 208 msec. ($SD = 37$ msec.). Mean simple reaction time in the patients with lesions of the right hemisphere was 275 msec. ($SD = 82$ msec.) and that in the patients with lesions of the left hemisphere was 308 msec. ($SD = 95$ msec.). The difference (67 msec.) between the mean scores of the control patients and the patients with lesions of the right hemisphere was significant ($p < .001$), as estimated by the t test applied to the speed scores. The difference (100 msec.) between the mean scores of the control patients and the patients with lesions of the left hemisphere was similarly significant ($p < .001$). The difference (33 msec.) between the mean scores of the patients with lesions of the right hemisphere and patients with lesions of the left hemisphere was nonsignificant but in the predicted direction.

Choice reaction time

The relations between the right hand and the left hand performance in the three groups of patients are illustrated in Figure 6. It will be seen that in the control patients the trend of reaction time from the right to the left hand approximates a horizontal line. On the other hand, the two groups of brain-damaged patients show trends which are opposite in direction, as hypothesized, and which cross each other.

Twelve control patients showed faster reaction times with the left hand and 8 showed faster reaction times with the right hand. Six patients with lesions of the right hemisphere showed faster reaction times with the left hand, 13 showed faster reaction times with the right hand and, in 1 patient, reaction time was equal in both hands. Sixteen patients with lesions of the left hemisphere showed faster reaction times with the left hand while 4 showed faster reaction times with the right hand. The difference (30 per cent vs. 80 per cent) in the proportions of patients in the two brain-damaged groups who showed faster reaction times with the left hand was found to be significant $(p < .05)$.

In the control patients, mean choice reaction time was 312 msec. for the right hand and 309 msec. for the left hand, the slight difference in means obviously being nonsignificant. In the patients with lesions of the right hemisphere, mean choice reaction time was 384 msec. for the right hand and 401 msec. for the left hand. The difference between the means was significant $(p < .05)$, as estimated by the t test for related measures applied to the speed scores. In the patients with lesions of the left hemisphere, mean choice reaction time was 411 msec. for the right hand and 391 msec. for the left hand. However, the difference between the means, which was in the predicted direction, did not attain an adequate level of significance $(p < .10)$.

The difference between the differences in the reaction times of the right and left hands in the two groups of brain-damaged patients was investigated to determine whether a significant difference in pattern of performance existed. In the group with lesions of the right hemisphere, the right hand reactions were faster than the left hand reactions by 17 msec.; in the group with lesions of the left hemisphere, the right hand reactions were slower than the left hand reactions by 20 msec. Hence there was a difference of 37 msec. between these mean differences in the two groups. This difference was significant $(p < .02)$, as estimated by the t test applied to the differences in the speed scores.

Influence of intra-hemispheric location of lesion

The pattern of choice reaction times in the right and left hands was examined with particular reference to the location of the lesions within each hemisphere. For the purposes of this analysis, the cases in each group were divided into post-rolandic subgroups (8 cases in the right hemisphere group, 7 cases in the left hemisphere group) and subgroups in which the lesion compromised the frontal lobe, either alone or with concurrent involvement of a post-rolandic area (12 cases in the right hemisphere group, 13 cases in the left hemisphere group).

The findings are presented in Table 11, which shows the right hand and left hand choice reaction times in each subgroup. It will be seen that the post-rolandic subgroups show the same trends that were found in the total groups, i.e., trends which are opposite in direction and which cross each other. The cases in which the lesion involved the frontal lobe, either alone or in combination with post-rolandic areas, appear to present a somewhat different picture. The left hemisphere subgroups show the hypothesized trend in that the right hand reactions are slower than those of the left hand by 22 msec. On the other hand, the trend of the right hemisphere subgroup, while in the predicted direction, is almost horizontal. These findings were somewhat unexpected. One might have predicted that the frontal cases would show the hypothesized opposition in trends more clearly than the post-rolandic cases on the ground that in the frontal cases there would be a greater possibility of encroachment on the motor areas.

Table 11. Mean choice reaction times (milliseconds) in different subgroups

Post-rolandic lesions		
	Left hand	*Right hand*
Left hemisphere	402	417
Right hemisphere	410	377
Frontal lesions		
	Left hand	*Right hand*
Left hemisphere	385	407
Right hemisphere	394	389

No statistical evaluation of these data was attempted because of the small number of cases in each subgroup. The findings must be regarded as inconclusive and further exploration of the possibility of a differential influence of lesions in different parts of the hemisphere is indicated.

Summary of findings

1. The hypothesis that patients with lesions of the right hemisphere would be slower than control patients in a simple reaction involving the right hand was confirmed.

2. The hypothesis that patients with lesions of the right hemisphere would be faster than patients with lesions of the left hemisphere in a simple reaction involving the right hand was not confirmed, although the observed difference was in the predicted direction.

3. The hypothesis that control patients would show no difference in speed between the right hand and the left hand in a choice reaction task was confirmed.

4. The hypothesis that patients with lesions of the right hemisphere would be faster in reactions involving the right hand than in those involving the left hand in a choice reaction task was confirmed.

5. The hypothesis that patients with lesions of the left hemisphere would be slower in reactions involving the right hand than in those involving the left hand in a choice reaction task was not confirmed, although the observed difference was in the predicted direction.

6. The hypothesis that the pattern of performance in a choice reaction task of patients with lesions of the right cerebral hemisphere would differ from the pattern shown by patients with lesions of the left cerebral hemisphere was confirmed.

DISCUSSION

The finding that patients with cerebral lesions confined to a single hemisphere show retardation in the speed of reactions involving the ipsilateral, as well as the contralateral, hand supports the conception that simple reaction time reflects overall cerebral status. Apparently these focal lesions impair a general organismic capacity ("vigilance," "maintenance of set," "readiness to react") which is an important determinant of the quality of simple high-speed performances.

However, within this setting of a general effect leading to retardation in reactions involving both the contralateral and ipsilateral sides, a specific effect which is related to the locus of the lesion is also discernible. Patients with cerebral lesions restricted to one hemisphere and with no apparent motor deficits on the side contralateral to that of the lesion tend to show a more marked retardation in the reactions of the contralateral hand as compared with that shown by the ipsilateral hand. This specific effect is suggested by intra-individual comparisons of right and left hand performances in patients with lesions of one or the other cerebral hemisphere and is shown most clearly when the two types of patients are compared on an inter-individual basis with respect to the pattern of performance shown by the right and left hands.

Judging from the relative size of the differences among the several groups and the levels of confidence associated with these differences, the general bilateral effect of a focal lesion on reaction time is clearly the major one. The specific unilateral effect is of secondary importance. Nevertheless the fact that such a specific effect is demonstrable in patients without clinically apparent motor deficits is worthy of note and conceivably could be of some clinical significance.

SUMMARY

The purpose of this study was to investigate the effects of lesions localized within a single cerebral hemisphere on reaction time in brain-damaged patients. The subjects were: (1) brain-damaged patients with lesions apparently restricted to the right cerebral hemisphere; (2) brain-damaged patients with lesions apparently restricted to the left cerebral hemisphere; (3) patients without known brain damage.

All patients had normal use of the upper extremities, as judged by the usual clinical criteria.

It was found that the brain-damaged patients were significantly slower than the control patients in a simple reaction time task involving the hand which was ipsilateral, as well as contralateral, to the side of the lesion. Control patients showed approximately equal reaction times in both hands in a choice reaction task. Patients with lesions of the right hemisphere showed significantly faster reactions with the right hand than with the left hand. Patients with lesions of the left hemisphere showed slower reactions with the right hand than with the left hand but the observed difference failed to attain statistical significance. There was a significant difference in the patterns of right hand–left hand performance in the two groups of brain-damaged patients.

The findings are interpreted as indicating that focal lesions have both a general bilateral and a specific unilateral effect on reaction time in patients without clinically apparent motor deficits.

REFERENCES

1. Benton, A. L. & Blackburn, H. L.: Practice effects in reaction-time tasks in brain-injured patients. J. abnorm. soc. Psychol. 54: 109–113 (1957).

2. Blackburn, H. L. & Benton, A. L.: Simple and choice reaction time in cerebral disease. Confin. neurol. 15: 327–338 (1955).

3. Smith, K. U.: Bilateral integrative action of the cerebral cortex in man in verbal association and sensori-motor coordination. J. exp. Psychol. 37: 367–376 (1947).

16.

The Crossmodal Retardation in Reaction Time of Patients with Cerebral Disease*

The question with which this investigation was concerned is whether, under a condition of serial presentation of stimuli, brain-damaged patients would show changes in simple reaction time as a function of changes in the stimulus and, if so, whether these changes differ from those shown by individuals without cerebral damage. The impetus for the study was provided by the results of similar investigations by Sutton et al. (6, 7) who found that schizophrenic patients showed a retardation in reaction time to auditory stimuli which had been preceded by a visual stimulus, as compared to their reaction time to auditory stimuli which had been preceded either by an identical or by a different auditory stimulus. Normal subjects also showed this "crossmodal" retardation in auditory reaction time, but its size was significantly greater in schizophrenic patients. The same trend toward a greater retardation in reaction

* A. L. Benton, S. Sutton, J. A. Kennedy, and J. R. Brokaw, *Journal of Nervous and Mental Disease*, 1962, 135, 413–418. Copyright 1962, Williams & Wilkins. Reproduced by permission.

time to visual stimuli preceded by auditory stimuli in schizophrenic patients as compared with normal subjects was also observed, but the differences between the two groups were not statistically significant.

The significance of this type of study and the procedure it employs is that is seems to provide a measure on a basic sensorimotor level of the behavioral capacity which has been called "capacity to shift set," "ability to respond appropriately to disparate environmental events," "behavioral flexibility," and the like. A deficit in this capacity (very often designated as "rigidity") has been postulated to be a determinant of the behavior of brain-damaged patients, mental defectives, schizophrenics, some types of neurotics and some types of normal individuals. Mettler (4) has reported that animals with experimentally produced lesions of the "striatum" (i.e., caudate nucleus and putamen) show a characteristic incapacity to react appropriately to changing environmental events. He has likened this behavioral deficit to that observed in schizophrenic patients and has suggested the possibility that the disease involves "striatal" dysfunction. In view of both Mettler's theoretical position and the positive results of the comparison of schizophrenic and normal subjects by Sutton et al. with respect to crossmodal retardation effects in reaction time, an extension of this type of study to the performances of patients with cerebral disease seemed indicated.

An attempt was made in the present investigation to determine whether brain-damaged patients would also show an excessive susceptibility to the crossmodal retardation effect. In addition, attention was directed to the questions of whether the effect was more pronounced in the auditory than in the visual modality and whether there were differences in performance between patients with diffuse lesions and those with focal lesions.

METHOD

The general procedure followed that of Sutton et al. The patient was seated before the reaction time apparatus with his right index finger resting lightly on the reaction key. He was familiarized with the four stimuli to be presented (red light, green light, 1000 cps tone, 400 cps tone) and instructed to press the key as quickly as possible when any of the four stimuli was presented. No warning stimulus was given.

The apparatus provided for the programming of the stimuli so that an equal number of each of several types of stimulus sequence was presented, viz. (I) 32 trials in which the stimulus was identical with the preceding stimulus, e.g., red light preceded by red light; (II) 32 trials in which the stimulus was preceded by a different stimulus in the same modality, e.g., red light preceded by green light; (III) 64 trials in which a stimulus was preceded by

a stimulus in a different modality, e.g., light preceded by tone (32 trials) or tone preceded by light (32 trials). Four successive blocks of 32 trials each were programed so that each of 16 possible sequence pairs classifiable into the three categories occurred twice within each block, thus equalizing positive and negative practice effects. The intertrial interval (controlled by a random noise generator) was two to four seconds. The stimuli were response-terminated and reaction time was recorded in milliseconds (msec) on an electronic counter. Since the program of stimulation was random within the constraint of presenting a certain number of each type of stimulus sequence, it was essentially unpredictable to the subject. The program is illustrated in Figure 7.

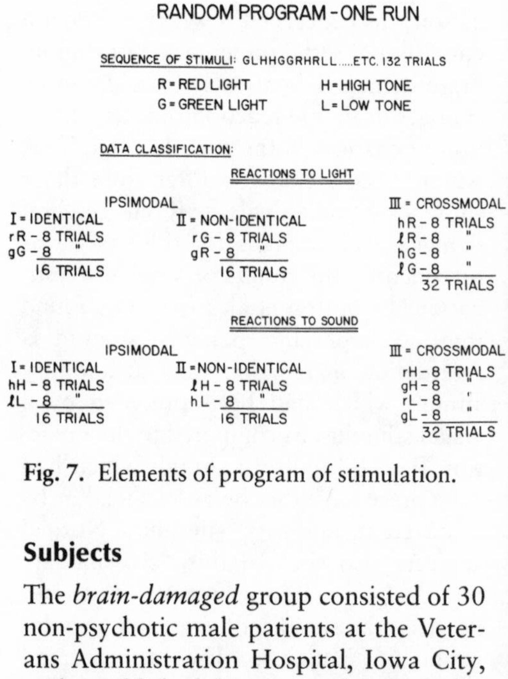

Fig. 7. Elements of program of stimulation.

Subjects

The *brain-damaged* group consisted of 30 non-psychotic male patients at the Veterans Administration Hospital, Iowa City, with established diagnoses of organic disease involving the cerebral hemispheres. Thirteen patients had focal disease in the sense that the identified lesion occupied a part of one hemisphere, while the other 17 patients had diffuse or bilateral disease. A variety of diagnoses was represented in the group, the most frequent being diffuse degenerative disease, neoplasm and cerebrovascular disease. Mean age of the group was 43.1 years (range: 25–62) and mean educational level was 10.3 years (range: 4–16). Age and educational level were not significantly related ($r = -.12$).

The *control* group consisted of 30 non-psychotic male patients at the same hospital who showed no evidence or history of cerebral disease, head trauma or epilepsy, and were hospitalized for a variety of disorders, the most frequent diagnosis being herniated intervertebral disc. Mean age of the group was 42.3 years (range: 26–62) and mean educational level was 10.1 years (range: 5–16). Age and educational level were not significantly related ($r = -.22$).

RESULTS

The median reaction time of each patient for each of the three classes of stimuli (i.e., identical—I, ipsimodal non-identical—II or crossmodal—III) was computed separately for reactions to light and sound stimuli. All the analyses to be reported were based on these individual median reaction time scores.

Overall reaction times

The means and standard deviations of the median scores for the control and brain-damaged patients are shown in Table 12. It will be seen, as has been shown in previous studies (1, 2, 5), that the brain-damaged patients are slower and more variable than the control patients. This holds for reactions both to sound and to light stimuli. It will also be noted that the reaction times of both groups are shorter to the sound stimuli than to the light sti-

muli, a finding which is in accord with long-standing observation (cf. 3). However, an unusual feature in the data is that inter-individual variability, as estimated by the standard deviations, was greater for the reactions to the sound stimuli than to the light stimuli. This was true for both diagnostic groups but the difference was particularly marked for the brain-damaged patients.

Reaction times to different classes of stimuli

With respect to reaction time as a function of stimulus class, it appears evident from inspection of Table 12 that the reaction times of both the brain-damaged and control patients to Class II stimuli are longer than those to Class I stimuli, and that their reaction times to Class III stimuli are longer than those to the other two classes. This holds for reactions to both sound and light. Reaction times to the several types of stimuli were found to be very closely related in both brain-damaged and control groups, the Pearson product-moment correlation coefficients ranging from .85 to .95.

The mean differences in reaction time to the different types of stimuli are shown in Table 13. The II–I differences reflect the retardation in reaction time which results from a change of stimulus within the same sensory modality (i.e., ipsimodal retardation) while the III–II differences reflect the retardation due to a change in sensory modality (i.e., crossmodal retardation). Examination of these differences in the control and brain-damaged patients shows that in three out of four comparisons the ipsimodal retardation was greater in size than the crossmodal retardation, the exception being the reactions to light of the brain-damaged patients, in which the crossmodal retardation was considerably greater than the ipsimodal

Table 12. Means and standard deviations (milliseconds) for reactions to different classes of stimuli

	Controls		Brain-damaged		Focal		Diffuse	
N	30		30		13		17	
	Mean	S.D.	Mean	S.D.	Mean	S.D.	Mean	S.D.
Light								
Class I (Identical)	310	44	351	64	350	60	351	61
Class II (Ipsimodal non-identical)	323	39	355	61	355	58	355	62
Class III (Crossmodal)	328	41	371	63	371	67	371	60
Sound								
Class I (Identical)	247	47	285	78	275	64	293	85
Class II (Ipsimodal non-identical)	264	64	318	96	289	57	340	113
Class III (Crossmodal)	271	65	332	110	299	79	358	122

retardation. Three of the four ipsimodal retardations were statistically significant, as determined by the t-test for correlated means. In contrast, only one of the four crossmodal retardations, that for reactions to light in the brain-damaged patients, was statistically significant.

Table 13. Mean differences (milliseconds) between reactions to different classes of stimuli

	Controls	Brain-damaged
Light		
II–I	13[a]	4
III–II	5	16[a]
Sound		
II–I	17[a]	33[b]
III–II	7	14

[a] $p < .001$.
[b] $p < .01$ (t-test for correlated means).

Retardation effects in brain-damaged and control patients

As Table 13 indicates, the crossmodal retardation effect appears to be greater for the brain-damaged than for the control patients. On the other hand, the ipsimodal retardation effect is apparently greater for the brain-damaged patients only with respect to reactions to sound stimuli. Covariance analyses were carried out to test the hypothesis that the brain-damaged patients showed significantly greater retardation in reaction time as a function of shift in stimulation than did the control patients (8). The use of this type of analysis appeared necessary because of the extremely high correlations between the reaction times to the different classes of stimuli. In these analyses, the brain-damaged patients were compared with the controls with respect to their performance on a given class of reactions (e.g., Class III reactions to light stimuli) while their performance on another class of reactions (e.g., Class II reactions to light stimuli) was held constant.

The results of these covariance analyses are shown in Table 14. It will be noted that the crossmodal retardation in reaction time to light stimuli (i.e., the comparison with respect to Class III reaction times when performance on Class II reactions is held constant) significantly discriminated the brain-damaged and control groups. The crossmodal retardation in reaction time to sound stimuli did not discriminate the two groups. The ipsimodal retardation in reaction time was not discriminative for either sound or light stimuli.

Table 14. Comparisons of brain-damaged and control groups by use of covariance analysis (*F*-ratios)

	Controls vs. brain-damaged	Controls vs. focal	Controls vs. diffuse
Light			
II (I held contant)	0.29	0.10	0.27
III (II held constant)	5.57[a]	2.98	4.95[a]
Sound			
II (I held constant)	1.11	0.10	2.80
III (II held constant)	0.43	0.04	1.13

[a] $p < .05$.

Comparison of patients with focal and diffuse lesions

Table 12 shows the mean reaction times of the 13 patients with focal lesions and the 17 patients with diffuse or bilateral lesions to the various classes of stimuli. It will be seen that the reaction times of the two subgroups to the light stimuli are almost identical. In contrast, the reaction times to the sound stimuli of the patients with diffuse lesions are consistently slower than those of the patients with focal lesions. Analysis of covariance (Table 14) showed that the crossmodal retardation for reactions to light (III–II) significantly discriminated the patients with diffuse lesions from the controls. The same crossmodal retardation did not significantly discriminate the patients with focal lesions from the control patients. However, the trend for the patients with focal lesions is in the same direction as for the patients with diffuse lesions, and the adjusted means from the covariance analysis show only a two-millisecond greater retardation for the diffuse group. None of the other types of reaction time retardation significantly discriminated between the control patients and either of the brain-damaged subgroups.

DISCUSSION

The findings show that retardation in simple reaction time as a function of a change in the stimulus will generally be shown by human subjects, whether normal or pathological. Moreover, the retardation is evident, whether the change in the stimulus involves a shift in sensory modality or not. Comparison of brain-damaged and control patients with respect to the magnitude of these retardation effects disclosed one significant difference, namely, in the crossmodal reaction to light stimuli. The brain-damaged patients showed a significantly greater retardation in reaction time to light stimuli preceded by sound stimuli than did control patients. Further analysis indicated that the greater susceptibility to crossmodal retardation effects in reaction to light stimuli was shown more clearly by the patients with diffuse cerebral disease.

The studies of Sutton et al. on schizophrenic patients have shown a significantly greater crossmodal retardation effect in the reactions of these patients to sound stimuli as compared with normal subjects. That is to say, the schizophrenic patients and normal subjects were found to be unequally retarded under the condition of change from visual to auditory stimuli. In the present study, the brain-damaged and control patients were found to be unequally retarded in their reaction times to visual stimuli, i.e., under the condition of change from auditory to visual stimuli. While the apparent difference in the "locus" of the crossmodal retardation effect in the two types of patients is most interesting, it would be wise first to determine whether the difference is in fact a stable one before speculating about its basic nature. The present experiment was a conventionally "exact" replication of the previous studies on schizophrenics in that it was done under similar conditions. However, there were some uncontrolled factors which made the experimental conditions far from identical. (One known uncontrolled factor is the intensity of the visual and auditory stimuli.) In order to verify the observed difference in the "locus" of the crossmodal retardation effect, it would seem desirable to compare brain-damaged and schizophrenic patients within the framework of a single study in the same laboratory. If the difference were confirmed, it would then be justifiable to consider it as a "real" one and to consider what might account for it.

Notwithstanding the apparent difference in the "locus" of the effect, it is nevertheless clear that patients with cerebral disease and schizophrenic patients show excessive susceptibility to one or another type of crossmodal retardation effect in the performance of a simple high-speed task. No explanation for this phenomenon can be advanced as yet. The conditions of the experiment were such that "easy" explanations which invoke factors such as mental dulling, lack of motivation, fatigue and the like, can be ruled out, since these variables would be expected to affect reaction times in general and not merely those to certain classes of stimuli as defined in this experiment. Nor can the concept of "set," in the usual sense of the term, be invoked to account for it because the experimental procedure involves no "build-up" of stimulus-response connections with repeated trials. It seems likely that there is a neurophysiological basis for this behavioral phenomenon, but knowledge of the nature of the neurophysiological deficit responsible for excessive crossmodal retardation in reaction time must wait upon further study.

SUMMARY

Comparison of the simple reaction times of brain-damaged and control patients to three classes of stimuli under a condition of serial presentation of stimuli gave the following results.

Both groups of patients showed slower reaction times to stimuli that had been preceded by a different stimulus than to stimuli that had been preceded by an identical stimulus. The degree of retardation in reaction time to stimuli preceded by a different stimulus in the same sensory modality (ipsimodal retardation effect) was not different in the two groups of patients.

The degree of retardation in reaction time to auditory stimuli preceded by a visual stimulus (crossmodal retardation effect) was also not different in the two groups. The degree of retardation in reaction time to visual stimuli preceded by an auditory stimulus was significantly greater in the brain-damaged than in the control patients, however. Patients with diffuse or bilateral cerebral disease showed a significantly larger crossmodal retardation than control patients; patients with focal lesions did not.

Comparison of the results of the present investigation with those of previous studies on schizophrenic patients indicates that both brain-damaged and schizophrenic patients show excessive susceptibility to the crossmodal retardation effect. There is an apparent difference in the "locus" of the effect in the two groups of patients, however, since schizophrenic patients have been found to show particularly marked retardation in reaction to sound stimuli preceded by visual stimuli. Further critical investigation of this apparent difference is indicated.

It is concluded that both patients with cerebral disease and schizophrenic patients show excessive susceptibility to the crossmodal retardation effect in simple high-speed performance tasks. The phenomenon cannot be explained in terms of lack of motivation, fatigability or failure to maintain set. It is likely that there is a neurophysiological basis for this behavioral deficit.

REFERENCES

1. Blackburn, H. L. Effects of motivating instructions on reaction time in cerebral disease. J. Abnorm. Soc. Psychol. **56:** 359–366, 1958.

2. Blackburn, H. L. & Benton, A. L. Simple and choice reaction time in cerebral disease. Confin. Neurol., **15:** 327–338, 1955.

3. Howell, W. C. & Donaldson, J. E. Human choice reaction time within and among sense modalities. Science, **135:** 429–430, 1962.

4. Mettler, F. A. Perceptual capacity, functions of the corpus striatum and schizophrenia. Psychiat. Quart., **29:** 89–109, 1955.

5. Shankweiler, D. P. Effects of success and failure instructions on reaction time in patients with brain damage. J. Comp. Physiol. Psychol., **52:** 546–549, 1959.

6. Sutton, S. Reaction times in schizophrenia. Paper presented at New York Academy of Sciences, October 16, 1961.

7. Sutton, S., Hakerem, G. & Zubin, J. The effect of shift in sensory modality on serial reaction time: A comparison of schizophrenics and normals. Amer. J. Psychol., **74:** 224–232, 1961.

8. Walker, H. M. & Lev, J. *Statistical Inference.* Holt, New York, 1953.

17.

Interactive Effects of Age and Brain Disease on Reaction Time*

This report discusses the results of an analysis of reaction time (RT) in younger and older patients with brain disease as compared to age-matched control patients. The question posed was whether or not evidence of an interactive effect of age and brain disease would be found. Data for the analysis came from an earlier study of simple visual and auditory RT in brain-diseased and control patients.[1]

PATIENTS AND METHODS

Twenty-four patients in the neurological and neurosurgical services of the University of Iowa Hospitals with a final diagnosis of hemispheric brain disease were studied. Group BY consisted of 12 patients ranging in age from 17 to 44 years (mean age, 35.5 years). Group BO consisted of 12 patients ranging in age from 46 to 63 years (mean age, 55.5 years). Six patients (50%) in each group had cerebrovascular disease. Four patients

(33%) in each group had neoplasms. Two patients in group BY had convulsive disorders, one associated with right temporal lobe abnormality, the other with left temporal lobe abnormality. Two patients in group BO had convulsive disorders, one associated with left temporal lobe abnormality, the other with generalized cerebral dysfunction. Seven patients (58%) in group BY and eight (67%) in group BO had lesions confined to the left hemisphere. Five patients (42%) in group BY and two (17%) in group BO had lesions confined to the right hemisphere.

Since there was this imbalance with respect to side of lesion in the two groups, smaller samples consisting of eight pairs of younger and older patients individually matched for both type and side of lesion were also formed. These samples consisted of three pairs of patients with neoplasm in the left hemisphere, three pairs with cerebrovascular disease of the left hemisphere, one pair with neoplasm in the right hemisphere, and one pair with cerebrovascular disease of the right hemisphere. The mean age of sample MY was

* A. L. Benton, *Archives of Neurology*, 1977, 34, 369–370. Copyright 1977, American Medical Association.

38.0 years (range, 23 to 44 years). The mean age of sample MO was 56.0 years (range, 46 to 63 years).

The control groups consisted of 24 patients in the neurological, neurosurgical, and medicine services who showed no history or evidence of brain disease. Group CY consisted of 12 patients ranging in age from 16 to 43 years (mean age, 31.4 years). Group CO consisted of 12 patients ranging in age from 47 to 63 years (mean age, 55.0 years).

The small differences in mean age of the three younger groups were not significant as estimated by *t* tests, i.e., the mean age of group BY was not significantly different from that of groups MY or CY, and the mean age of group MY was not significantly different from that of group CY. Similarly, the differences in the mean ages of groups BO, MO, and CO were not significant.

Sixty warned simple visual RTs and 60 warned auditory RTs were obtained on each patient. The warning was a verbal "ready" signal by the experimenter that was followed 2 to 5 seconds later by presentation of the visual or auditory stimulus. Patients without motor impairment used their preferred hand, while those with hemiparesis used the hand ipsilateral to side of lesion. The median score for each set of 60 trials was determined for each patient. The group means of these individual median scores were then computed.

RESULTS

The mean visual and auditory RTs of groups BY, BO, CY, and CO are presented in Figure 8. The older control patients showed a slight retardation (14 to 20 msec) in both auditory and visual RT as compared to the younger controls. In contrast, the older brain-diseased patients showed a much greater retardation (66 to 84 msec) as compared to the younger brain-diseased patients. The difference in mean RT between the younger brain-diseased and control groups was 24 msec for visual RT and 23 msec for auditory RT. These differences were substantially greater for the older brain-diseased and control groups (94 msec for visual RT; 68 msec for auditory RT).

These indications of an interactive effect of age and brain disease on RT were evaluated statistically by analyses of variance assessing the main effects of age and diagnosis and their interactions for visual RT and auditory RT. For visual RT, the main effect of age was significant ($p < .01$) and the main effect of diagnostic category was highly significant ($p < .001$), reflecting the slower RTs of the brain-diseased patients. The age by diagnosis interaction was also significant ($p < .04$), reflecting a stronger effect of brain disease on RT in older than in younger patients. Separate *t* tests indicated that the difference in mean visual RT was not significant ($p > .20$) for the younger and older control patients but was significant ($p < .01$) for the younger and older brain-diseased patients.

The results of the analysis of variance for auditory RT were similar. The main effect of age was significant ($p < .04$) and the main effect of diagnostic category was also significant ($p < .03$). The age by diagnosis interaction was not significant ($p > .20$). Separate *t* tests indicated that the difference in auditory RT was not significant ($p > .20$) for the younger and older control patients but approached significance ($p < .07$) for the younger and older brain-diseased patients.

Matched subsamples

The mean visual and auditory RTs of MY and MO subsamples were similar to those of the parent groups. The mean visual RT of the younger patients was 264 msec and

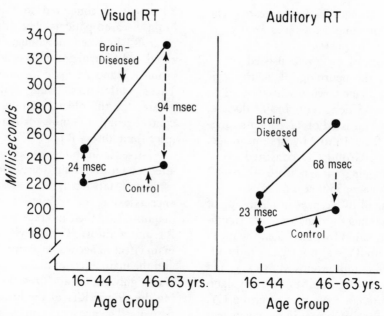

Fig. 8. Visual and auditory reaction times (RTs) in control and brain-diseased patients.

that of the older patients was 334 msec. The difference of 70 msec may be compared to the difference of 14 msec found for the younger and older control patients. The mean auditory RT was 236 msec for the younger patients and 280 msec for the older patients, the difference of 44 msec being substantially larger than the comparable difference of 20 msec for the younger and older control patients. The difference in mean RT between the younger brain-diseased and control groups was 39 msec for visual RT and 44 msec for auditory RT. The older brain-diseased and control groups showed larger differences in mean score: 95 msec for visual RT and 68 msec for auditory RT.

Analysis of the variance of the performances of the matched subsamples and the control groups yielded results similar to those found in the parent groups. For visual RT, the main effect of age was significant ($p < .04$), and the main effect of diagnostic category was highly significant ($p < .001$). The age by diagnosis interaction was also significant ($p < .025$). For auditory RT, the main effect of age was not significant ($p > .20$), but the main effect of diagnostic category was significant ($p < .002$). However, the age by diagnosis interaction was not significant ($p > .20$).

COMMENT

These indications of a differential effect of brain disease on RT as a function of age are based on a comparison of groups of younger and older patients who were matched for type but not for locus or size of lesion. However, the fact that analysis of the performances of smaller samples of younger and older patients who were individually matched for type and side of lesion (but not for size or intrahemispheric locus) yielded the same results as those found in the larger groups suggests that the failure to control for all lesional variables was not an important determinant of the observed relationships. Thus, the findings do suggest that there is an interactive effect of age and brain disease on simple RT. However, the evidence is not strong and the study is best viewed as having generated an interesting hypothesis that requires more rigorous testing. Moreover, in view of the evidence that multiple-choice RT is disproportionately slow as compared to simple RT in both older normal persons and patients with brain disease,[2-6] this interaction hypothesis also should be investigated for multiple-choice RT.

The slowing of psychomotor processes seen in older normal subjects is often interpreted as reflecting diffuse cerebral changes characterized by neuronal degeneration and loss. The findings of the present study suggest that an acquired lesion in an older brain leads to more pronounced retardation in RT than does a comparable lesion in a young brain. In this respect, they are in accord with the results of many studies assessing the effects of experimentally produced lesions in immature and mature animals, the tenor of which is that focal lesions sustained in early life have less severe effects than do comparable lesions in maturity.[7-11]

Whether the same pattern of results would be found for more complex cognitive abilities, particularly those more directly related to educational background, remains to be determined. Retardation in psychomotor functions is surely the most prominent behavioral change associated with aging. Thus, it may be that the execution of high-speed responses is a performance that is particularly vulnerable to the interactive effects of aging and an acquired brain lesion.

REFERENCES

1. Boehnert J. B.: *Auditory and Visual Reaction Time in Cerebral Disease*, thesis. University of Iowa, Iowa City, 1964.

2. Norman B. Svahn K.: A follow-up study of severe brain injuries. *Acta Psychiatr Scand* 37: 236–264, 1961.

3. Simon J. R.: S–R processing time as a function of aging. *J. Exp Psychol* 78: 76–80, 1968.

4. Miller E.: Simple and choice reaction time following severe head injury. *Cortex* 6: 121–127, 1970.

5. Dirken J. M. (ed): *Functional Age of Industrial Workers*. Groningen, Wolters-Noordhoff, 1972.

6. Dee H. L., Van Allen M. W.: Speed of decision-making processes in patients with unilateral cerebral disease. *Arch Neurol* 28: 163–166, 1973.

7. Kennard M.: Relation of age to motor impairment in man and subhuman primates. *Arch Neurol Psychiatry* 44: 377–397, 1940.

8. Benjamin R. D., Thompson R. F.: Differential effects of cortical lesions in infant and adult cats on roughness discrimination. *Exp Neurol* 1: 305–321, 1959.

9. Scharlock D. P., Tucker T. J., Strominger N. L.: Auditory discrimination by the cat after neonatal ablation of temporal cortex. *Science* 141: 1197–1198, 1963.

10. Akert K., Orth O. S., Harlow H. F., et al: Learned behavior of rhesus monkeys following neonatal bilateral prefrontal lobotomy. *Science* 132: 1944–1945, 1965.

11. Tucker T. J., Kling A., Scharlock D. P.: Sparing of photic frequency and brightness discrimination after striatectomy in neonatal cats. *Neurophysiology* 31: 818–832, 1968.

VI.
The Gerstmann Syndrome

18.

An Early Description of the Gerstmann Syndrome*

In 1924 Josef Gerstmann described "finger agnosia," an apparently hitherto unrecognized behavioral deficit appearing as a consequence of cerebral disease.[1] In this and subsequent papers, he called attention to the frequent association of finger agnosia with right-left disorientation, dyscalculia, and dysgraphia.[2,3] His observations were soon confirmed by other investigators, and the tetrad of symptoms has come to be known as the Gerstmann syndrome.

While right-left disorientation, dyscalculia, and dysgraphia were phenomena that had long been familiar to clinicians, it is generally believed that finger agnosia, that is, the inability to localize fingers subjected to tactual stimulation or to name or otherwise indicate them upon verbal command, was not known before the appearance of Gerstmann's communication. This impression is not altogether correct. In 1888 the French ophthalmologist, Jules Badal, published a detailed case report[4]

* A. L. Benton and R. Meyers, *Neurology*, 1956, 6, 838–842.

describing a female patient who, during a considerable period of study following severe eclampsia characterized by edema, convulsions, coma, and anemia, showed a variety of behavioral deficits including finger agnosia and the other elements of the Gerstmann syndrome. Other deficits, sometimes considered to be associated with the syndrome, such as constructional apraxia and spatial and temporal disorientation, were also present.

Badal's case report was evidently not unknown to neurologists 50 years ago. In a monograph published in 1898 Pick quoted rather extensively from it, and in a communication 10 years later he referred to it as "the well known case of Badal."[5,6] However, this early contribution appears to have been overlooked in recent years, for it is not mentioned in the reasonably complete historical surveys included in current monographs.[7-10] Hence, it seems worthwhile to recall attention to this once "well known" case report, both as a matter of intrinsic historical interest and because it poses a problem which is still unsettled.

The case of Valerie Clem . . .

Badal's patient was a 31 year old married woman who entered his clinic in Bordeaux complaining of rather peculiar visual disturbances and exhibiting "a strange combination of bizarre and incoherent phenomena." Her medical history prior to a recent first pregnancy had been unremarkable. The pregnancy itself had been uneventful until the eighth month when edema developed, initially involving the lower extremities and progressing rapidly to implicate the thigh and abdomen. One morning she suffered from copious epistaxis, which was followed by four major eclamptic attacks within an hour. At the obstetric clinic, to which she had been brought in an unconscious state, it was noted that the edema was severe, involving the labia and the abdominal wall as well as the lower limbs. The convulsions were controlled after use of chloroform for three hours. Consciousness was regained during the next hour. Variable amounts of albumin (1 to 7 gr./1,000 cc.) were found in the urine during the next week. No visual disturbances were observed.

Eight days after admission she delivered two living female infants, the first weighing 900 gm. and the second, a breech delivery accomplished 90 minutes after the first, weighing 2,200 gm. There was extensive hemorrhage after the birth of the second infant. The edema now receded rapidly. During the following week she showed mild delirium and confusion with hallucinatory activity and occasionally refused food. A paralysis of the left levator palpebrae superioris was apparent and persisted for some eight days. The pupils were dilated and sluggish. Vision appeared to be profoundly disturbed, but ophthalmoscopic examination was negative. At one time during this period she ran a temperature of 104° F. Anemia was severe. Neither motor nor speech difficulty was ever manifested, although a general asthenia was apparent.

The confusional state and the blepharoptosis disappeared, and the patient returned home. However, the visual difficulties persisted during the next six weeks, at the end of which period she entered Badal's clinic. Her principal complaint was visual disorientation.

Despite apparently excellent visual acuity, she could not find her way about the house. She had difficulty in locating objects, and when found she would reach past or to the side of them in attempts at apprehension. There was no diplopia, strabismus, or other disturbance of the extraocular movements. The pupils were not considered remarkable and their reactions to accommodation were intact.

Color vision was intact and color naming fluent. Central visual acuity was normal, but perimetric study indicated both a bilateral inferior hemianopsia and significant constriction of both upper visual fields. There was complete loss of topographic orientation. The patient could not find her way about the neighborhood, nor was she able to answer simple questions about the spatial relations of the main streets of Bordeaux although she had long been thoroughly familiar with them.

She could read letters and numbers, but only the simplest and most familiar words. She could not read other simple words and seemed to have lost all sense of directional orientation with respect to the printed material. "She could name isolated characters without difficulty but when several letters were placed, one after the other, she could not follow the order in which they were arranged . . . It was impossible for her to say whether such and such a letter was placed before or after another and consequently she could not make out the simplest syllable or determine where the line began or ended." She found it quite impossible to spell even those words which she was able to read.

She appeared to have an absolute agraphia. She could not write, either from dictation or a model, single letters which she could name and visualize. Thus, asked if she could imagine the letter, "a," she would close her eyes and say, "Yes, I see it. It has a round part and a stroke." Asked to write it, she would draw a line in some direction but was unable to continue. When the examiner drew the letter on the board, she quickly recognized it but could not copy the model. There was also virtually complete inability to draw even the simplest designs either from memory or from a model. Thus, given a square to copy, she drew something resembling a "Z." She also showed severe impairment in estimating the size, distance, location, and spatial relations of objects. In attempting to localize objects in space, there was no tendency to transpose them laterally, that is, no visual allochiria. Also there was no evidence of metamorphopsia.

In short, Badal's patient showed visual disorientation within the setting of intact visual acuity, a condition that was a topic of much clinical investigation and discussion in the 1890s. However, on the basis of further observation, Badal believed that his patient suffered from a spatial disorientation which affected all modalities, by no means being restricted to vision. Thus, while auditory acuity appeared to be intact, she found it difficult to indicate the directional source of sounds. There were no consistent lateral trends in this regard and thus no evidence of auditory allochiria.

Evidence for a disturbed spatial sense also appeared in the tactual-kinesthetic realm. She could no longer distinguish the right and left sides of her body. "In order to make this discrimination, and even then she sometimes made errors, she had to make the sign of the cross; she knew that she used the right hand for this." Esthesiometric testing indicated slight generalized hypesthesia and a rise in the two-point threshold. But Badal felt that this was not sufficient to explain such "bizarre phenomena" as the following: "It happended frequently that the patient was not able to say which of her fingers had been touched or pricked and, for example, would report the index finger when the ring finger had been pricked . . . Sometimes the same errors were made even when the eyes were allowed to remain open so that they could guide the tactual impressions; moreover, if one asked Valerie to name the five fingers of the hand, one after the other and in the order in which they were placed, it was rare for her not to commit some error, either in naming them or in classifying them from 1 to 5." Badal believed that these deficits "were due chiefly to a profound alteration of the sense of space" and were not explicable in terms of impaired tactual or kinesthetic sensitivity. There were no disturbances in position sense. "The patient had perfect awareness of the movements which she executed, had a correct idea of the position

in which her extremities might be placed and, with her eyes closed, could reproduce this position with the homologous member fairly exactly." Pain and thermal sensitivity appeared to be intact. No areas of cutaneous anesthesia could be discovered.

She also showed a moderate but definite dyscalculia. She could count, do very simple additions, and serial addition by two's was easily accomplished. However, in serial addition by three's, she would invariably fail beyond 24, despite repeated attempts by a variety of methods to combine 24 and 3. Her concept of the basic number series was defective as shown, for example, by her inability to say what number was placed between 14 and 16.

Two further behavioral deficits may be noted. She showed impairment in the execution of a number of skilled acts, including a dyspraxia for dressing. She could not put up her hair without assistance and such familiar skills as knitting or threading a needle were now beyond her capabilities. She was no longer able to dress herself. For example, she put garments on in the wrong order and slipped her arm into the wrong sleeve. She also showed some time disorientation. She could not say confidently what year (1888) it was, but tended to hesitate between 1885 and 1888.

DISCUSSION

Badal considered the question whether the symptoms shown by his patient were organic or functional in nature, but reached no definite conclusion. He did not incline to the view that she was an "hysteric." In describing her premorbid history he stressed that she had never shown any signs of nervous disturbance, and in discussing some aspects of the symptomatology he contrasted them with those shown by hysterical patients. However, it is perhaps worthy of note that Badal described the following characteristics: "The ocular mucosa had not lost any of its sensibility; in contrast, that of the auditory canals and of the nasal chambers was dulled; one could tickle them without eliciting reflexes. There was complete anesthesia of the pharyngeal mucosa, and the finger could be introduced into the back of the throat without eliciting the least reaction. A sudden pressure on the epigastrium, a shock strong enough to give any other person a particularly painful sensation, was easily tolerated."

Looking back at this early case report, it now seems probable that the patient suffered a cerebrovascular insult of rather diffuse nature with significant parieto-occipital involvement as a consequence of the severe eclampsia. As has been mentioned, Badal was inclined to interpret most of the symptoms as expressions of a single basic deficit, namely, a loss of the sense of space.

The fact that Badal described finger agnosia some 70 years ago does not detract from the significant contribution of Josef Gerstmann in "rediscovering" it, so to speak, in describing its relations to other behavioral deficits and, above all, in elucidating its neuropathologic significance. Nevertheless, Badal's report merits consideration not merely for its historic interest, but also because its author's theoretic interpretation still possesses relevance for current thinking about the nature of the Gerstmann syndrome.

Badal's patient showed all the elements of the Gerstmann syndrome—finger agnosia, right-left disorientation, dysgraphia, dyscalculia—and a good deal more, for example, visual disorientation, as manifested in her inability to fixate, locate objects in the environment, and order objects along a visuospatial continuum; constructive apraxia, expressed in an inability to draw and a particular type of dressing dyspraxia; and some degree of temporal disorientation. All of these deficits have been found at times associated with the Gerstmann syndrome. On the other hand, she did not show color agnosia, a sympton that has been mentioned as

an "accompaniment" of the Gerstmann syndrome more frequently than has any other.

The clinical picture presented by Badal's patient might be interpreted as a "Gerstmann syndrome," unrecognized as such. However, as it happens, the clinical picture fits equally well the combination of symptoms for which Critchley[8] has suggested the designation of "Leonhard's syndrome,"[11] that is, dysgraphia, dyscalculia, constructive apraxia, and temporal disorientation. Clearly, if the one syndrome was missed, so was the other. Moreover, Badal created his own more comprehensive syndrome of loss of the "sense of space" to account for the observed aggregation of symptoms, a conception which is quite similar to that of later writes, notably Lange.[12]

The situation presented by clinical observation relating to the Gerstmann syndrome since the time of Badal would seem to be about as follows. A relatively large number of behavioral deficits are frequently shown by patients with parieto-occipital lesions. A given patient is more likely than not to exhibit a combination of these deficits. Necessarily some patients will show the same combination of deficits, and this circumstance of combination has led to a search for an underlying unitary factor. Moreover, certain combinations of symptoms which have impressed clinical observers have been abstracted and given the special status of "syndromes," for example, Gerstmann and Leonhard. Once these special categories have been established, there is a tendency not only to use them in the observation and description of subsequent case material, but also to allow them to determine to some extent which behavioral events are selected for study and report and which are not.

Obviously, there is nothing inherently wrong about this process of selection and abstraction of symptoms. Indeed, this is a necessary component of the scientific approach to disease. However, it is also obvious that not all syntheses are equally valuable. The "correctness" of any classification is determined only by its meaningfulness. In the case of the Gerstmann syndrome, the cogency in selecting this combination of symptoms would seem to depend upon whether, as a matter of phenomenologic fact, the four deficits do show a distinctively close mutual association, as compared with the degree of their association with other allegedly "parietal" deficits, and also whether the use of this descriptive category possesses special value for diagnostic inference.

At the present time the meaningfulness of the syndrome in either the phenomenologic or inferential sense remains an open question.[8,13,14] From the phenomenologic standpoint, "incomplete" forms of the Gerstmann syndrome are not rare and more often than not the patient shows other deficits (for example, color agnosia, constructive apraxia, and so on) that have been suggested by one writer or another as properly belonging to the syndrome. Thus it is not known whether the four Gerstmann symptoms show a particularly close association with each other as compared to their "associative bonds" with the other symptoms. Nor is there cogent evidence that the syndrome, considered as a unit, possesses a neuropathologic or psychopathologic significance not furnished by its component elements or by the associated behavioral deficits.

One possible approach to this problem of the combination of symptoms of the "parieto-occipital" type is to make a careful quantitative assessment of the degree of relationship occurring among the several deficits through systematic and relatively unbiased study of an adequate sample of patients. Almost certainly, such an inquiry would show that in general the various deficits are significantly related to one another, thus supporting the tenability of the current hypothesis of a broad "parieto-occipital" syndrome. More importantly, the analysis would show whether or not there are significant differences in the degree of relationship of the several deficits and whether specific subgroups of symptoms that are characterized by strong intragroup associative bonds can be isolated. If such clusters of deficits do appear, it could then be determined whether or not they possess particular significance from a neuropathologic, psychopathologic, or general psychologic standpoint. Similarly, it would be possible to determine whether or not they correspond to those syndromes (Gerstmann, Leonhard) that have already been isolated on a more or less impressionistic basis.

REFERENCES

1. Gerstmann. J.: Fingeragnosie; eine umschriebene Störung der Orientierung am eigenen Körper. Wien. klin. Wchnschr. 37:1010, 1924.

2. Gerstmann, J.: Fingeragnosie und isolierte Agraphie: ein neues Syndrom. Ztschr. Neurol. u. Psychiat. 108:152, 1927.

3. Gerstmann, J.: Zur Symptomatologie der Hirnläsionen im Übergangsgebiet der unteren Parietal und mittleren Occipitalwindung. Nervenarzt 3: 691, 1930.

4. Badal, Jules: Contribution à l'étude des cécités psychiques: alexie, agraphie, hémianopsie inférieure, trouble du sens de l'space. Arch opht. 8:97, 1888.

5. Pick, A.: Beiträge zur Pathologie und pathologischen Anatomie des Centralnervensystems. Berlin, S. Karger, 1898, 324 pp.

6. Pick. A.: Arbeiten aus der deutschen psychiatrischen Universitäts-Klinik in Prag. Berlin, S. Karger, 1908, 143 pp.

7. de Ajuriaguerra, J., & Hécaen, H.: Le cortex cérébral. Paris, Masson, 1949, 413 pp.

8. Critchley, M.: The Parietal Lobes. London, Edward Arnold, 1953, 480 pp.

9. Hécaen, H., & de Ajuriaguerra, J.: Méconnaissances et hallucinations corporelles. Paris, Masson, 1952, 382 pp.

10. Nielsen, J. M.: Agnosia, Apraxia, Aphasia; Their Value in Cerebral Localization. New York, Hoeber, 1946, 292 pp.

11. Leonhard, K.: Rechen- und zeitliche Orientierungsstörung bei Agraphie und konstruktiver Apraxie. Arch. Psychiat. 188:504, 1952.

12. Lange, J.: Fingeragnosie und Agraphie.

Monatsschr. Psychiat. u. Neurol. 76:129, 1930.

13. Benton, A. L., Hutcheon, J. F., & Seymour, E.: Arithmetic ability, finger-localization capacity and right-left discrimination in normal and defective children. Am. J. Orthopsychiat. 21:756, 1951.

14. Benton, A. L. & Abramson, L. S.: Gerstmann symptoms following electroshock treatment. Arch. Neurol. & Psychiat. 68:248, 1952.

19.

The Fiction of the "Gerstmann Syndrome"*

The problem with which this study is concerned can be stated as follows. A patient with parieto-occipital disease may show one or more of a relatively large number of diverse behavioural deficits. When he presents with two, three, or more of these symptoms, the latter may be viewed by the clinical observer as forming a naturally occurring combination of deficits and given the status of a syndrome, this status implying that the concurrence of deficits is not a chance one, that there is an underlying factor responsible for it, and that it possesses a distinctive neuropathological significance. Once such a special combination or syndrome is established, not only is it used in the observation and description of subsequent cases but it may also determine which aspects of a patient's behaviour are selected for study and which are not. The "Gerstmann syndrome" represents such a combination of behavioural deficits. The study to be reported examines the question of

* A. L. Benton, *Journal of Neurology, Neurosurgery and Psychiatry*, 1961, 24, 176–181.

whether, as is usually assumed, this "assembly of unlikely and unexpected symptoms" (Critchley, 1953) is a naturally occurring combination or whether it is only one of a very large number of more or less fortuitous combinations of behavioural deficits which may be encountered in patients with cerebral disease.

The history of the Gerstmann syndrome has been recounted in detail elsewhere (cf. Critchley, 1953; Benton, 1959); only a few major points need be mentioned to introduce the present investigation. Before the end of the nineteenth century, the four behavioural deficits comprising the syndrome—right-left disorientation, acalculia, agraphia, and finger agnosia—had been described as occurring in patients with cerebral disease. The first three were well-known symptoms but the description of finger agnosia in 1888 by Jules Badal had escaped the attention of neurologists, a fact which is not altogether surprising in view of the circumstances that the Bordeaux eye specialist published in an ophthalmological journal, and the finger agnosia which he quite clearly described was only one of a large number of deficits shown by his patient. In 1924, Gerstmann once again described finger agnosia, designating it as "a circumscribed disorder of orientation to one's own body." In 1927, he advanced the idea that finger agnosia and agraphia formed "a new syndrome." However, in 1930 he enlarged the syndrome to include right-left disorientation and acalculia and proposed that it had a highly specific neuropathological significance. At the same time, he discussed the question of the *Grundstörung* responsible for this presumably "natural" concurrence of behavioural deficits.

Clinical experience appeared to confirm the real existence of the syndrome; case reports of patients manifesting it appeared in the literature and speculations regarding the basic impairment underlying its occurrence were offered. However, it was certainly not rare to encounter patients who showed one, two, or three deficits but not the full syndrome. While such observations were often interpreted as simply representing *formes frustes* of the syndrome, they did indicate at least that the four symptoms did not necessarily occur together in every case and they did have implications regarding the cogency of those theoretical formulations which had been advanced to account for an obligatory concurrence of the deficits. On the other hand, a wide variety of other deficits were also observed to occur in connexion with any or all of the four symptoms. These were given a subordinate status as accompanying symptoms which might or might not be manifested. Among them were general mental impairment, aphasic disorders, colour agnosia, visual disorientation, dyslexia, and constructional apraxia. Indeed, the last-named deficit, constructional apraxia, has been observed so often to accompany one or more of the four deficits that some

authors have come to consider it, explicitly or implicitly, as part of the syndrome. For example, Ajuriaguerra and Hécaen (1960), discussing the interrelations of the elements of the syndrome and the connexions with other symptoms, remark that "the most frequent and most important association is that between finger agnosia and constructional apraxia. We have seen that such an association cannot be considered to be simply fortuitous or anatomically conditioned."

If the "Gerstmann syndrome" is a naturally occurring combination of interrelated deficits, all of which are expressions of a single basic impairment, and not merely the product of selective attention and observation, the four behavioural deficits which comprise it should show stronger "associative bonds," so to speak, among themselves than they do with symptoms which are considered to be outside of the syndrome. If unbiased analysis should show this to be the case, the findings could be reasonably interpreted as evidence for a special coherence of the four symptoms and both the designation of the combination as a syndrome and a search for the common factor responsible for the coherence are justified. On the other hand, if such analysis should disclose that this is not the case, the findings could be reasonably interpreted as indicating that this particular combination of deficits is no more or less likely to occur in patients with cerebral disease than a great many similar combinations and that, unless it can be shown to have a distinctive neuropathological significance, neither its designation as a syndrome nor the postulation of a common psychoneurological factor to account for it (as distinguished from other combinations) is justified.

It might be thought that a comprehensive survey of the pertinent clinical literature would provide the answer to this question of the phenomenological reality of the Gerstmann syndrome. However, the literature proves to be virtually without value in this respect. The methods and criteria utilized for making clinical judgments regarding the presence or absence of defect in the performances investigated are so diverse that the findings from one case to another are not comparable. Not infrequently the criteria employed in making judgments of deficit are not mentioned and notations such as "slight finger agnosia," "questionable right-left disorientation," or "no noteworthy constructional apraxia" are made. Moreover, the majority of case reports fail to mention the presence or absence of one or more pertinent accompanying deficits and hence must be excluded from a systematic analysis. Finally, the factor of selective attention and observation when one is dealing with an already established entity, such as the Gerstmann syndrome, may introduce a bias in the original observations for which the reviewer cannot correct.

It seems evident that the question of the status of the Gerstmann syndrome as a behavioural phenomenon can be answered only by an investigation which has been deliberately designed to answer it and which employs explicitly described procedures for assessment and criteria for judgment. The present paper reports such an investigation.

CASE MATERIAL AND METHODS

The case material consisted of 100 non-psychotic patients with unequivocal diagnoses of disease or injury involving the cerebral hemispheres who had been seen in the neurological and neurosurgical services of the University Hospitals and Veterans Administration Hospital, Iowa City. Any patient who was suffering from acute illness, whose behaviour raised the question of psychosis, who had a history of treatment in hospital for a psychiatric disorder, or whose history was suggestive of a state of mental defect dating back to childhood, was excluded from the study. All the patients were between the ages of 16 and 64 years and were clearly capable of understanding directions, cooperating in the test procedures and undergoing one to two hours of examination without discomfort. The mean age of the group was 42 years. The mean educational level was 10 years (range: 5 to 16 years). A variety of cerebral conditions, focal and diffuse, was represented in the group. The performances of 12 right-handed patients with focal disease involving the left parietal lobe were analysed separately, in addition to the main analyses of the total group of 100 patients of which they formed a part.

A control group of 100 non-psychotic patients from the neurological, neurosurgical, and medical services who showed no evidence or history of cerebral disease or injury were also examined, their performances being utilized to establish objective normative standards on the basis of which the presence or absence of impairment could be defined. The mean age of this group was 41 years (range: 16 to 65 years) and mean educational level was 10 years (range: 5 to 14 years).

All the patients were given a battery of seven tests designed to provide objective and comprehensive assessments of the following capacities: (1) right-left orientation; (2) finger localization; (3) arithmetic calculation; (4) writing; (5) constructional praxis; (6) reading; (7) visual memory. The testing procedures were as follows:

Right-left Orientation. This test battery (32 items) required the patient to execute localizing movements to oral command and assessed the following aspects of right-left orientation: (A) with the aid of vision, identification of single lateral body parts on one's own body; (B) with the aid of vision, execution of double uncrossed and crossed commands with respect to lateral body parts on one's own body, e.g., left hand on right eye; (C) without the aid of vision, identification of single lateral body parts; (D) without the aid of vision, execution of double commands; (E) identification of single lateral body parts on a front-view representation of a man; (F) execution of double commands involving identification of lateral body parts of both the patient and the representation, e.g., patient's right hand on a man's right eye. The details of this test battery may be found in a paper by Benton and Kemble (1960). Level of performance was defined as the number of correct localizations made by the patient.

Finger Localization. This test battery (80 items) assessed the following aspects of finger identification: (A) with the aid of vision, presentation of single fingers on oral command; (B) identification of single fingers on schematic drawings of the hands; (C) with the aid of vision, identification of single fingers which had been touched; (D) without the aid of vision, identification of single fingers which had been touched; (E) without the aid of vision, identification of pairs of fingers subjected to simultaneous tactile stimulation. (For details regarding the arrangements for tactile stimulation of the fingers, see Benton, 1959.) Level of performance was defined as the number of correct localizations made by the patient.

Arithmetic Calculation. This untimed 16-item written test consisted of simple problems in addition, subtraction, multiplication, and division involving one- and two- digit numbers. Level of performance was defined as the number of correct solutions.

Writing. The patient was asked to write his name, copy two simple sentences, write two simple sentences to dictation, and write down anything that came into his mind. Unlined $5\frac{1}{2} \times 8$ in. paper was used. Each specimen of writing was independently rated by two examiners on the basis of the following factors: alignment of lines; elisions and omissions; formation of letters; spelling; substitutions and additions. Each of these factors was rated from 0 (poor) to 2 (within normal limits). Level of performance was defined in terms of an overall rating consisting of the sum of the two examiners' ratings on each of these factors. However, in the case of patients with sensorimotor deficits of the preferred hand, the "formation of letters" factor was excluded from consideration and a weighted sum of the examiners' ratings on the other factors was computed.

Constructional Praxis. Both two-dimensional and three-dimensional praxis was assessed. The two-dimensional task consisted in having the patient copy six "stick" designs presented by the examiner while the three-dimensional task consisted in having him copy four models made of rectangular blocks of various sizes and dimensions. The patient was allowed to use only one hand in arranging the sticks or blocks. Level of performance was defined as the number of sticks and blocks correctly placed.

Reading. The patient read four short paragraphs and, with the paragraphs in view, answered questions which assessed his understanding of them. Level of performance was defined as the number of questions correctly answered. No time limit was enforced.

Visual Memory. Multiple choice form G of the visual retention test (Benton, 1953) consisting of 15 designs was used. Each

Table 15. Second-order correlation coefficients (age and education "partialled out") in 100 brain-damaged patients

	Finger localization	Writing	Calculation	Constructional praxis	Reading	Visual memory
Right-left	.62	.48	.46	.51	.48	.57
Finger localization		.52	.35	.60	.42	.50
Writing			.46	.44	.57	.52
Calculation				.51	.60	.58
Constructional praxis					.42	.47
Reading						.56

design was presented to the patient for 5 sec., after which he was required to identify the design on a card containing it and three similar designs. Level of performance was defined as the number of correct choices made by the patient.

Distributions of the scores of the 100 control patients on each of the seven tests were made and inspected. For each distribution, a score which was equalled or exceeded by 91 to 94% of the patients was selected as a "cutting score" and scores below this level were considered to indicate significantly defective performance. Natural "breaks" which occurred in the lower ends of some of the distributions were utilized in establishing these cutting scores, a circumstance which accounts for the slight variation in the percentage values of the various scores.

THE INVESTIGATION

Relationships among performances

The intercorrelations among the seven performances for the total group of 100 brain-damaged patients are shown in Table 15. These are "second-order" correlation coefficients, from which the effects of variation in age and educational level on performance have been eliminated. Inspection of this matrix suggests that the correlations among the elements of the syndrome are neither higher nor lower than those between these elements and the performances which presumably

do not belong to the syndrome. Thus, while the highest correlation coefficient in the matrix (.62) is between two syndrome performances (right-left orientation vs. finger localization), it will be seen that the lowest correlation coefficient (.35) is also between two syndrome performances (finger localization vs. calculation). The mean correlation coefficient of the performances within the syndrome (derived from averaging the six relevant correlation coefficients) is .48. This may be compared with the mean correlation coefficient between the syndrome performances and those performances which are outside of the syndrome. This statistic (derived from averaging the 12 relevant correlation coefficients) is .52, indicating that the syndrome performances show no closer relationship among themselves than they do with performances outside of the syndrome.

A more detailed analysis of the strength of the relationships existing among elements of the syndrome as compared with that existing between them and the other performances is presented in Table 16, which shows the mean correlation coefficient of each syndrome performance with the other three syndrome performances and of each extra-syndrome performance with the four syndrome performances. The findings indicate quite clearly that constructional praxis, reading, and visual memory are as closely related to the elements of the syndrome as the latter are among themselves, i.e., that the elements of the syndrome do not show particularly close associative bonds.

Cohesiveness of syndromes

As has already been noted, the mean inter-correlation among the elements of the syndrome is .48, which may be inter-preted as an index of its "cohesiveness", i.e., of the tendency of elements to vary concurrently. Thirty-five combinations of four performances each can be formed from the seven "parietal" performances investigated in this study. Each combi-nation will include one or more elements of the syndrome, one of them being the syndrome. If there is a special tendency for the elements of the syndrome to vary concurrently, its observed mean intercor-relation of .48 should be higher than those derived from combinations consisting of mixtures of syndrome and non-syndrome elements. The mean correlation coeffi-cient (derived from the six relevant corre-lation coefficients) of each of the 34 mixed combinations was computed. They ranged in size from .48 to .54. Two coeffi-cients were as high as .54 and four were as low as .48. It is clear from these findings that all 35 combinations of elements show about the same degree of cohesiveness and that the syndrome is not at all distinctive in this respect.

The incidence of significant deficit in performance (as defined above, i.e., per-formances which fell within the lowest 6

to 9% of the scores of the control group) was computed for each patient. Twenty-nine showed no significant deficits and 23 showed only one deficit. The remaining 48 patients showed two to seven deficits, 10 of them showing four deficits. Examin-ation of these 10 sets of four deficits dis-closed that all involved combinations of syndrome and non-syndrome perfor-mances. The pure Gerstmann syndrome did not appear. The combination of defi-cits in finger localization, writing, reading, and constructional praxis appeared twice. Eight other combinations appeared once. Again the findings indicate no particularly strong tendency for the symptoms of the Gerstmann syndrome to appear concur-rently.

Performances of patients with left parietal lesions

It might be argued that assumptions about the essential unity of the elements of the Gerstmann syndrome hold only for patients with parieto-occipital disease of the dominant hemisphere and that a study involving patients with various types of lesion cannot provide cogent evidence about these assumptions. The contention is quite debatable. The explanations which have been advanced to account for the supposedly obligatory concurrence of the symptoms have been of a broad psy-chological or psychoneurological nature and have no necessary reference to a specific locus of the responsible lesion.

Table 16. Mean correlation coefficients between individual performances and the syndrome in 100 brain-damaged patients

	r
Right-left vs. finger localization — writing — calculation	.52
Finger localization vs. right-left — writing — calculation	.51
Writing vs. right-left — finger localization — calculation	.49
Calculation vs. right-left — finger localization — writing	.42
Constructional praxis vs. right-left — finger localization — writing — calculation	.52
Reading vs. right-left — finger localization — writing — calculation	.52
Visual memory vs. right-left — finger localization — writing — calculation	.54

Table 17. Mean correlations between individual performances and the syndrome in 12 patients with left parietal lobe disease

	r
Right-left vs. finger localization — writing — calculation	.53
Finger localization vs. right-left — writing — calculation	.38
Writing vs. right-left — finger localization — calculation	.21
Calculation vs. right-left — finger localization — writing	.51
Constructional praxis vs. right-left — finger localization — writing — calculation	.53
Reading vs. right-left — finger localization — writing — calculation	.61
Visual memory vs. right-left — finger localization — writing — calculation	.44

Thus such concepts as the importance of intact finger gnosis for writing and calculation, of intact right-left orientation for calculation, or of intact spatial thinking for all the performances have been applied to all situations in which the deficits appear, e.g., developmental deficit, and are not dependent upon the presence of a specified lesion. Nevertheless, it seemed worthwhile to make a separate analysis of the performances of the 12 right-handed patients in the group who had disease of the left parietal lobe to determine the nature of the relationships of the syndrome performances among themselves and with the other performances.

The mean correlation coefficient of each of the syndrome performances with the other three syndrome performances and of each extra-syndrome performance with the four syndrome performances is shown in Table 17. It is evident from

inspection of this table that constructional praxis, reading, and visual memory are as closely related to the elements of the syndrome as the latter are to each other. Thus in this group of patients with focal disease of the left parietal lobe there is also no evidence that the elements of the syndrome show any noteworthy strength of association.

The significant deficits in performance shown by these 12 patients are shown in detail in Table 18. It will be seen that no patient showed the full Gerstmann syndrome. Four patients (E.H., R.K., A.P., D.T.) presented with three Gerstmann symptoms but in each case these appeared in association with other deficits.

DISCUSSION

This investigation represents an attempt to determine whether the four beha-

Table 18. Incidence of deficits in patients with left parietal lobe disease

No.	Patient	Right-left	Finger localization	Writing	Calculation	Constructional praxis	Reading	Visual memory
1	N.F.	0	0	0	0	+	0	+
2	E.H.	+	+	0	+	+	0	+
3	V.H.	0	0	0	0	0	0	0
4	R.K.	+	+	0	+	+	+	+
5	E.K.	0	0	0	0	+	0	0
6	A.P.	+	+	0	+	+	+	0
7	D.T.	+	0	+	+	0	+	0
8	E.H.	0	0	0	0	0	0	0
9	R.M.	0	0	0	0	0	0	0
10	E.M.	0	0	0	0	0	0	0
11	J.C.	+	+	0	0	+	0	0
12	J.D.	0	0	0	0	0	0	0

+ = deficit; 0 = no deficit.

vioural deficits comprising the so-called "Gerstmann syndrome" form a distinctive constellation. A variety of analyses, which provided evidence concerning the strength of the relationships existing among these elements and that existing between the elements and performances which do not belong to the syndrome, were done. These analyses, made both on a large group of patients with diverse types of cerebral disease and a smaller group of right-handed patients with focal disease of the left parietal lobe, consistently indicated that the particular combination of behavioural deficits which form the syndrome show no stronger internal associative bonds than do a score of other combinations of behavioural deficits. A large number of combinations of four behavioural deficits may be presented by patients with cerebral disease. The analyses of the present study suggest that there is about an equal probability of occurrence for any one of them, including the combination known as the Gerstmann syndrome.

These results provide a reasonable explanation of the frequent reports in the clinical literature of so-called incomplete forms of the syndrome as well as the even more frequent reports of symptoms which are observed to "accompany" it. Such behavioural pictures are simply other combinations of deficits which tend not to be accepted in their own right because of the predilection of clinical observers to look first for elements of the Gerstmann combination and to use these elements as an anchoring point to which accompanying symptoms may be attached. The findings also indicate that theoretical speculations concerning the basic impairment which must underlie the so-called Gerstmann syndrome are hardly warranted. There is no obligatory concurrence of deficits to account for and, in any case, if it is necessary to explain this particular combination of deficits, it is equally necessary to explain the existence of a score of other combinations of behavioural deficits.

A tenable conclusion from these results is that, judged from the standpoint of behavioural analysis, the Gerstmann syndrome is a fiction; it is simply an artifact of defective and biased observations. Objective, unbiased observation discloses a large number of combinations of parietal deficits. Since all these combinations appear to be about equally strong with respect to their internal associative bonds and frequency of occurrence, either all or none should be designated as syndromes.

This study has not been concerned directly with the question of the possible neuropathological significance of the combination of deficits known as the Gerstmann syndrome. Despite the fact that this combination of deficits does not seem to be any different from many other combinations of parietal symptoms, there is the possibility that when it is manifested in pure form it does possess the highly specific focal diagnostic significance which has been claimed for it, namely a lesion of "that nodal area which corresponds to the angular gyrus in its transition to the second occipital convolution" (Gerstmann, 1957). However, Critchley (1953), reviewing the clinical literature, was inclined to conclude that the syndrome was more reasonably interpreted as a sign of parietal disease in general rather than specifically indicating a lesion of the angular gyrus. Similarly, Heimberger, DeMyer, and Reitan (1957) found that when patients manifested the full syndrome, the responsible lesion, even when restricted to the dominant hemisphere, was invariably an extensive one. Finally, there are case reports, such as the recent one by Brusa, Rossi, and Tartarini (1960), of the occurrence of the syndrome in patients with lesions apparently restricted to the frontal lobes. Thus those analyses of the question as have been done throw considerable doubt on the assertion that the syndrome has a highly specific focal diagnostic import. If it does possess such a significance, it might be expected that the other 34 of the 35 syndromes investigated in this study would also have a similarly specific significance. But the weight of clinicopathological evidence gathered over the last 60 years makes it extremely unlikely that such "punctate" localization of functions or deficits exists.

In directing the attention of neurologists both to certain disorders of the body schema and to the unusual variety of combinations of behavioural deficits which a brain-damaged patient may show, the Gerstmann syndrome has perhaps been a useful fiction during the past 30 years. Now that these purposes have been accomplished, adherence to the fiction may well operate to retard further advances in the understanding of the patterns of behavioural deficit which may occur as a consequence of cerebral disease, for it tends to prejudice clinical observation and to produce a distorted picture of the organization of abilities and disabilities in brain-damaged patients.

SUMMARY

Systematic, objective analysis of the performances of patients with cerebral disease on seven "parietal" tasks (right-left orientation, finger localization, writing, calculation, constructional praxis, reading, visual memory) indicates that many combinations of deficits, including that known as the "Gerstmann syndrome," may be observed. The syndrome appears to be no different from the other combinations in respect to either the strength of the mutual interrelationships among its elements or the strength of the relationships between its elements and performances not belonging to it. These results hold both for patients with diverse cerebral conditions and for those with focal lesions of the dominant parietal lobe.

The findings are interpreted as indicating that the Gerstmann syndrome is an artifact of defective and biased observation. Further, a review of the pertinent clinical literature offers little support for its alleged focal diagnostic significance. The general conclusion is that the syndrome is a fiction which has perhaps served a useful purpose in the past in certain respects, but which now carries the hazard of retarding advances in the understanding of the organization of abilities and disabilities in patients with cerebral disease.

REFERENCES

Ajuriaguerra, J. de, and Hécaen, H. (1960). *Le Cortex Cérébral.* Masson, Paris.

Badal, J (1888). *Arch. Ophtal. (Paris),* **8,** 97.

Benton, A. L. (1953). *Manuel pour l'Application clinique du Test de Rétention Visuelle.* Editions du Centre de Psychologie Appliquée, Paris.

――― (1959). *Right-Left Discrimination and Finger Localization: Development and Pathology.* Hoeber, New York.

――― & Kemble, J. D. (1960). *Psychiat. et Neurol. (Basel),* **139,** 49.

Brusa, A., Rossi, R., & Tartarini, E. (1960). *Encéphale,* **49,** 319.

Critchley, M. (1953). *The Parietal Lobes.* Arnold, London

Gerstmann. J. (1924). *Wien klin. Wschr.,* **37,** 1010.

――― (1927). *Z. ges. Neurol. Psychiat.,* **108,** 152.

――― (1930). *Nervenarzt,* **3,** 691.

――― (1957). *Neurology (Minneap.),* **7,** 866.

Heimberger, R. F., DeMyer, W., & Reitan, R. M. (1957). Implications of Gerstmann's syndrome. *Journal of Neurology, Neurosurgery and Pychiatry,* 1964, *27, 52–57.*

20.

Reflections on the Gerstmann Syndrome*

The aims of this paper are to make an analysis of recent studies concerned with the aggregate of behavioral deficits called the "Gerstmann syndrome" and to offer an assessment of its neuropsychological significance. The deficits with which we are concerned are, of course, finger agnosia, right-left disorientation, acalculia, and agraphia. During the past decade there has been much debate, not always free from acrimony, about whether or not the aggregate is in any meaningful sense a "syndrome." On the one hand, a number of investigators have marshalled empirical evidence supporting the conclusion that the syndrome is essentially an artifact of selective observation and that its nuclear component, finger agnosia, is a nonspecific performance deficit reflecting more pervasive cognitive impairment and lacking the neurological implications originally claimed for it. On the other hand, the syndrome has its staunch defenders who have attacked the methods and logic

of the empiricists and have insisted that the constellation of symptoms described by Gerstmann some 50 years ago is a valuable index of focal brain disease.

My own studies, which were initiated about 25 years ago, were the first to cast serious doubt upon the reality and significance of the Gerstmann syndrome. Hence, although I *think* that I am free from bias, I can scarcely make that claim. However, I have tried to be impartial and to give equally careful consideration to the merits of the opposing positions on the basic issue. Only the occurrence of the syndrome in adult patients with acquired brain disease will be considered. The "developmental Gerstmann syndrome" is a question with its own specific problems and one that is best examined independently.

A BIT OF HISTORY

The final formulation of his syndrome was the product of the evolution of Gerstmann's thought on the topic over a number of years. In 1924, he described

* A. L. Benton, *Brain and Language*, 1977, 4, 45–62. Copyright 1977, Academic Press.

"finger agnosia" in a nonaphasic but mentally dulled patient and he interpreted the symptom as a reflection of a circumscribed defect in the most differentiated aspect of the body schema. The patient showed agraphia, acalculia, and slight impairment in right-left orientation, but these were, at the time, not linked by him to the disturbance in finger recognition. However, in 1927, he described two more patients with finger agnosia and agraphia and, at that time, he postulated that the two deficits constituted "a new syndrome," the underlying basis of which remained unclear. Further clinical observation led him, in 1930, to the description of the full syndrome, all the elements of which he now regarded as expressions of a disturbance of the body schema attributable to focal disease of the parieto-occipital area of the dominant hemisphere.

Shortly after Gerstmann's first publication in 1924, Herrmann and Pötzl (1926) described a second patient with finger agnosia and agraphia. They interpreted their patient's inability to show his fingers on command, as well as his awkward finger movements, to be a form of apraxia. Gerstmann (1927) contested this view, arguing that the impairment in fine finger movements, which he himself had also observed, was a consequence of the primary agnosic defect.

Some years later, Schilder (1931) took up the question in a larger context and concluded that there existed a number of independent defects associated with the naming, recognition, and movement of the fingers. He distinguished five types of defect, each with its specific lesional localization. One was the inability to show individual fingers on command, which he equated with the "finger agnosia" of Gerstmann and which, he agreed, corresponded to a lesion in the territory of the angular gyrus. On the other hand, the inability to name the fingers, which he called "finger aphasia," corresponded to a lesion in Wernicke's area, and the inability to identify the examiner's fingers, which he called "visual finger agnosia," corresponded to a more posteriorly placed occipital lesion. He distinguished between the inability to move the individual fingers on command ("apraxia of finger choice") and the inability to imitate finger postures ("constructive finger apraxia"), but ascribed both defects to lesions in the region of the supramarginal gyrus.

Once formulated, the Gerstmann syndrome was generally recognized by neurologists as a clinical entity. Many case reports describing patients who exhibited the four symptoms (always in combination with other deficits, such as constructional apraxia or aphasic disorder) appeared in the 1930s and early 1940s. Its localizing implication as a sign of disease of the posterior parietal area of the dominant hemisphere was also generally accepted.

Nevertheless, from the very beginning, some theoretically oriented neurologists who had devoted serious thought to the question tended to reject Gerstmann's view that the symptoms were the outcome of a partial dissolution of the body schema. Instead, they marshalled evidence in favor of broader conceptions that extended beyond the body schema by showing that "Gerstmann" patients invariably showed other types of perceptual or cognitive defects. Lange (1930, 1933) spoke of an impairment in directional sense, Conrad (1932) spoke of defects in configurational thinking, and Stengel (1944) spoke of a loss of spatial orientation. Stengel was particularly insistent in his emphasis that the Gerstmann syndrome should be considered a part of a more pervasive disorder of spatial disorientation rather than as an autonomous entity.

Thus, the early history of the syndrome shows two features that are relevant to the current controversy. The first was Schilder's analysis of performances having to do with the fingers into discrete types with differential neurological implications. The second was the forwarding of explanatory concepts that were broader than Gerstmann's body-schema hypothesis and that viewed the Gerstmann symptoms as part of a more general syndrome encompassing other types of impairment.

THE COMPONENTS OF THE SYNDROME

A meaningful analysis of recent developments in thought about the Gerstmann syndrome required that each of its individual elements be subjected to scrutiny. In reality, each "symptom" in the aggregate refers not to a single disability but to a range of performance deficits of differing scope and complexity and making different demands on cognitive capacity.

Finger agnosia

Although Schilder (1931) did not present empirical evidence to support his classification of specific types of impairment in finger recognition and praxis, his general conception that a variety of performance deficits may be observed has been fully validated. For example, Ettlinger (1963) studied the performances of patients with parietal lobe disease on 12 tests of finger recognition. Some tests required a naming response; others called for a nonverbal localizing response. Some required the patient to identify his own fingers; others required identification on a model or the examiner's hand. He found a fairly high degree of specificity in performance pattern, with failure on one test having only limited predictive significance with respect to failure on the other tests. He also found that the frequency of failure differed

according to the nature of the test. Those requiring identification on the basis of tactile stimulation without vision and those requiring identification on the fingers of the examiner or a model elicited more frequent failure than did those performed under vision or calling for localization on the patient's own hand. Similarly, in developing their own tests to assess finger recognition, Kinsbourne and Warrington (1962) emphasized that "essential to finger agnosia is the manner of testing for it" and their case material included instances of dissociation between levels of performance on verbal tests of finger recognition and their nonverbal tests.

Poeck and Orgass (1969) assessed diverse aspects of finger recognition in an unselected group of patients with brain disease with verbal and nonverbal tests. Their results indicated that the tests could not be considered to form a homogeneous set of measures. Tests requiring naming or identification by name formed a cluster and failure on them was closely associated with aphasic disorder and a low WAIS Verbal Scale IQ. In contrast, nonverbal finger identification was more closely correlated with low WAIS Performance Scale IQ and was unrelated to aphasic disorder.

The findings of these studies lead to the conclusion that there is no such entity as a unitary "finger sense" or its pathological counterpart, a unitary "finger agnosia." Specific finger recognition tasks make distinctive demands on cognitive capacity. Verbal tasks obviously call on linguistic skills and it is not surprising that performance on them should be closely associated with aphasic disorder. Successful finger identification on the basis of tactile stimulation alone calls for intersensory integrative operations to the degree that tactile information must be translated into visual terms in order to make the localization in visual space. Identification of fingers on a model implies some capacity for representational thinking (cf. Lefford, Birch, & Green, 1974).

This conclusion implies that performance level on a battery of diverse tests designed to measure finger recognition can have only a nonspecific neuropsychological significance. The point can be illustrated by the findings of a study in which I gave an 80-item battery consisting of verbal and nonverbal tests assessing finger recognition capacity to groups of control and brain-diseased patients, matched for age and educational background (Benton, 1961). Only 31% of the control group made perfect scores and 19% made 5 or more errors on this rather demanding test. However, only 8% made as many as 9–12 errors. In contrast, no less than 23% of the brain-diseased patients performed at a level below that of the poorest control patient and another 18% made 9–12 errors, i.e., they performed at a level exceeded by 92% of the controls. These results suggest that performance on a comprehensive test battery designed to measure diverse aspects of finger recognition is itself a rather sensitive measure of the presence of brain disease. But, to interpret the findings as indicating that about 25% of patients with brain disease suffer from a specific "finger agnosia" seems rather farfetched. A more plausible explanation is that, since this battery of finger recognition tests makes demands on diverse abilities as well as on the capacity for sustained attention, the overall performance level of a substantial proportion of patients with brain disease is likely to be significantly below expectations.

The localizing significance of disturbances in finger recognition also may be considered. Traditionally, these disturbances, whether indexed by verbal or nonverbal test performance, have been associated with disease of the left hemisphere. The study of Sauguet, Benton, and

Hécaen (1971) supported this assumption. Restricting consideration to patients with unilateral disease and without evidence of general mental impairment, they found that a substantial proportion (19–67%) of left-hemisphere-damaged patients with receptive language deficit performed defectively on finger recognition tests. In contrast, the incidence of defective performance in nonaphasic patients with either left or right hemisphere disease was negligible. However, the recent study of Gainotti, Cianchetti, and Tiacci (1972) of the performances of *unselected* groups of patients with unilateral disease produced a different pattern of results. Bilateral impairment in finger recognition was as frequently encountered in patients with right hemisphere disease as in those with left hemisphere lesions (16 vs. 18%). But most of the right hemisphere patients with "finger agnosia" showed evidence of general mental deterioration, while most of the left hemisphere patients were aphasic. Thus, the findings of the two studies are not in disagreement. Considered together, they suggest that defects in finger recognition are related to different disabilities, depending upon side of lesion, and they confirm the emphasis placed by Poeck and Orgass (1969) on the overriding importance of aphasia and general mental impairment as primary determinants of failing performance.

Right-left disorientation

"Right-left disorientation" is an equally broad concept that covers failure on tasks of different levels of complexity and of a diverse qualitative nature (cf. Benton, 1959, 1968; Poeck & Orgass, 1967). The patient may be required to name lateral body parts, to execute movements to verbal command or to imitate the examiner's movements. He may be required to execute a single command (e.g., show the left hand) or a double command (e.g., touch the left eye with the right hand). He may be requested to identify his own lateral body parts or those of the examiner's, the latter task assessing whether or not he understands the relativistic nature of right-left orientation. He may be required to execute commands that involve both the "own body" and "confronting person" systems of right-left orientation, as when asked to touch the *examiner's* right ear with *his* left hand. Failure in all of these tasks, with the possible exception of imitation, is closely associated with the presence of receptive aphasic disorder (Head, 1926; Benton, 1959; Poeck & Orgass, 1967; Sauguet, Benton, & Hécaen, 1971). On the other hand, patients with right hemisphere disease often fail on imitation tasks, while performing adequately on verbal tasks, perhaps because of the presence of a more general visuospatial disability (Sauguet, Benton, & Hécaen. 1971). A recent case study by Dennis (1976) describes a striking dissociation in performance on verbal and nonverbal right-left discrimination tasks on the part of a patient who had undergone a left temporal resection for relief of seizures 3 years prior to examination.

Here again, one deals with a set of tasks that makes demands on expressive language, receptive language, conceptual thinking, somatosensory schemata, spatial thinking, and capacity for sustained attention. The same patients who had been given the finger localization test were also given a 32-item test assessing a number of aspects of right-left orientation (cf. Benton, 1959). Twenty-three percent of the brain-diseased patients performed on a level exceeded by 99% of the control group. It is surely more plausible to interpret these failing performances as reflecting any of a number of diverse disabilities than to infer that such a large number of brain-damaged patients show mild or severe impairment of a single specific function.

Agraphia

Disturbances in writing associated with brain disease are often divided into two major types. "Aphasic" agraphia is characterized by misspelling, omissions and intrusions, word and letter substitutions and nonsense words with passable calligraphy; in severe cases, the result is jargon agraphia, in which individual letters and words are recognizable but no meaningful message is conveyed. "Apraxic," "parietal," or "spatial" agraphia is characterized by faulty formation of letters and words and inability to keep to the line of writing; in severe cases, the result is an unintelligible scrawl. Copying as well as writing to dictation is disturbed in "apraxic" agraphia, while copying is generally superior to writing to dictation in "aphasic" agraphia and, indeed, may be quite intact. This typological classification provides a useful framework within which the writing performances of patients may be evaluated. However, there is no doubt that it is an oversimplification and does not do justice to the diverse forms that writing disturbances may take or to the relationships between these disturbances and performances with which they share common elements, such as block writing and oral spelling.

Gerstmann's (1924) first case and Conrad's (1932) case showed a primarily "apraxic" agraphia with inability to hold to the line of writing and with impairment in copying as well as writing to dictation. In contrast, the two cases reported by Gerstmann in 1927 showed relatively intact ability to copy. Critchley (1953) states that the Gerstmann patient "typically" is able to copy and hence does not present the characteristic features of a "parietal" dysgraphia. However, he also considers it plausible that "Gerstmann's agraphia is really a writing dyspraxia, and so bears no closer affinity to speech loss than does, say an articulatory dyspraxia" (Critchley, 1953, p. 211). Kinsbourne and Warrington (1962, 1964) emphasize the prominence of errors of letter order in both the writing and oral spelling of Gerstmann patients in contrast to the intrusions or extraneous letter errors found in the writing of aphasic patients. However, they also report difficulties in forming letters, as well as in copying, in these patients. Absolute agraphia, i.e., inability to write even a single letter or digit, has also been described in patients with a presumed Gerstmann syndrome (cf. Pedersen, 1936).

Thus, it appears that diverse types of agraphia may be shown by patients with the Gerstmann syndrome. Kinsbourne and Warrington believe that failure to take account of the qualitative features of the writing of Gerstmann patients (i.e., the prominence of letter order errors) and those of aphasic patients is in part responsible for contradictory findings regarding the relationship between the syndrome and aphasia.

Acalculia

Like the other elements of the syndrome, "acalculia" represents performance failure that may arise from diverse sources and take a number of forms (cf. Grewel, 1952; Hécaen, 1962, 1972; Benson & Weir, 1973). It is often found in association with aphasic disorders where the difficulty appears to be loss of the ability to understand or to read numbers. A "spatial" acalculia, characterized by difficulty in aligning numbers in the proper columns, carrying numbers, and shifting attention from one point to another, and reflected more clearly in written than in oral calculation, has also been described. Finally, a purer type of disability, "anarithmetria," consisting of impairment in one or another type of computation with presumed ability to remember, read, and carry numbers, has been postulated. "Aphasic" acalculia is, of course, associated primarily with left hemisphere disease. "Spatial" acalculia is found rather more often in cases of right hemisphere disease, typically in association with other visuoperceptive and visuospatial defects. Anarithmetria is encountered in demented patients where it may reflect impaired concentration and short-term memory. In nondemented patients with focal brain disease, it is usually associated with left hemisphere disease.

Is the acalculia of the Gerstmann syndrome of a specific type? Both Critchley (1953) and Hécaen (1972) state that the form of acalculia most likely to be encountered in patients with the Gerstmann syndrome is the spatial type, more evident in written than in oral calculation and with faulty alignment of numbers as a prominent difficulty. On the other hand, Gerstmann (1940) himself emphasized that it was the purer "anarithmetric" type of calculation difficulty which was found in association with the other elements of the syndrome rather than either the "aphasic" or, as he termed it, the "apractic" type. His opinion is, of course, understandable in view of his theoretical assumption of "an intimate relationship between differentiation of fingers and calculation." From their description, it appears that the patients of Kinsbourne and Warrington (1962) showed features of both "aphasic" and "spatial" acalculia. "Adding and subtracting double figures was nearly impossible. On paper, the columns of figures were hopelessly muddled. Reading or writing down compound figures was very poor." (pp. 54–55.) In another context, Kinsbourne and Rosenfield (1974) write that milder impairment in written, as compared to oral, calculation is typical of the Gerstmann syndrome.

Given this diversity in opinion, one must conclude that it is not at all clear that a particular type of acalculia is characteristic of the Gerstmann syndrome.

A summing up

It is quite evident that the elements of the Gerstmann syndrome do not correspond to well-defined specific disabilities, but rather to impairment in one or more of the diverse mental operations involved in finger recognition, lateral orientation, writing, or calculation. Some authors have tried to identify the specific deficits underlying failing performance in one or another area. For example, as has been seen, Kinsbourne and Warrington implicate letter order errors as the cardinal feature of the agraphia of Gerstmann patients, and Critchley and Hécaen indicate that the impairment in calculation is of the "spatial" type. But these distinctions are based on clinical impression and lack a solid empirical foundation. At the same time, studies of the Gerstmann syndrome generally have not taken account of them. Consequently, *if* these distinctions are valid, the failure to respect them must be a potent source of confusion.

THE IMPACT OF RECENT STUDIES

Two major studies in the early 1960s cast serious doubt on the neurological significance of the Gerstmann syndrome and, indeed, on its actual existence. One was my study of the interrelations among the elements of the syndrome and other symptoms referable to parietal lobe disease (Benton, 1961). The second was the clini-copathological investigation of Heimburger, DeMyer, and Reitan (1964).

My study addressed the question of whether the syndrome is a naturally occurring combination of symptoms or "only one of a very large number of more or less fortuitous combinations of behavioural deficits which may be encountered in patients with cerebral disease." (Benton, 1961, p. 176). It was pointed out that a variety of other deficits had been observed to occur in association with each of the four symptoms, most notably aphasic disorder, general mental impairment, constructional apraxia, alexia, and visuoperceptual deficits. I had previously advanced the hypothesis that both bilateral finger agnosia and right-left disorientation in patients with left hemisphere disease are expressions of impairment of language function, i.e., of an aphasic disorder (Benton, 1959).

The study assessed the interrelations among seven performances—right-left orientation, finger recognition, calculation, writing, constructional praxis, reading, and nonverbal visual memory—in 100 patients with hemispheric disease. The results were unequivocal in their indications that the three non-Gerstmann performances correlated as closely with the Gerstmann performances as the latter did with each other. A second analysis, restricted to the performances of the 12 patients in the group with left parietal lobe disease, generated the same results. The mean correlation coefficient between finger recognition and the other three components of the syndrome was .38 and that between right-left orientation and the other three components was .53, but constructional praxis and reading correlated as closely with the four components of the syndrome (mean r = .53 and .61, respectively). Inspection of the performance patterns of these patients with left parietal lobe disease disclosed that three of the four patients who showed three Gerst-mann symptoms also showed at least two of the three non-Gerstmann deficits. The remaining case was that of a woman with impaired right-left orientation, writing, and calculation (but absolutely perfect finger recognition), who showed only the additional symptom of defective reading. She was seen 4 years after removal of a clot and a considerable amount of necro-tic tissue from the left posterior parieto-temporal area, and one could view her as an example of a relatively pure partial Gerstmann syndrome with appropriate localizing implications if it were not for the fact that the lady was clinically aphasic. She had word-finding difficulties and limitations in understanding conver-sational speech. Formal testing disclosed defective visual and tactile naming, defec-tive understanding of oral language, impaired repetition, and severe defects in reading and writing.

Thus, it seemed clear that the particu-lar combination of deficits forming the syndrome showed no stronger internal associative bonds than did a variety of other combinations of deficits and I drew the conclusion that "judged from the standpoint of behavioural analysis, the Gerstmann syndrome is a fiction; it is simply an artifact of defective and biased observations" (Benton, 1961, p. 180).

The implications of the study of Heimburger, DeMyer, and Reitan (1964) were equally destructive of the concept of an autonomous Gerstmann syndrome with a distinctive neurological signifi-cance. Of a total sample of 456 patients, 111 were found to have one or more com-ponents of the syndrome, as defined by objective assessment procedures, and 23 showed all four components. Every patient in the latter subgroup was aphasic, as judged from their performance on stan-dardized tests. Among the 23 patients who showed three Gerstmann symptoms,

22 were aphasic. From a neuropathologi-cal standpoint, the lesions in the patients with the full syndrome were invariably large and generally of a progressive or recurrent nature. Forty-eight percent were known to be dead 5 years after the initial work-up. In the majority of cases, the left angular gyrus was involved, but in no case was the lesion restricted to that area, and the left superior temporal gyrus and supramarginal gyrus were as frequently compromised by these extensive lesions. Heimburger, DeMyer, and Reitan there-fore concluded that the "syndrome is not to be regarded as an autonomous entity, but merges with numerous other neurolo-gical deficits, notably aphasia."

Subsequently, a series of studies by Poeck and Orgass (1966, 1967, 1969) on the relationship of the Gerstmann syn-drome and its elements to aphasia and mental deterioration strongly reinforced this negative conclusion. In their investi-gation of 50 unselected patients with hemispheric disease, they identified 9 who showed either the full syndrome or at least three components of it. Eight of these 9 patients were aphasic and all showed at least one other concomitant deficit, such as constructional apraxia and impairment in verbal memory. All 9 patients had either left hemisphere or bilateral disease. In contrast, patients showing only one or two components of the syndrome were as likely to have right hemisphere lesions as left.

The impact of these studies was, in effect, to destroy the autonomy of the Gerstmann syndrome and its alleged localizing significance. Briefly stated, they indicated the following. The full Gerst-mann syndrome is invariably associated with aphasia and/or general mental impairment; it does not appear in isola-tion from more general linguistic or cogni-tive defects, and to abstract these particular deficits from their matrix and give it the status of a syndrome is both arbitrary and meaningless; the full Gerstmann syndrome does indeed imply left hemisphere disease, but this implication cannot be considered in isolation from the deficits with which it is so intimately associated, most notably, aphasic disorder which also implies left hemisphere disease.

We may turn now to two major studies that defend the autonomy and localizing significance of the syndrome. The first is by Kinsbourne and Warrington (1962), which may be considered to be a direct response to the implications of my 1961 study. The second is a case report by Strub and Geschwind (1974; Geschwind & Strub, 1975) which describes a patient with the Gerstmann syndrome and which includes a critique of the negative studies.

The study of Kinsbourne and Warrington dealt with 12 patients who were selected because they exhibited one or more elements of the Gerstmann syndrome; 8 patients showed the complete syndrome and two showed three deficits. In these 10 cases, the lesion was left-sided in 4, right-sided in 2, and bilateral in 4 cases. Constructional apraxia was present in all cases. All but 1 patient were judged to have some degree of intellectual deterioration. However, only 3 cases were clinically aphasic. A heterogeneous control group of 20 patients with brain disease who did not show impairment in finger recognition, as assessed by nonverbal tests, was also formed. Five of these patients were moderately or severely aphasic and 3 were minimally aphasic. All but 1 showed some degree of intellectual deterioration.

Kinsbourne and Warrington drew two major conclusions from these observations. The first was that, since the majority of their Gerstmann patients were not aphasic and, conversely, since there were eight aphasic patients in their control group, impairment in language function is not essential for the appearance of finger agnosia. Their second conclusion was that, since the majority of their Gerstmann patients showed the full syndrome, the "conjunction of symptoms is more than coincidental."

Strub and Geschwind (1974) present a case of the full Gerstmann syndrome without aphasia and use this case as a springboard for discussion of the problems involved in assessing whether or not the Gerstmann aggregate is, in fact, a syndrome. The case was that of a 52-year-old woman who was referred to the neurosurgical service of Charity Hospital in New Orleans because of progressive impairment in writing and calculation, both of which were confirmed on examination. She showed intact right-left orientation both on her own body and on that of the examiner. However, she failed badly when she had to use both systems of orientation concurrently, e.g., when she was asked to touch the *examiner's* left hand with *her* left hand. She named her own fingers accurately, but could neither identify the examiner's fingers by name nor touch a finger on the examiner's corresponding to one touched on her own hand. She was not aphasic. Her speech was fluent, accurate, and with normal prosody, with only an occasional phonemic paraphasia when she had to pronounce an unfamiliar word. Oral language comprehension and reading comprehension were essentially intact. Her WAIS Verbal Scale IQ was 101, which was only about 10 points below expectations for this rather bright lady. She showed a marked constructional apraxia and her WAIS Performance Scale IQ was only 67. She showed geographic disorientation and a mild dyspraxia for dressing. She had a normal EEG, echogram, brain scan, and angiogram, but cortical atrophy was evident on the pneumoencephalogram. The presumptive diagnosis was presenile dementia.

In summary, this was allegedly a patient with agraphia, acalculia, finger agnosia, right-left disorientation, and constructional apraxia with practically completely intact spoken language. Hence, it is marshalled as evidence against the view that the Gerstmann syndrome is merely an expression of aphasic disorder.

The more important part of Strub and Geschwind's (1974) paper is the authors' discussion of the conceptual aspects of the question and the shortcomings of empirical studies purporting to show that the Gerstmann aggregate is not a syndrome in any meaningful sense. Their first point is that intercorrelational studies, such as my own, demonstrating that the elements of the syndrome do not have particularly strong internal associative bonds, are based on a misunderstanding of the concept of "syndrome" and, hence, are not relevant to the issue.

In general, a syndrome is a collection of signs and symptoms which, in fact, have a low intercorrelation, but which, when present together in a single patient, strongly suggest the presence of a specific disease. For example, consider the triad of skin pigmentation, liver disease, and diabetes. In most cases, a patient with any of these findings will not manifest the other two. On the other hand, when all three occur together there is a strong chance that one is dealing with hemochromatosis. Indeed, if the intercorrelation among the elements of a syndrome were very high, only one component would be required for the physician to make the correct diagnosis and a search for the other components would be unnecessary. The appropriate question about the Gerstmann syndrome is whether the presence of all four components does predict with high accuracy damage in the left parietal area. (Strub & Geschwind, 1974, p. 378)

Their second point is that the case

reported, as well as others in the series of Heimburger, DeMyer, and Reitan (1964) and Poeck and Orgass (1966), offer examples of the occurrence of the Gerstmann syndrome without aphasia. Therefore, despite the empirically established close correlation between the syndrome and aphasia, one cannot consider aphasic disorder to be the factor underlying the appearance of the syndrome.

Their third point is that the Gerstmann syndrome, when it occurs in the absence of aphasic disorder, does have a specific localizing significance in implicating dysfunction of the left posterior parietal area and they cite the findings of Heimburger, DeMyer, and Reitan and of Poeck and Orgass, as well as the Strub-Geschwind case, to support this contention.

REFLECTIONS

We have reviewed the major studies underlying the controversy about the autonomy of the Gerstmann syndrome and its neuropsychological significance. Each may be critically evaluated in terms of the information bearing on the question that it has generated.

First, we may consider my 1961 study, which was of a purely behavioral nature. It assessed the intercorrelations both within the Gerstmann symptoms and between these symptoms and other "parietal" symptoms and found that the Gerstmann symptoms appeared to be part of a larger syndrome. There was no evidence that the "syndrome" formed a coherent and autonomous unity. The conclusion was drawn that the singling out of the Gerstmann aggregate out of the 35 possible aggregates that could be formed from the seven deficits which were assessed was arbitrary and unjustified. Admittedly, the conclusion is vulnerable to the criticism leveled by Strub and Geschwind that a statistical determination of the degree of concurrence of symptoms without reference to underlying pathology is not relevant to the concept of the "syndrome" in medical thought.

The findings of the Heimburger-DeMyer-Reitan study were clear enough. Dealing with a large case material, they never encountered the Gerstmann syndrome in isolation. In 45 out of 46 cases an aphasic disorder was present. In all cases, other "parietal" deficits such as constructional apraxia were in evidence. The responsible lesions did indeed involve the left posterior parietal area, but they were always extensive and never of a limited focal character. They also found that, in the majority of cases, the lesions were of a "destructive" character, as they termed it, in that a large mass of tissue was involved, progression or recurrence was the rule, and the outlook for survival was not good. I think it is hard to discount the implications of this study that the Gerstmann aggregate is part of a larger assemblage of symptoms reflecting extensive disease of the left hemisphere. Strub and Geschwind state that Heimburger, DeMyer, and Reitan reported cases of the Gerstmann syndrome without aphasia, but this is an overstatement. It can apply only to patients showing one or two components and not to those showing three components or the full syndrome.

In contrast to my 1961 study, Poeck and Orgass (1966) used quite simple tests to assess Gerstmann and non-Gerstmann performance. Hence, their confirmation of my findings that the elements of the Gerstmann syndrome are as closely associated with other deficits as they are with each other is particularly important, because it mitigates the criticism that variation in general intellectual competence may have been responsible for the essential equal degree of correlation among all of the performances. Poeck and Orgass also confirmed the finding of Heimburger, DeMyer, and Reitan that aphasic disorder is seen virtually always in patients with either the full syndrome or three elements of it. Again, the statement by Strub and Geschwind that they encountered Gerstmann patients who were not aphasic, although literally accurate, is somewhat misleading. Only one of their nine patients with three or four Gerstmann symptoms was not aphasic. The incidence of aphasic disorder in their patients who showed only one or two symptoms was lower, but it is, of course, quite questionable whether or not such patients should be considered as having a "Gerstmann syndrome".

The findings reported by Kinsbourne and Warrington (1962) are somewhat difficult to intepret because of the selection procedures employed and some apparent inconsistencies. Only three of their Gerstmann patients were judged to be clinically aphasic. However, as Heimburger, DeMyer, and Reitan (1964) have noted, some of their nonaphasic patients are described as having at least mild difficulties in reading, naming, and oral language understanding. Moreover, most showed some degree of mental deterioration. There seems to be little basis for the conclusion that the elements of the Gerstmann syndrome form an autonomous entity, since the patients were selected in the first place on the basis of showing the syndrome. Poeck and Orgass (1975) have pointed out that neither they nor I maintained that the degree of correlation among the Gerstmann symptoms is low, but rather that the correlation between the Gerstmann symptoms and other deficits is as close as that among the Gerstmann deficits themselves. Nevertheless, Kinsbourne and Warrington have shown clearly that many aphasic patients perform adequately on finger recognition tasks that do not require producing or understanding the names of the fingers.

The case report of Strub and Geschwind exemplifies the ambiguities that bedevil discussion of the Gerstmann syndrome. Their patient is said to have shown the syndrome and yet to have been completely free of aphasic disorder, although an at least moderate degree of general mental impairment was quite evident. She showed a clear "aphasic" agraphia and severe impairment in calculation. However, that she showed "finger agnosia" in the Gerstmann sense is quite questionable, since she could name her own fingers accurately and failed only when required to identify the fingers of the examiner. In other words, she showed the "visual finger agnosia" of Schilder rather than the classic "finger agnosia" of Gerstmann. As Poeck and Orgass (1975) have pointed out in a trenchant critique of the case report, the disability fits in well with the pervasive visual disorientation that this patient showed. Nor did the patient show right-left disorientation to a clinically significant degree. She could localize lateral body parts both on herself and the examiner. It was only when she was required to utilize both systems of orientation concurrently that she failed. But this is a type of failure in conceptual thinking that is shown regularly by patients who are mentally impaired and, indeed, by many normal subjects. Thus, the case report does not stand up well as an example of a "Gerstmann syndrome without aphasia."

We turn now to their analysis of the conceptual aspects of the problem. In my view, their reasoning and logic are sound. A syndrome is a combination of signs and symptoms that permits a valid inference about underlying pathology or pathogenetic mechanisms and there is no necessity for the elements of a syndrome to occur always, or even frequently, in conjuntion with each other.

But I do not believe that the logic applies to the aggregate of deficits known as the Gerstmann syndrome. There is, first of all, the fact that there is not in the entire literature on the topic a single "pure" case of the full Gerstmann syndrome unaccompanied by other deficits such as constructional apraxia or aphasia. Certainly, the Strub-Geschwind case would not fit in this category. Moreover, there is no evidence that the *specific* combination of symptoms called the "Gerstmann syndrome" possesses a neurological significance different from other combinations of symptoms that might be assembled to form a "syndrome" from which left posterior parietal lobe disease might be inferred. Critchley (1966) mentions a number of such combinations to which the appellation "syndrome" might be applied. Finally, assuming that relatively pure instances of the Gerstmann syndrome referable to focal posterior parietal disease are identified, one must ask whether it is the syndrome as a whole or only certain components of it that give the combination a localizing significance. It seems to me extremely probable that the localizing implications are carried neither by the aggregate as a whole nor by its nuclear component, finger agnosia, but by agraphia and acalculia, which, both singly and in combination, always raise the question of focal posterior left hemisphere disease.

CONCLUSION

This review of the recent literature on the reality and significance of the Gerstmann syndrome seems to me to indicate that the case for it is even weaker than when I first raised the question 25 years ago (Benton & Abramson, 1952). Both large-scale investigation and intensive case study have failed to generate evidence that this aggregate is anything more than an arbitrary grouping of deficits without a distinctive neuropsychological significance. Its localizing significance appears to be related, on the one hand, to its very close association with aphasic disorder and, on the other hand, to the circumstances that two of its components are agraphia and acalculia. Finger agnosia, its nuclear component, appears to have a nonspecific neurologic significance, carrying only the implication of either aphasic disorder or general mental impairment.

Yet, some areas of uncertainty deserve further consideration. As has been pointed out, the components of the Gerstmann aggregate are, in reality, collective terms for diverse types of disability of a perceptual, praxic, linguistic, and conceptual nature. It is possible that, if studies in the area defined these disabilities more carefully, a clearer understanding of the Gerstmann aggregate would be achieved. It is unlikely that this will lead to a resurrection of the "syndrome," but such analytic study might identify those aspects of impaired finger recognition and right-left disorientation that possess specific neurological implications.

A second point that merits scrutiny is the nature of the relationship of defective finger recognition and right-left orientation to aphasia, general mental impairment, and visual disorientation. That these defects are practically dependent upon the broader linguistic and intellectual impairment has been well established (Poeck & Orgass, 1966; Sauguet, Benton, & Hécaen, 1971). But, although receptive aphasic disorder and general mental impairment are necessary conditions for the appearance of finger agnosia and right-left disorientation, they are not sufficient conditions for these failures in performance. As the Kinsbourne-Warrington (1962) and Benton-Sauguet-Hécaen (1971) studies showed, many patients with significant receptive aphasic disorder

perform adequately on finger recognition and right-left orientation tasks. Benton (1959) and Selecki and Herron (1965) have suggested that aphasic disorder interacts with another factor, such as somatosensory impairment or a primary disturbance of the body schema, to produce defective performance in these areas. The finding of Gainotti, Cianchetti, and Tiacci (1972) that finger agnosia is significantly related to the presence of contralateral sensory impairment in patients with left hemisphere disease (but not in those with right hemisphere lesions) provides some support for this suggestion. More detailed investigation of this possibility might well yield further insight into the neurological significance of defective finger recognition and right-left orientation.

REFERENCES

Benson, D. F., & Weir, W. F. 1972. Acalculia: Acquired anarithmetria. *Cortex*, 8, 465–472.

Benton, A. L. 1959. *Right-left discrimination and finger localization: Development and pathology.* New York: Hoeber-Harper.

Benton, A. L. 1961. The fiction of the "Gerstmann syndrome." *Journal of Neurology, Neurosurgery and Psychiatry*, **24**, 176–181.

Benton, A. L. 1968. Right-left discrimination. *Pediatric Clinics of North America*, **15**, 747–758.

Benton, A. L., & Abramson, L. S. 1952. Gerstmann symptoms following electroshock treatment. *Archives of Neurology and Psychiatry*, **68**, 248–257.

Conrad, K. L. 1932. Versuch einer psychologischen Analyse des Parietalsyndroms. *Monatsschrift für Psychiatrie und Neurologie*, **84**, 28–97.

Critchley, M. 1953. *The parietal lobes.* London: Arnold.

Critchley, M. 1966. The enigma of Gerstmann's syndrome. *Brain*, 89, 183–198.

Dennis, M. 1976. Dissociated naming and locating of body parts after left anterior temporal lobe resection. *Brain and Language*, 3, 147–163.

Ettlinger, G. 1963. Defective identification of fingers. *Neuropsychologia*, 1, 39–45.

Gainotti, G., Cianchetti, C., & Tiacci, C. 1972. The influence of hemispheric side of lesion on non-verbal tasks of finger localization. *Cortex*, 8, 364–382.

Gerstmann, J. 1924. Fingeragnosie: eine umschriebene Störung der Orientierung am eigenen Körper. *Wiener klinische Wochenschrift*, 37, 1010–1012.

Gerstmann, J. 1927. Fingeragnosie und isolierte Agraphie: ein neues Syndrom. *Zeitschrift für die gesamte Neurologie und Psychiatrie*, 108, 152–177.

Gerstmann, J. 1930. Zur Symptomatologie der Hirnläsionen im Übergangsgebiet der unteren Parietal- und mittlerem Occipitalwindung. *Nervenarzt*, 3, 691–695.

Gerstmann, J. 1940. Syndrome of finger agnosia, disorientation for right and left, agraphia and acalculia. *Archives of Neurology and Psychiatry*, 44: 398–408.

Geschwind, N., & Strub, R. 1975. Gerstmann syndrome without aphasia: A reply to Poeck & Orgass. *Cortex*, 11, 296–298.

Grewel. F. 1952. Acalculia. *Brain*, 75, 397–407.

Head, H. 1926. *Aphasia and kindred disorders and speech*. Cambridge, England: The University Press.

Hécaen. H. 1962. Clinical symptomatology in right and left hemispheric lesions. In V. B. Mountcastle (Ed.), *Interhemispheric relations and cerebal dominance*. Baltimore: Johns Hopkins Press.

Hécaen. H. 1972. *Introduction a la neuropsychologie*. Paris: Larousse.

Heimburger, R. F., DeMyer, W. C., & Reitan, R. M. 1964. Implications of Gerstmann's syndrome. *Journal of Neurology, Neurosurgery and Psychiatry*, 27, 52–57.

Herrmann, G., & Pötzl, O. 1926. *Über die Agraphie und ihre lokaldiagnostischen Beziehungen*. Berlin: Karger.

Kinsbourne, M., & Rosenfield, D. 1974. Agraphia selective for written spelling: An experimental case study. *Brain and Language*, 1: 215–226.

Kinsbourne, M., & Warrington, E. K. 1962. A study of finger agnosia. *Brain*, 85, 47–66.

Kinsbourne, M., & Warrington, E. K. 1964. Disorders of spelling. *Journal of Neurology, Neurosurgery and Psychiatry*, 27, 296–299.

Lange, J. 1930. Fingeragnosie und Agraphie. *Monatsschrift für Psychiatrie und Neurologie* 76, 129–188.

Lange, J. 1933. Probleme der Fingeragnosie. *Zeitschrift für die gesamte Neurologie und Psychiatrie*, 147, 594–610.

Lefford, A., Birch, H. G., & Green, G. 1974. The perceptual and cognitive bases for finger localization and selective finger movement in preschool children. *Child Development*, 45, 335–343.

Pederson, O. 1936. Zur Kenntnis der Symptomatologie der parietoccipitalen Übergangsregion. *Archiv für Psychiatrie*, 105, 535–549.

Poeck, K., & Orgass, B. 1966. Gerstmann's syndrome and aphasia. *Cortex*, 2, 421–427.

Poeck, K., & Orgass, B. 1967. Über Störungen der Rechts-Links Orientierung. *Nervenarzt*, 38, 285–291.

Poeck, K., & Orgass, B. 1969. An experimental investigation of finger agnosia. *Neurology*, 19, 801–807.

Poeck, K., & Orgass, B. 1975. Gerstmann syndrome without aphasia: Comments on the paper by Strub and Geschwind. *Cortex*, 11, 291–295.

Sauguet, J., Benton, A. L., & Hécaen, H. 1971. Disturbances of the body schema in relation to language impairment and hemispheric locus of lesion. *Journal of Neurology, Neurosurgery and Psychiatry*, 34, 496–501.

Schilder, P. 1931. Fingeragnosie, Fingerapraxie, Fingeraphasie. *Nervenarzt*, 4, 625–629.

Selecki, B. R., & Herron J. T. 1965. Disturbances of the verbal body image: A particular syndrome of sensory aphasia. *Journal of Nervous and Mental Disease*, 141, 42–52.

Stengel, E. 1944. Loss of spatial orientation, constructional apraxia and Gerstmann's syndrome. *Journal of Mental Science*, 90, 753–760.

Strub, R., & Geschwind, N. 1974. Gerstmann syndrome without aphasia. *Cortex*, 10, 378–387.

VII.
Hemispheric Dominance and Vision

21.

Stereoscopic Vision in Patients with Unilateral Cerebral Disease*

Carmon and Bechtoldt[1] have recently reported a striking impairment in stereoscopic vision in patients with disease of the right hemisphere; in contrast, patients with left hemisphere disease performed on the same level as did control patients without cerebral disease. Random-letter stereograms, generated from an IBM 7044 computer program[2] and representing a slight modification of the random-dot stereograms developed by Julesz,[3] were employed to assess capacity for stereoscopic vision. These stereograms provide an almost ideal method for the investigation of binocular depth perception, since they eliminate monocular figure-ground contours and other monocular cues that could be utilized to achieve stereoscopic vision. They also possess the advantage of permitting the experimenter to vary in a systematic manner such factors as matrix density and degree of retinal disparity which may influence level of performance of this type of task.[4,5] Car-

mon and Bechtoldt interpret their results as supporting the hypothesis that, in the absence of monocular cues of form and depth, the right hemisphere is "dominant" for stereopsis in human subjects.

These remarkable findings and their far-reaching theoretical and practical implications led us to undertake an independent replication of the Carmon-Bechtoldt study on a group of patients in another clinical setting. We employed the same test materials (supplied by Dr. Bechtoldt) and, with certain modifications, the same procedure as in the original study.

MATERIALS AND METHODS

Subjects

Two groups of right-handed patients (nine with lesions of the left hemisphere and eight with lesions of the right hemisphere) on the neurological service of the Centre Neurochirurgical Sainte-Anne, Paris, were studied. Pathological and clinical characteristics of these patients were detailed in Table 19.

* A. L. Benton and H. Hécaen, *Neurology*, 1970, 20, 1084–1088.

Table 19. Pathological and clinical characteristics of subjects

Patients with lesions of the left hemisphere

1. MAZ 68–0104, male, age 28; traumatic lesion of parietotemporal area, verified at operation; aphasic, of conduction type; no visual field defect. Test score, 24.
2. BAR 68–0227, male, age 66; glioma of temporo-occipital area, verified at operation; aphasic; right homonymous hemianopia. Test score, 23.
3. GRA 66–1027, male, age 18; astrocytoma of parieto-temporo-occipital region; aphasic; right homonymous hemianopia. Test score, 24.
4. MAL 67–1663, male, age 39; vascular accident; right hemiparesis and hemisensory defect; not aphasic; no visual field defect. Test score, 24.
5. DUP 68–0411, male, age 46; vascular disease; not aphasic; right homonymous hemianopia. Test score, 24.
6. PAR 68–0647, male, age 48; vascular disease; not aphasic; no visual field defect. Test score, 21.
7. LEB 67–0748, female, age 31; astrocytoma of temporal lobe; aphasic, of motor and amnesic types; right homonymous hemianopia. Test score, 24.
8. LHE N.S.7037, female, age 40; intracerebral hematoma of temporal lobe; aphasic, of conduction type; no visual field defect. Test score, 24.
9. DEL 67–1123, female, age 59; vascular disease; aphasic; right inferior quadrantanopia. Test score, 24.

Patients with lesions of the right hemisphere

1. THI 67–1468, male, age 48; thrombosis of middle cerebral artery; not aphasic; no visual field defect. Test score, 16.
2. ADJ 68–0236, male, age 53; metastatic epithelioma of temporal lobe; not aphasic; no visual field defect. Test score, 12.
3. TET 68–0329, male, age 64; glioblastoma of temporal lobe; not aphasic; left inferior quadrantanopia. Test score, 24.
4. MAU 68–0603, male, age 48; atrophy secondary to occlusive vascular disease; previously hemiplegic with spatial disorientation; not aphasic; no visual field defect. Test score, 24.
5. COU 68–0570, male, age 42; intracerebral hematoma of frontal lobe; not aphasic; no visual field defect. Test score, 16.
6. CAV 68–0616, male, age 57; glioma of frontal lobe; not aphasic; no visual field defect. Test score, 18.
7. ROZ 68–0163, female, age 57; astrocytoma of parieto-occipital area; not aphasic; left inferior quadrantanopia. Test score, 8.
8. KOR 68–0452, female, age 53; astrocytoma of temporal lobe; not aphasic; left inferior quadrantanopia. Test score, 4.

Left-handed patients

1. THE 68–0267, male, age 61; glioma of left temporal lobe; Wada test indicated bilateral representation of language functions; pronounced amnesic aphasia and alexia but intact language comprehension; right upper quadrantanopia. Test score, 15.
2. BOV 68–0482, male, age 32; right frontal lobe resection and clipping of right anterior cerebral artery after rupture of aneurysm of anterior communicating artery; not aphasic; no visual field defect; shows confabulation and temporal disorientation. Test score, 24.

Materials

The visual stimuli were computer-generated, 35-mm. random-letter stereograms as described by Carmon and Bechtoldt. The stereograms were presented in a Realist Electric Stereoviewer, Model 2062, supplied with a 44-mm. lens system, illumination level being set at 3.5-footcandles. Each slide presented a stereoscopic square field of 23.3° visual angle within which the patient was instructed to identify and locate a smaller square of 5° visual angle. The small square was distinguishable from the large square, in which it was embedded only by the presence of horizontal binocular disparity between the two half-images. Thus no monocular cue indicated the location of the small square in one of the four quadrants of the large square. Three levels of matrix density (defined as the ratio of the actual number of letters to the maximum possible number of letters in the slide) were used: 10, 40 and 100%. In addition, 2° of horizontal disparity were introduced: a nasal shift for the small square of one column of letters (15.5' of visual arc) and a nasal shift of three columns of letters (46.5' of visual arc). The effect of this shift in the nasal direction is to lead to a judgment that the small square is in front of the large square.

Procedure

The procedure was described to the patient as being a special examination of his vision. The patient held the stereo-viewer in front of his eyes, the examiner assisting him when necessary. The stereo-viewer was adjusted for interocular distance and focal clarity by the use of a number of slides from the Keystone Home Training series. After he had achieved satisfactory fusion and saw the figures clearly, the Keystone slide DB6D of Test 7 was presented to assess stereoscopic vision with defined forms. This slide consists of 12 rows of forms; when viewed stereoscopically, one form in each row appears to be in front of the others because of the introduction of binocular disparity; the degree of disparity introduced decreases systematically from the top to the bottom row.

Three patients showed essentially monocular vision, being unable to identify any of the forms which should appear in front of the others in a row because of binocular disparity, and they were excluded from the study. The remaining patients were able to identify the critical forms in at least 9 of the 12 rows.

Four random-letter stereograms with a nasal shift of 46.5' of arc and 40% matrix density, each with the small square in a different quadrant of the field, were presented twice to the patient to introduce him to the task and give him some practice in it. A square sheet of paper divided into numbered quadrants was provided so

that the patient had the option of indicating the location of the small square in any one of three ways: saying "upper right," "lower left," and so on; referring to the paper and calling the number of the quadrant; or referring to the paper and pointing to the quadrant (see Figure 9). All patients were able to respond correctly in at least 2 of the 8 trials in this practice series.

The series of 24 test slides was then presented to the patient in the order shown in Table 20. As will be seen, the series included an equal number of stimuli representing each of the six possible combinations of level of matrix density and degree of horizontal disparity, with each combination presented twice in the first half and twice in the second half of the series of 24 trials. Two patients with right homonymous hemianopia identified at least 11 of the 12 small squares located in the left quadrants but none in the right quadrants. When the slides presenting the small squares in the right quadrants were reversed in the stereoviewer, so that they

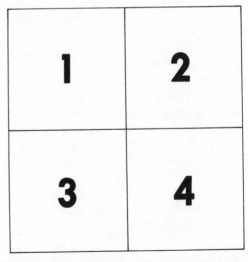

Fig. 9. Square sheet of paper on which patient could make his localizations by either pointing to a quadrant or calling its number. Actual size, 15-cm. sides.

Table 20. Sequence of stimuli

No.	Density level (percent)	Disparity (minutes of arc)	Location of small square
1	40	46.5	UR
2	10	15.5	UL
3	100	46.5	LL
4	40	15.5	LR
5	10	46.5	LR
6	100	15.5	LL
7	10	46.5	UL
8	100	15.5	UR
9	40	46.5	UL
10	10	15.5	LL
11	100	46.5	LR
12	40	15.5	UR
13	100	15.5	UL
14	40	46.5	LR
15	10	15.5	UR
16	100	46.5	UL
17	40	15.5	LL
18	10	46.5	LL
19	40	15.5	UL
20	10	46.5	UR
21	100	15.5	LR
22	40	46.5	LL
23	10	15.5	LR
24	100	46.5	UR

U = upper; L = lower; R = right; L = left.

were now located in the left quadrants, the patients identified all of them without difficulty. In these two cases, the performances were scored on the basis of the responses in the left field. A time limit of one minute was set for each trial, a failure being scored if the patient did not respond within this period.

No difficulty was encountered in explaining the procedure to the aphasic patients in the left hemisphere group; as suggested in Table 19, they showed primarily expressive disturbances of language. However, some of them found it necessary to point to the quadrant in which the small square appeared instead of giving a verbal response.

There were a number of major differences between the procedure in the present study and that of Carmon and Bechtoldt. Twenty-four trials were given in the present study as compared with 48 trials in the Carmon-Bechtoldt study. A time limit of one minute was established in the present study, while Carmon and Bechtoldt had set a time limit of thirty seconds. Carmon and Bechtoldt recorded the time taken to respond, but this was not done in the present study. Finally, the Keystone DB6D stereoscopic slide presenting defined forms was used as screening in this investigation but not in the Carmon-Bechtoldt study.

RESULTS

The distributions of the total number of correct responses in the 24 trials in the two groups of patients are shown in Table 21. A difference in the overall performance levels is quite obvious. All nine patients with left hemisphere disease performed on an adequate level, the poorest among them making only three errors. In contrast, 6 of the 8 patients with right hemisphere disease performed defectively, making 6 to 20 errors. The difference between the two score distributions is significant at the 0.0001 level, as estimated by the Mann-Whitney U test (using the formula appropriate for tied scores).

The mean number of errors made by the patients with left hemisphere disease was 0.44, while the mean number made by patients with right hemisphere disease was 8.75. Carmon and Bechtoldt obtained considerably higher mean scores, but responding time limits were so different results are not comparable.

Table 21. Distribution of number of correct responses

Group	23–24	21–22	19–20	17–18	15–16	13–14	11–12	9–10	7–8	5–6	3–4
Left hemisphere cases (N = 9)	8	1	—	—	—	—	—	—	—	—	—
Right hemisphere cases (N = 8)	2	—	—	1	2	—	1	—	1	—	1

Table 22. Number of errors for each combination of density level and degree of disparity

Density (percent)	Disparity (minutes of arc)	No. of errors
10	15.5	14
10	46.5	11
		25
40	15.5	7
40	46.5	6
		13
100	15.5	16
100	46.5	20
		36

An analysis of the effect of level of matrix density and the degree of binocular disparity on performance level was done by computing the sums of the errors made at each combination of density level and degree of disparity. The results are shown in Table 22. It is evident from inspection of the table that matrix density is a potent determinant of performance level. Almost three times as many errors were made at the 100% level of matrix density as at the 40% level. The 10% density level also appears to augment the difficulty of the task, approximately twice as many errors being made with stimuli at that level as compared with the 40% level. These findings are consistent with the results of normative studies by Bechtoldt and Bunge[4] and Geffen.[5] On the other hand, the two degrees of disparity did not appear to have a differential effect on performance level.

Observations on left-handed patients

Two left-handed patients, one with a left hemisphere lesion and the other with a right hemisphere lesion, were also examined and are listed in Table 19. Their performance showed a reversal of the relationship found in the two groups of right-handed patients. The patient with a lesion of the left hemisphere performed defectively, making a score of 15 with two errors in the right quadrants and seven errors in the left quadrants. The patient with a right hemisphere lesion made an errorless performance.

DISCUSSION

Our results completely confirm the findings of Carmon and Bechtoldt that a relatively high proportion of right-handed patients with disease of the right hemisphere show impairment in stereoscopic perception, while right-handed patients with left hemisphere disease perform on an essentially normal level. As Carmon and Bechtoldt point out, frank complaints of disturbances in stereopsis are mentioned in only a few case reports in the literature of clinical neurology. In this connection, it is worthy of note that in the present study even those patients who failed the random-letter stereoscopic task were able to perform adequately on a conventional test of stereoscopic vision (the Keystone slide) involving defined forms. Evidently a technique of the type developed by Julesz and Bechtoldt, in which monocular cues are excluded, is required to demonstrate the striking defect described by Carmon and Bechtoldt and in the present study. On the other hand, difficulty in estimating relative or absolute distance or size and mislocalization of objects in space have been described much more frequently.[6] The relationship of these disabilities to basic impairment in stereopsis, as assessed by Julesz-Bechtoldt technique, merits investigation.

Our observations on two left-handed patients can scarcely be the basis for any conclusions. Nevertheless, the finding that the left-handed patient with a left hemisphere lesion performed defectively while the one with a right hemisphere lesion performed errorlessly suggests that handedness and cerebral dominance for language in relation to stereopsis in patients with cerebral disease be explored.

Normal stereoscopic vision has consistently been reported to be a characteristic of patients with section of the corpus callosum.[7-9] These observations are in accord with the generally accepted concept that binocular integration is primarily mediated by subcortical mechanisms. The study of Carmon and Bechtoldt and the replication of it described here indicate that, in addition to these subcortical mechanisms, the right hemisphere plays an essential role in the realization of stereoscopic vision in man.

SUMMARY

The study of Carmon and Bechtoldt reporting that a significant proportion of patients with disease of the right hemisphere show impairment in stereoscopic vision while patients with left hemisphere lesions perform on a normal level was replicated with certain modifications. The results fully confirmed the findings of the Carmon-Bechtoldt study. A majority of right-handed patients with lesions of the right hemisphere performed defectively, and all patients with left hemisphere lesions, including those with aphasia, performed on a normal level. Two left-handed patients with unilateral lesions showed a reversal of this relationship. The results are interpreted as supporting the hypothesis that the right hemisphere plays a crucial role in the realization of stereoscopic vision in man.

REFERENCES

1. Carmon, A., & Bechtoldt, H. P.: Dominance of the right cerebral hemisphere for stereopsis. Neuropsychologia 7:29, 1969.

2. Bunge, J. V.: IBM 7044 program for generating artificial stereograms. Behav. Sci. 12:344, 1967.

3. Julesz, B.: Binocular depth perception without familiarity cues. Science 145:356, 1964.

4. Bechtoldt, H. P. & Bunge, J. V.: Speed of binocular form perception in random letter displays as a function of horizontal disparity, form rivalry, brightness rivalry, and field density. Paper presented at the annual meeting of the Psychonomic Society, Chicago. October 1966.

5. Geffen, J.: The relationship between age and response speed with random letter stereograms. Proc. Iowa Acad. Sci. 75:324, 1968.

6. Benton, A. L.: Disorders of spatial orientation. In: Handbook of Clinical Neurology. Vol. 3. Amsterdam: North-Holland Publishing Co., 1969.

7. Bridgman, C. S. & Smith, K. U.: Bilateral neural integration in visual perception after section of the corpus callosum. J. comp. Neurol. 83:57, 1945.

8. Sperry, R. W.: Some general aspects of interhemispheric integration. In: Interhemispheric Relations and Cerebral Dominance. Edited by V. B. Mountcastle. Baltimore: Johns Hopkins Press, 1962.

9. Gazzaniga, M. S., Bogen, J. E., & Sperry, R. W.: Observations on visual perception after disconnexion of the cerebral hemispheres in man. Brain 88:221, 1965.

22.

Visual Perception of Line Direction in Patients with Unilateral Brain Disease*

Two complementary approaches have been used to assess the role of the right hemisphere in spatial perception. One has been to compare patients with disease of the right or left hemisphere in respect to performance of appropriate perceptual or perceptuomotor tasks such as constructional praxis, the perception of direction, stereopsis, and maze learning.[1-8] The finding of impairment in patients with lesions of the right hemisphere provides a basis for ascribing special functional properties to that hemisphere in the mediation of these performances. A second approach has been to compare performance level on spatial tasks in the left and right visual fields or on the left and right sides of the body in normal right-handed subjects or in patients who have been subjected to section of the corpus callosum and other interhemispheric commissures.[9-11] Superior performance in the left visual field or on the left side of the body is interpreted as reflecting a rela-

tive dominance of the right hemisphere for these activities.

Both approaches have been used in studies of the perception of the direction of lines in the tactile and the visual modalities. Carmon and Benton[3] and Fontenot and Benton[8] showed that in a significant proportion of patients with right hemisphere disease, recognition of the direction of linear punctuate stimulation applied to the surface of the palms was bilaterally impaired, while patients with left hemisphere disease showed only the expected contralateral impairment. They interpreted their findings "as providing further evidence to support the concept that the right hemisphere plays a more important role than the left in the mediation of behavior requiring the apprehension of spatial relations and as extending this evidence to a test situation involving the tactile modality."[3] In a complementary study, Benton, Levin, and Varney[11] assessed the accuracy of tactile perception of direction on the left and right palms of normal right-handed subjects and found significantly superior performance on the

* A. L. Benton, H. J. Hannay, and N. R. Varney, *Neurology*, 1975, 25, 907–910.

left palm. The results were interpreted as supporting the inference drawn from the earlier observations of patients with unilateral brain disease.

Analogous studies of visual perception of direction have been done both in patients with brain disease and in normal subjects. Warrington and Rabin[7] compared the performance of patients with unilateral brain disease in judging whether or not pairs of lines differed in slope, and found that the mean error score was significantly higher in the group with right hemisphere lesions as compared with either the group with left hemisphere lesions or the control group. The two latter groups did not differ in performance level. Patients with right parietal lesions showed particularly severe impairment. Fontenot and Benton[10] assessed the accuracy of identification of lines tachistoscopically exposed in the left and right visual fields of normal right-handed subjects, and found a significantly higher level of accuracy in the left field.

Thus, the results to date consistently indicate that the tactile as well as the visual perception of the directional characteristics of stimuli is mediated primarily by the right hemisphere in right-handed subjects. The purpose of the present investigation was to pursue this line of inquiry further by studying the performances of patients with unilateral brain disease in a somewhat more complex task that required accurate identification of two simultaneously presented lines of different slope on a subsequently presented multiple-choice display. The questions raised were whether or not this more demanding perceptual task would separate unilateral groups more effectively than the standard task of identifying the direction of a single line and also whether the findings would be sufficiently impressive to encourage the development of a diagnostic procedure for clinical use.

METHOD

Subjects

Three groups of patients from the neurologic services of University Hospitals, Iowa City, were studied. One group consisted of 21 right-handed patients with lesions confined to the left hemisphere, as determined by clinical examination and the findings from angiography, radioactive brain scan, and computerized tomography. Twelve patients in this group had some type of aphasic disorder. A second group consisted of 22 right-handed patients with lesions confined to the right hemisphere. None of these patients was aphasic. A third group consisted of 22 right-handed patients who had no history or evidence of brain disease.

The mean ages of patients in the left hemisphere, right hemisphere, and control groups were 52 years (SD = 13.2), 55 years (SD = 11.4), and 49 years (SD = 15.3), respectively. None of the differences between groups in respect to mean age was significant. The proportion of men and women in the left hemisphere and control groups was approximately equal (11 men, 10 women; 12 men, 10 women, respectively), but there was a predominance of men in the right hemisphere group (16 men, six women). Cerebrovascular disease was the most frequent diagnosis in both groups with brain disease (48 percent in the left hemisphere group, 50 percent in the right hemisphere group), and neoplasm was the second most frequent diagnosis (33 percent in the left hemisphere group, 45 percent in the right hemisphere group). All the patients with neoplasms were studied before surgery.

Procedure

Stimuli were presented through a three-channel tachistoscope, which was described to the patient as a viewer. The patient was shown a white card with a single horizontal line on it and told that it would appear on the screen of the viewer for a very short time. The patient then looked into the tachistoscope while the card was exposed for 300 msec and reported whether or not he saw the line. After he had reported seeing the line, a second card (Figure 10) showing 11 lines in different directional orientations was presented for viewing. The patient was requested to say how many lines there were and to read the numbers above them. He was shown the horizontal line again and informed that it corresponded in respect to slope and position to one of the lines on the multiple-choice response card. He was then given a practice trial in which the single line was presented for 300 msec to central vision; following this, a blank field was presented for 2 seconds and then the response card for 6 seconds. The patient was asked to give the number of the line that was in the same position as the previously exposed single line. If he responded incorrectly, the explanation

was repeated and a second trial given. Patients who failed to respond correctly on the second trial were excluded from the study. Five patients, four of whom were aphasic, showed evidence of not understanding the instruction.

Following the practice trial(s), the first part of the experiment was carried out. This consisted of the sequential presentation of 11 lines, one in each of the 11 positions shown on the response card (Figure 11A). The second part of the experiment consisted of the simultaneous presentation of 22 pairs of lines (Figure 11B) representing 22 different combinations from the 55 possible combinations. The patient was shown an example of this type of stimulus and instructed to give the numbers of the same lines on the response card. Exposure durations and the temporal sequence were the same as in the first part of the experiment.

The lines on the stimulus and response cards for both tasks were 5 cm long and were presented at a distance of 123 cm.

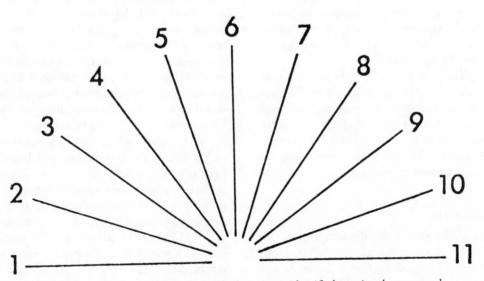

Fig. 10. Multiple-choice card on which patients identified previously presented stimuli.

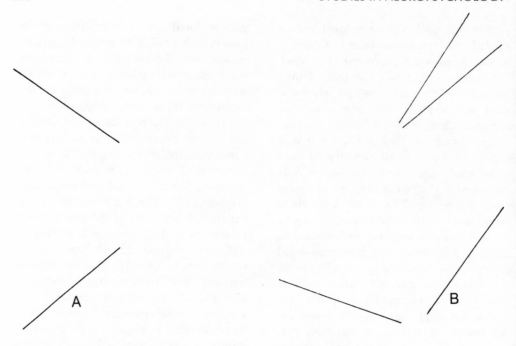

Fig. 11. Examples of stimuli presented to patients. (*A*) Single-line stimuli. (*B*) Double-line stimuli.

The screen in the viewer was 16 cm horizontally and 11 cm vertically. Illumination was maintained at 49.7 cd per square meter during the presentation of stimuli and the response card and at 65.1 cd per square meter during the intervening 2 second blank interval.

Two aphasic patients experienced difficulty in saying the numbers of the lines, and the procedure was modified to permit them to point to the numbers on a separate response card. This, of course, required them to look away from the tachistoscope on each trial.

RESULTS

Table 23 shows the distributions of the scores of the three groups for the total task and for parts 1 and 2 (single and double lines) separately. The performance of the patients with right hemisphere disease obviously differs from that of the other two groups. On the other hand, the score distributions of the control patients and those with left hemisphere disease appear to be fairly similar. The mean score of the patients with left hemisphere disease was slightly lower than that of the controls for each task (combined task, single lines, double lines), but in no instance was the difference between the means of the two groups significant.

In contrast, a substantial proportion of patients with right hemisphere lesions performed at a level below that represented by the lowest score in either the control or the left hemisphere group. This proportion was 59 percent for the total task (33 trials), 18 percent for the single lines (11 trials), and 50 percent for the double lines (22 trials). The observed difference of 32 percent between the proportions of patients with right hemisphere

Table 23. Distribution of scores

Combined task (33 trials)			
Score	Control	Left lesion	Right lesion
31–33	1	1	—
28–30	6	3	1
25–27	12	7	3
22–24	1	8	2
19–21	2	2	3
16–18	—	—	7
< 16	—	—	6

Single lines (11 trials)			
Score	Control	Left lesion	Right lesion
11	15	10	4
10	5	6	4
9	1	3	5
8	—	2	4
7	1	—	1
6	—	—	2
< 6	—	—	2

Double lines (22 trials)			
Score	Control	Left lesion	Right lesion
21–22	—	1	—
19–20	3	1	1
17–18	6	3	1
15–16	9	7	2
13–14	3	6	3
11–12	1	2	1
9–10	—	1	3
7–8	—	—	6
< 7	—	—	5

disease who performed defectively on the single-lines and double-lines tasks suggests that the latter task discriminated between the right and left hemisphere groups more effectively than the easier single line task. This impression was confirmed by statistical test, the difference in proportions being significant at the .005 probability level, as estimated by a correlated proportions test.[12]

Correlates of performance

Since there was a predominance of men in the right hemisphere group while the number of men and women in the left hemisphere group was approximately equal, the question of whether this imbalance in the sex composition of the two groups might have contributed to the interhemispheric difference in performance was investigated. Four (67 percent) of the six women in the right hemisphere group performed defectively as compared with nine (56 percent) of the 16 men. Clearly, the predominance of men in that group was not responsible for the generally poor performance. Nor was the presence of visual field defect correlated with performance level. Only five patients in the right hemisphere group (three of whom had parietal lesions) had demonstrable field defects. Three (60 percent) performed defectively as compared with an overall relative frequency of 59 percent for the entire group. Nine patients (43 percent) in the left hemisphere group had demonstrable visual field defects. Their mean score (25.1) was almost identical to the mean score (25.2) of the 12 patients without field defects. Similarly the mean score (24.7) of the 12 aphasic patients in the left hemisphere group did not differ significantly from the mean score (25.8) of the 10 nonaphasic patients in that group. Five patients were aphasic and had visual field defects; their mean score (23.8) did not differ significantly from the mean score (25.0) of the five nonaphasic patients without field defects. Age was not significantly related to performance level in any of the groups, the three correlation coefficients ranging from −.21 to +.15.

Locus of lesion and performance level

It was possible to infer the locus of the lesion by means of radiographic techniques in 15 of the 22 patients with right hemisphere disease. Four patients had neoplasms involving the right prefrontal area; all performed within normal limits, although 1 made a borderline score of 21. In contrast, all 5 patients with lesions involving the posterior frontal, anterior temporal and/or anterior parietal area performed defectively, their scores ranging from 13 to 18. Three of the 6 patients with lesions involving the posterior parietal or parieto-occipital area performed defectively. The frequency of defective performance (50 percent) in this subgroup was essentially the same as that for the right hemisphere group as a whole.

DISCUSSION

The results confirm those of Warrington and Rabin.[7] Patients with disease of the right hemisphere were significantly less accurate in perceiving the direction of lines than either control patients or those with left hemisphere disease. The latter groups did not differ significantly from each other in this respect. The findings are also in accord with those of Fontenot and Benton[10] demonstrating a left field superiority for the perception of line direction in normal right-handed subjects. Since the experimental task is primarily of a spatial nature, the findings further support the concept that the right hemisphere plays a peculiarly important role in mediating the appreciation of spatial relations in right-handed individuals.

The experimental task identified a remarkably high proportion of patients with right hemisphere disease as performing defectively. It is not possible to precisely compare the findings in this respect with those of Warrington and Rabin, but it appears that the two hemispheric groups were differentiated more sharply in the present study. The probable reasons for this are (1) the limitation of exposure time to 300 msec and (2) the introduction of the more complex task of identifying the slopes of pairs of lines instead of only single lines. The frequency of defective performance by the patients with right hemisphere disease was significantly higher in the double-lines task than in the single-lines task.

Warrington and Rabin reported that as a group, patients with lesions of the posterior parietal region of the right hemisphere performed most defectively. Our own data are too sparse to investigate in any detail this question of the influence of the intrahemispheric locus of lesion on performance. The indications are that patients with right prefrontal lesions may be expected to perform normally. On the other hand, a trend toward particularly poor performance on the part of patients with right parieto-occipital lesions was not apparent. Rather unexpectedly, the frequency of defective performance was highest in patients with posterior frontal-anterior temporal and posterior frontal-anterior parietal lesions.

The remarkably high frequency of defective performance of this visuospatial task on the part of patients with right hemisphere disease, in contrast to essentially normal performance by patients with left hemisphere disease, suggests that it may be helpful to develop the procedure for clinicodiagnostic use. Parametric studies are planned to identify the optimal exposure duration and optimal interval between the presentations of the stimulus and response cards for diagnostic differentiation.

REFERENCES

1. Benton A. L.: Disorders of spatial orientation. In Vinken P. J., Bruyn G. W. (Editors): Handbook of Clinical Neurology. Amsterdam, North Holland Publishing Company, 1969, vol. 3, pp. 212–228.

2. Carmon A., Bechtoldt H. P.: Dominance of the right hemisphere for stereopsis. Neuropsychologia 7:29–39, 1969.

3. Carmon A., Benton A. L .: Tactile perception of direction and number in patients with unilateral cerebral disease. Neurology (Minneap) 19:525–532, 1969.

4. Newcombe F., Russell W. R.: Disso-

ciated visual perception and spatial deficits in focal lesions of the right hemisphere. J Neurol Neurosurg Psychiatry 32:73–81, 1969.

5. Warrington E. K., Constructional apraxia. In Vinken P. J., Bruyn G. W. (Editors): Handbook of Clinical Neurology. Amsterdam. North Holland Publishing Company, 1969, vol. 4, pp. 67–83.

6. Benton A. L., Hécaen H.: Stereoscopic vision in patients with unilateral cerebral disease. Neurology (Minneap) 20:1084–1088, 1970.

7. Warrington E. K., Rabin P.: Perceptual matching in patients with cerebral lesions. Neuropsychologia 8:475–487, 1970.

8. Fontenot D. J., Benton A. L.: Tactile perception of direction in relation to hemi-spheric locus of lesion. Neuropsychologia 9:83–88, 1971.

9. Gazzaniga M. S.: The Bisected Brain. New York, Appleton-Century-Crofts, 1970.

10. Fontenot D. J., Benton A. L.: Perception of direction in the right and left visual fields. Neuropsychologia 10:477–452, 1972.

11. Benton A. L., Levin H. S., Varney N. R.: Tactile perception of direction in normal subjects: Implications for hemispheric cerebral dominance. Neurology (Minneap) 23: 1248–1250, 1973.

12. Dixon W. J., Massey F. J: Introduction to Statistical Analysis. Ed. 3. New York, McGraw-Hill Book Company, 1969, pp. 250–251.

23.

Facial Recognition 1984*

Impairment in facial recognition was a topic that engaged the interest of Henri Hécaen over the course of many years. As early as 1952, he published a case report of a patient with prosopagnosia and discussed the nature of the disorder and its underlying mechanisms (Hécaen, Ajuria-guerra, Magis, & Angelergues, 1952). In 1957, he described two additional cases with special reference to the question of different forms of facial agnosia (Hécaen, Angelergues, Bernhardt, & Chiarelli, 1957). In 1962, he wrote a comprehensive review of the literature that was influential in stimulating the interest of investigators in facial recognition and its disturbances (Hécaen & Angelergues, 1962). At that time, the papers dealing with prosopagnosia were still relatively few in number, of variable quality, and sometimes contradictory in their implications. With characteristic acumen,

* Paper presented by A. L. Benton in a session honoring the memory of Henri Hécaen, Seventh European Meeting, International Neuropsychological Society, Aachen, Germany, June 15, 1984.

Hécaen analyzed the material and formulated a clear statement of what was then known about the salient features, correlates, and determinants of this rather bizarre disability. Subsequently, a number of studies of both prosopagnosia and impairment in the capacity to discriminate unfamiliar faces were reported from his unit (Hécaen & Tzavaras, 1969; Rondot & Tzavaras, 1969; Tzavaras, Hécaen, & Le Bras, 1970; Tzavaras, Merienne, & Masure, 1973).

In his 1962 paper, Hécaen defined prosopagnosia as failure on the part of a patient "to recognize people known to him on the basis of visual perception of their faces." When identification is achieved, it is based on the person's voice, size, clothes, gait, or even on an adventitious facial feature or accessory, such as a scar or blemish, a moustache, or eyeglasses. But the more essential features, such as facial structure, eyes, nose, and mouth cannot be utilized for identification. The majority of prosopagnosic patients appear to have a clear percept of a familiar face, in that they can describe its features accurately, even though they cannot identify the person. However, some patients experience visuoperceptive distortions (i.e., metamorphopsia), and they describe faces as torn, warped, contorted, lifeless, or lacking in expression— the affective tone of the experience always being unpleasant.

Hécaen considered facial agnosia to be a specific disability in the sense that it could not be conceived to be simply an expression of a pervasive visuoperceptual deficit. However, he did not accept the extreme view of Bodamer (1947) that it represented derangement of an innate mechanism concerned solely with recognition of the human face. The impairment can extend to the perception of the faces of animals, where inspection may not permit identification of the species, much less the individual animal, and can even extend to the identification of particular places or automobiles. In addition, there may be failure to grasp the symbolic import of abstract figures, such as a red cross or a plus sign.

Reviewing the clinical findings reported in the literature and the records of patients seen in his own unit, Hécaen noted the positive association of facial agnosia with signs and symptoms of right-hemisphere disease (e.g., left visual field defect, left lateral neglect, and visuoconstructive disability) as well as the lack of correlation with deficits reflecting left-hemisphere disease (e.g., disturbances in speech, calculation, and praxis). He commented that "There is much evidence to support the hypothesis that a lesion of the right hemisphere is a sufficient antecedent condition" for the appearance of the disability. He further noted that Faust (1947, 1955) had called attention to the extraordinarily high frequency of left superior visual-field defects in prosopagnosic patients, and he agreed with Faust's conclusion that a basal occipital lesion was a crucial underlying factor. Nevertheless, he acknowledged that the lack of autopsy data prevented drawing a definitive conclusion: "While the available evidence is strongly in favor of a lesional localization in the right hemisphere, one is still not altogether certain of this" (Hécaen & Angelergues, 1962, p. 97).

It is just as well that Hécaen expressed this reservation, for subsequent analyses of the anatomical findings in prosopagnosic patients have indicated that bilateral disease is a necessary precondition for the appearance of the abnormality. Study of the 12 patients who have come to autopsy discloses bilateral disease in every case, including some whose clinical symptoms during life suggested the presence of a lesion confined to the right hemisphere (Nardelli et al., 1982; Benton, 1984). In almost all instances, bilateral inferior occipitotemporal lesions have been found, with the exceptional cases showing inferior occipitotemporal changes in the right hemisphere in combination with lesions in another area of the left hemisphere.

Computerized tomography findings also support the inference that bilateral occipital disease is the basis for a persisting prosopagnosia. Of 14 reported cases known to me, the CT scan showed bilateral occipital abnormality in 11 cases and a right-hemisphere lesion in 3 cases. Of the latter 3 cases, 1 exhibited only a transient prosopagnosia following removal of a glioma in the occipitoparietal territory of the right hemisphere (Whitely & Warrington, 1977, Case 3). With respect to the other 2 cases (Whitely & Warrington, 1977, Case 2; Boudouresques et al., 1979), there are grounds for suspecting that the CT scans did not disclose the full extent of cerebral change.

If we accept the conclusion that bilateral disease is the necessary context for the occurrence of a persisting prosopagnosia, we still should address the question of why the disability is more often accompanied by clinical signs of disease of the right hemisphere than of the left hemisphere. Particularly impressive is its association with loss of vision in the left superior visual field, indicative of right inferior occipital lobe disease. This was first observed by Faust (1947, 1955) and subsequently documented by Meadows (1974), who pointed out that the functional effect of a lesion so situated is to block the transmission of visual information to other areas of the brain, primarily the middle temporal, inferior temporal and hippocampal gyri as well as the left occipitotemporal territory. Despite their apparent importance, unilateral lesions directly compromising the right lingual and fusiform gyri and hippocampus do not cause prosopagnosia, although they may produce other visuoperceptual defects (cf. Lhermitte et al., 1972; Lhermitte & Pillon, 1975; Damasio, Damasio, & Van Hoesen, 1982). Indeed, even complete right cerebral hemispherectomy does not seem to produce prosopagnosia (cf. Smith, 1969; Damasio, Lima, & Damasio, 1975). This puzzle, which has been discussed by Lhermitte and his coworkers (1972, 1975), has yet to be solved.

Over the years, there has been a fair amount of discussion of the nature of the cognitive disability underlying failure to identify familiar faces and a number of proposals have been advanced. The simplest (and, in a way, the most parsimonious) explanation is that facial agnosia is only the most prominent expression of more general visuoperceptive impairment. The statement is tenable for a few cases but does not fit the majority of cases, and it is not generally accepted. Other proposals are: (1) the disability reflects a failure to identify individuality within a class of objects (e.g., faces, buildings, automobiles); (2) the failure to identify individu-

ality within a class of objects is material specific (i.e., restricted to faces); (3) the deficit reflects nonverbal memory impairment wherein the perceived face, automobile, or building cannot be placed in its appropriate context; and (4) the deficit reflects partial, material-specific memory impairment restricted to faces.

It is not difficult to find cases for which each formulation holds, but it is equally easy to demonstrate that a given formulation is untenable if applied to other cases. Indeed, the generalizations do not go very far beyond the observed findings in particular cases, and they scarcely qualify as true explanations. The chances are that there are different types of prosopagnosia. Better stated, there are a number of reasons why a patient may fail to identify familiar faces. Certainly, there is a difference between the patient who says that people look strange and ugly with faces "like fish heads" (Whitely & Warrington, 1977, Case 3) or the patient who sees a schematic drawing of a face as an apple with the eyes being "two worm holes" (Teuber, 1975) and the patient who experiences a clear, unremarkable percept of a face but who canot identify the person. Severe perceptual derangement must play a role in the first two patients' performances, whereas the last patient's failure in identification almost surely reflects a disorder of memory.

The task of isolating distinctive types of prosopagnosia is complicated by two factors. First, although facial agnosia is not as rare as was once thought, it is still a relatively uncommon disability. Consequently, there is not a large body of information available for analysis such as one has for the aphasic disorders or visuoconstructional disability. Second, the case reports published in the literature vary so widely in respect to method of examination that it is difficult to put together a body of comparable data. The question of types and determinants of prosopagnosia will be resolved only when an adequate number of patients are assessed according to a standard protocol specifically designed to test various hypotheses about the nature of the disorder.

The prosopagnosic patients described in case reports suffer from an impairment in facial recognition that is severe, that is obvious to themselves and others, and that impels them to seek medical help. Does the disability occur in milder form where it is not a subject of complaint by the patients and perhaps not even noticed by them or their relatives? Here, the disability would be manifested not by failure to recognize persons who are most familiar to the patient but by the patient's failure to identify acquaintances who are seen only occasionally or people who are encountered under unusual circumstances (e.g. a person in a swimsuit, a physician without his white coat, or a man without his moustache). General observation suggests that this mild form of impaired facial identification does occur both in patients with brain disease and in older persons. In fact, there may be significant individual differences in the normal population with respect to the capacity for facial recognition.

Hécaen used both family photographs and pictures of public personages to assess facial identification in patients in whom there was a suspicion of a prosopagnosic difficulty. Subsequently, pictures of public and historical figures have been used by investigators to evaluate both facial identification and remote memory. In an early study, Warrington and James (1967) found that impairment in the identification of well-known public figures was associated with right-hemisphere disease. More recently Albert, Butters, and Levin (1979) have utilized a similar test to assess remote memory in Korsakoff patients.

However, it is important to keep in mind that these picture tests are not necessarily measures of facial identification and that designations such as "famous faces" are not altogether accurate because, in fact, many items are full-length or half-length photographs of, for example, Charles Chaplin, Benito Mussolini, or Charles de Gaulle in their characteristic dress. In these instances, a prosopagnosic patient might be able to achieve identification on the basis of extra facial features. On the other hand, an amnesic patient's performance on such a test would depend on the extent of his or her retrograde amnesia.

The task of developing an adequate test of identification of public figures on the basis of their facial characteristics is a difficult one. There are wide individual differences in the fund of general and historical knowledge in normal subjects of the same age and educational level. Moreover, one finds that when the test items are simply faces without extra facial cues, many well-known and historical figures are not easily identified by normal subjects. Despite their imperfections, these picture tests have proven to be of value in investigative work. We should try to devise more refined instruments for assessing facial recognition in the patient without frank prosopagnosia.

I have already mentioned that Hécaen's 1962 paper provided the impetus for a number of investigators to undertake studies of facial recognition. Because prosopagnosia itself was such an uncommon disorder, this generally took the form of developing what was assumed to be an experimental model of prosopagnosia, one in which the recognition and discrimination of unfamiliar faces were evaluated. Consequently, several tests that yielded quantitative measures of the capacity to discriminate unfamilar faces were devised in a number of laboratories, including Hécaen's own unit (Warrington & James,

1967; Benton & Van Allen, 1968; De Renzi, Faglioni, & Spinnler, 1968; Tzavaras, Hécaen, & Le Bras, 1970).

The results of these studies are well known. Impairment in facial discrimination is a fairly frequent occurrence in patients with brain disease, certainly far more frequent than is prosopagnosia. Nor is there any necessary association between the two disabilities. There are prosopagnosic patients who show adequate discrimination of unfamiliar faces. Of course, the marked difference in the relative frequency of the two disabilities indicates that most patients who are impaired in the discrimination of unfamiliar faces are not prosopagnosic (Rondot, Tzavaras, & Garcin, 1967; Assal, 1969; Benton & Van Allen, 1972; Tzavaras, Merienne, & Masure, 1973; Malone, Morris, Kay, & Levin, 1982). Moreover, Warrington and James (1967) found that, although both the identification of well-known public figures and the discrimination of unfamiliar faces were impaired in patients with right-hemisphere disease, the two performances were not correlated with each other in this group of patients.

Among nonaphasic patients, defective facial discrimination is shown far more frequently by those with right-hemisphere disease than those with left-hemisphere lesions (cf. Benton, 1980, 1984; Lezak, 1983). However, there is a subgroup of aphasic patients (most of them of the Wernicke type but, in any case, always showing impairment in oral verbal comprehension) who perform defectively on tests of facial discrimination (Hamsher, Levin, & Benton, 1979). But not all aphasic patients with receptive language impairment perform defectively on the task, and the reason why some do is obscure. One would be inclined to ascribe their failure to their lack of understanding of task requirements were it not for the fact that many of them perform quite ade-

quately on visuoconstructional and other visuoperceptive tests. In any case, the outcome of these studies has been to bring to light a perceptual deficit that is independent of the symptom of facial agnosia and, indeed, that has proved to be of broader significance from a clinical standpoint.

In passing, we should note that performance on tests requiring the discrimination of unfamiliar faces decreases with advancing age. Beginning at about the age of 55 years, mean performance level declines and by the age of 75 years about 20 percent of ostensibly normal oldsters perform defectively as defined by the distribution of scores of younger subjects (Benton, Eslinger, & Damasio, 1981; Benton, Hamsher, Varney, & Spreen, 1983). But there is a concomitant increase in inter-individual variability with some subjects in their late 70s and 80s who still perform on a superior level. This raises the question of whether the defective performances of some older subjects should not be interpreted as indicative of some pathologic change rather than being viewed as simply a reflection of the overall decline in cognitive efficiency to be expected of persons in the 70s and 80s. As might be anticipated, demented patients show a relatively high frequency of failure on tests of facial discrimination (Eslinger & Benton, 1983). However, a striking preservation of the capacity is sometimes seen in grossly deteriorated patients, and this testifies to the rather specific nature of the facial discrimination process. Patients with closed head injuries, particularly those with evidence of right-hemisphere damage, often show impairment in facial discrimination (Levin, Grossman, & Kelly, 1977).

It was the complaint of prosopagnosia that led to studies of impairment in the discrimination of unfamiliar faces in patients with focal brain disease. In turn, these clinical studies provided the impetus for intensive study of facial recognition in normal subjects through the technique of tachistoscopic visual half-field stimulation. As with the clinical studies, this research effort has addressed the question of the hemispheric contribution to performance. However, it has also gone beyond clinical studies to probe the nature of the cognitive processes underlying the recognition of both familiar and unfamiliar faces; in brief, this research has been more functionally oriented than the earlier clinical studies, which, for the most part, were concerned solely with the relationship of performance to locus of lesion. The outcome of this effort has been a complex set of findings that are not easy to integrate. I shall focus attention on those issues that are most closely related to the findings of clinical studies and the questions raised by them.

The employment of lateralized tachistoscopic stimulation to investigate hemispheric asymmetry in visual perception is, of course, not new. In the 1950s, investigators demonstrated a right visual-field advantage in the perception of letters and words, indicative of the specialization of the left hemisphere for verbal information processing. In 1966, Kimura adduced evidence for a left visual-field advantage in the perception of certain types of nonverbal stimulus material, indicative of the specialization of the right hemisphere for nonverbal information processing, and her findings were generally confirmed.

The first studies of lateral differences in facial perception, those of Geffen, Bradshaw, and Wallace (1971) and of Rizzolati, Umiltà, and Berlucchi (1971), were clearly inspired by the earlier clinical investigations on patients with unilateral brain disease. Both studies reported faster reaction times for left visual-field presentations of unfamiliar faces than for right-field presentations. Subsequent studies

demonstrated a left-field superiority in accuracy as well as speed of perception (Hilliard, 1973; St. John, 1981).

Thus, the overall findings of these experimental studies of normal right-handed subjects were quite consistent with those on brain-lesioned patients, indicating a right-hemisphere specialization for facial discrimination. However, they also brought out some facts about individual differences in performance that generally had been ignored in the clinical studies where, in the search for valid generalizations, little attention had been paid to deviant cases, that is, the patient with right-hemisphere disease who did *not* show impairment in facial discrimination and the left-hemisphere damaged patient who *did* show impairment. This approach was reflected in the utilization of parametric statistics in these clinical studies, which resulted in findings that were presented in terms of comparisons of mean scores and analyses of variance.

The parametric statistical approach, in which deviant cases are treated as part of "error variance," has also been the rule in experimental studies. But the fact that (within the context of an overall left-field superiority in facial perception), there are carefully selected young right-handed subjects who show either no field difference or a right-field superiority did not escape attention. The proportion of such subjects is not negligible, ranging from 10 percent to 35 percent in different studies, and the phenomenon has become a topic of investigation and considerable discussion.

The first comment that may be made about this finding is that it is, in fact, congruent with clinical observations. Deviant cases are certainly not a rare occurrence. A recent comparison of the relative frequency of defective facial discrimination in right-handed brain-diseased patients found a 42 percent frequency in patients with right-hemisphere lesions and a 20 percent frequency in those with left-hemisphere lesions (cf. Hamsher, Levin, & Benton, 1979; Benton, 1980). Among the right-hemisphere damaged patients, the highest frequency of impairment, 58 percent, was found in those with posterior lesions and visual-field defects. It is tenable to assume that the 32 percent in this subgroup who performed adequately did not have lesions that compromised the neural mechanism in the right hemisphere that mediates facial perception. But it is also possible that the reason for sparing of the ability is that at least some of these patients employed a neural mechanism in the left hemisphere in effecting the performance. More important, 20 percent of the patients with left-hemisphere disease performed defectively. Obviously, their presumably intact right hemisphere was not sufficient to permit normal facial perception, and it seems reasonable to conclude that derangement of a mechanism in the left hemisphere led to impaired performance.

A second point that needs to be made concerns the role of instability in performance when determining the occurrence of supposedly deviant cases. We know that indexes of ear advantage in dichotic listening tests show only a limited degree of stability, with about 30 percent of normal subjects showing a change in ear advantage in responding to digits or consonants from test to retest (Pizzamiglio, De Pascalis, & Vignati, 1974; Blumstein, Goodglass, & Tartter, 1975). The reversals in visual-field advantage that have been observed to occur over trials and the inconsistent findings of different studies make it highly probable that this instability also holds for tachistoscopic facial perception in normal subjects.

What are the determinants of these individual differences in respect to visual-field advantage and of the oscillations in performance that almost certainly contribute to them? Experimental studies have implicated a variety of factors.

On the one hand, we have the finding that women show a smaller field advantage or none at all under conditions in which men show a significant field difference (cf. McGlone, 1980). However, some studies have found no evidence for such a sex difference (Leehey, Carey, Diamond, & Cahn, 1978; Hannay & Rogers, 1979). In any case, one looks for relevant sex-related factors rather than simply class membership to elucidate what essentially amounts to greater inter-individual variability in the performances of women. One such factor is cognitive style as reflected in performance on the Witkin tasks (Oltman, Ehrlichman, & Cox, 1977; Zoccolati & Oltman, 1978; Rapaczynski & Ehrlichman, 1979; Pizzamiglio & Zoccolati, 1981). Field independence is associated with a stronger left-field advantage in both men and women; when this factor is controlled, the between-sex difference disappears. Conversely, language facility (as reflected in vocabulary test scores) has been found to be associated with a right-field advantage in performance (Hannay & Rogers, 1979).

On the other hand, diverse experimental conditions and task requirements have been found to influence the presence and degree of field differences. The inconsistency in the outcomes of different studies (which, it seems, are never exact replications of each other) make it difficult to integrate the findings into a coherent picture. In their thoughtful review of the present status of the question of hemispheric asymmetry in facial perception, Sergent and Bindra (1981) remind us that the term *facial recognition* is used in an indiscriminate way to denote at least three different cognitive processes: (1) perceptual discrimination, involving only the judgment of whether two simultaneously presented faces are the same or different;

(2) recognition, in which the judgment of same or different involves the memory trace of a previously *presented face*; (3) identification, where the subject must specify *whose* face has been presented.

Sergent and Bindra go on to point out that identification requires a more searching examination of facial features than does discrimination or recognition where two faces are presented for comparison and where perception of a single feature may suffice to reach a "difference" judgment. As we saw, clinical investigators distinguish clearly between the complaint of prosopagnosia and the impairment in the discrimination of unfamilar faces that is brought out by tests. But in their work with normal subjects, some experimentalists apparently have assumed that discrimination and identification involve the same cognitive processes. In any case, the overall left-field superiority that is found for the discrimination and recognition of unfamilar faces is not evident for the identification of public figures where experimental studies have generated a mass of contradictory results (cf. Sergent & Bindra, 1981; Young & Bion, 1981).

Experimental study has dealt with a variety of questions, for example, the role of memory, stimulus duration, level of difficulty, repeated stimulus exposure, and the opposition of holistic and analytic information processing in the production of visual half-field differences in performance (cf. Sergent & Bindra, 1981; Bryden, 1982). As I mentioned, it is difficult (at least for me) to integrate the findings of these studies and arrive at generalizations about the influence of specific factors (or their combinations) in the production of asymmetry in field performance. The reason is that each study seems to have its own distinctive set of experimental conditions so that the role of a single factor or set of factors cannot be isolated. We have in various combinations

photographs of actual faces and schematic faces, tasks with and without memory load, easy tasks and difficult tasks, and different response measures. Taken together, the approximately 50 papers published in the past 15 years still do not provide a large enough body of information to permit drawing firm conclusions.

But, of course, information will always be incomplete unless attention is focused on the specific questions that need to be answered. To do this, one must propose hypotheses to be tested by empirical study. This is what Sergent and Bindra (1981) have done in their review of the methodology of studies of facial perception. They conclude from their analysis that a number of experimental conditions operate to produce a left visual-field advantage. These include short stimulus duration, low task difficulty, familiarity, and simple task demands, that is, for discrimination or recognition rather than identification. All these factors favor the employment of an holistic, nonanalytic mode of information processing that appears to be mediated by right-hemisphere mechanisms. The converse situation—where the perceptual task is difficult, unfamiliar, and calling for a specific identification response—operates to favor a right visual-field advantage and the employment of an analytic mode of information processing that appears to be mediated by left-hemisphere mechanisms. Thus, each hemisphere appears to have the capability for facial perception and the preferential use of right- or left-hemisphere mechanisms is influenced by both experimental and subject variables. The extent of influence of these variables and of the interactions between them remains to be ascertained.

A comment about the meaning of the instability in performance that is observed in the course of a single session and that, in all probability, also occurs from one occasion to another is in order. It would be an error to view this instability as a reflection of unreliability, with its implication of imperfect measurement of a "true" fixed characteristic. Instead, it should be considered to be the valid expression of a dynamic state of affairs. Galper and Costa (1980) have shown that preexperimental information emphasizing either the physical or social attributes of faces influences the recognition of subsequently presented faces in each half-field in contrasting ways. Klein, Moscovitch and Vigna (1976) have reported that so-called hemispheric priming, that is, preexperimental performance of a verbal or a nonverbal task, influences subsequent patterns of visual-field performance. Turkewitz and Ross (1983) have plotted the changes in visual-field advantage that take place over the course of repeated presentations of a set of faces and adduced evidence that this reflects a corresponding shift in information processing strategy on the part of the subjects.

There is no reason to doubt that the same changes may occur independently of experimental manipulations in normal subjects. They may choose to attend to either the physical or social attributes of faces and to change their choice over trials. Even if they have a preference for the use of one or another cognitive style, they may adopt an analytic approach on one occasion and an holistic approach on another occasion, depending on their mood, physical condition, immediately preceding experiences or other factors. To put it in neurological (neuromythological?) terms, given an intact brain with the capacity for unimpeded interhemispheric interactions, the subjects may shift from one hemispheric operation to the other simply because their integrated brain is there to be used.

Finally, I should like to make a com-ment of a general nature about the relationship between clinical study of patients with brain disease and experimentation on normal subjects. Most of what we know about functional localization in the human brain has been gained from observations on brain-diseased patients. It is these "experiments of nature" (to use a hackneyed phrase), that have given us the most securely established facts about cerebral organization, such as the locus of the cortical sensory areas and the association of speech with the left hemisphere, of visuospatial behavior with the right hemisphere, and of memory with the mesial temporal lobes. Thus, there can be no doubt about the basic validity of making inferences about the normal brain from the study of pathological cases.

Nevertheless, making such inferences has to be done carefully and with reserve. Loss of tissue from disease is not (or may not be) simply a subtraction from a stable system, but, instead, may produce a change in the organization of the entire system. For example, a focal lesion will produce a retardation in reaction time not only for performances involving mechanisms that are compromised by the lesion but also for performances not involving these mechanisms (cf. Benton & Joynt, 1959). Or consider the findings of Sprague (1966) and Sherman (1974) that visual defect produced by occipital lobe ablation in the cat may be attenuated or even disappear if the superior colliculus or its commissures are subsequently destroyed. Observations such as these make it clear that a focal brain lesion can exert effects on the interactive components of a neural system and, thus, alter the structure of that system.

If we accept this formulation, then we should be prepared to find that the results with brain-diseased patients and those with normal subjects are not congruent in every respect. To the extent that a lesion has altered the neural system of the brain as a unit, neurobehavioral associations may be found in patients that are not apparent in subjects with intact brains and vice versa. Of course, our ultimate goal is to discover relationships that hold for all subjects, normal and pathological. But we are still quite far from that goal. It is reassuring that, so far as I can tell, no major inconsistency in the findings obtained in the two classes of subjects has emerged.

Clinicians and experimentalists, no doubt, will continue to pursue their respective lines of investigation. If each group of researchers will take the trouble to monitor developments in the other's field and try to make sense of the totality of findings coming from both areas, this would surely facilitate progress toward a deeper understanding of normal and deranged facial recognition.

REFERENCES

Albert, M. S., Butters, N., & Levin, J. Temporal gradients in the retrograde amnesia in patients with alcoholic Korsakoff's disease. *Archives of Neurology*, 1979, 36, 211–216.

Assal, G. Régression des troubles de la reconnaissance des physionomies et de la mémoire topographique chez un malade opéré d'un hématome intracérébral pariéto-temporal droit. *Revue Neurologique*, 1969, 121, 184–185.

Benton, A. L. The neuropsychology of facial recognition. *American Psychologist*, 1980, 35, 176–186.

Benton, A. L. Visuoperceptual, visuospatial and visuoconstructive disorders. In K. M. Heilman & E. Valenstein (Eds.), *Clinical Neuropsychology*, 2nd Edition. New York: Oxford University Press, 1984.

Benton, A. L., Eslinger, P. J., & Damasio, A. R. Normative observations on neuropsychological test performances in old age. *Journal of Clinical Neuropsychology*, 1981, 3, 33–42.

Benton, A. L., Hamsher, K., Varney, N. R., & Spreen, O. *Contributions to Neuropsychological Assessment*. New York: Oxford University Press, 1983.

Benton, A. L., & Joynt, R. J. Rection time in unilateral cerebral disease. *Confinia Neurologica*, 1959, 19, 247–256.

Benton, A. L., & Van Allen, M. W. Impairment in facial recognition in patients with unilateral cerebral disease. *Cortex*, 1968, 4, 344–358.

Benton, A. L., & Van Allen, M. W. Prosopagnosia and facial discrimination. *Journal of the Neurological Sciences*, 1972, 15, 167–172.

Blumstein, S., Goodglass, H., & Tartter, V. The reliability of ear advantage in dichotic listening. *Brain and Language*, 1975, 2, 226–236.

Bodamer, J. Die Prosop-Agnosie. *Archiv für Psychiatrie und Nervenkrankheiten*, 1947, 179, 6–54.

Boudouresques, J., Poncet, M., Ali Cherif, A., & Balzamo, M. L'agnosie des visages. *Bulletin de l'Académie Nationale de Médecine*, 1979, 163, 659–702.

Bryden, M. P. *Laterality: Functional Asymmetry in the Intact Brain*. New York: Academic Press, 1982.

Damasio, A. R., Damasio, H., & Van Hoesen, G. W. Prosopagnosia: Anatomic basis and behavioral mechanisms. *Neurology*, 1982, 32, 331–341.

Damasio, A. R., Lima, A., & Damasio, H. Nervous function after right hemispherectomy. *Neurology*, 1975, 25, 89–93.

De Renzi, E., Faglioni, P., & Spinnler, H. The performance of patients with unilateral damage on facial recognition tests. *Cortex*, 1968, 4, 17–34.

Eslinger, P. H., & Benton, A. L. Visuoperceptual performances in aging and dementia. *Journal of Clinical Neuropsychology*, 1983, 5, 313–320.

Faust, C. Partielle Seelenblindheit nach Occipitalhirnverletzung mit besonderer Beeinträchtigung des Physiognomieerkennungs. *Nervenarzt*, 1947, 18, 294–297.

Faust, C. *Die zerebralen Herdstörungen bei Hinterhauptsverletzungen und ihre Beurteilung*. Stuttgart: Thieme, 1955.

Galper, R. E., & Costa, L. Hemispheric

superiority for recognizing faces depends upon how they are learned. *Cortex*, 1980, 16, 21–38.

Geffen, G., Bradshaw, J., & Wallace, G. Inter-hemispheric effects on reaction time to verbal and non-verbal stimuli. *Journal of Experimental Psychology*, 1971, 87, 415–422.

Hamsher, K., Levin, H. S., & Benton, A. L. Facial recognition in patients with focal brain lesions. *Archives of Neurology*, 1979, 36, 837–839.

Hannay, H. J., & Rogers, J. P. Individual differences and asymmetry effects in memory for unfamiliar faces. *Cortex*, 1979, 15, 257–267.

Hécaen, H., Ajuriaguerra, J. de, Magis, C., & Angelergues, R. Le problème de l'agnosie des physionomies. *Encéphale*, 1952, 51, 322–355.

Hécaen, H., Angelergues, R. Agnosia for faces (prosopagnosia). *Archives of Neurology*, 1962, 7, 92–100.

Hécaen, H., Angelergues, R., Bernhardt, C., & Chiarelli, J. Essai de distinction des modalités cliniques de l'agnosie des physionomies. *Revue Neurologique*, 1957, 96, 125–144.

Hécaen, H. & Tzavaras, A. Etude neuropsychologique des troubles de la reconnaissance des visages humaines. *Bulletin de Psychologie*, 1969, 22, 754–762.

Hilliard, R. D. Hemispheric laterality effects on a facial recognition task in normal subjects. *Cortex*, 1973, 9, 246–258.

Klein, D., Moscovitch, M., & Vigna, C. Attentional mechanisms and perceptual asymmetries in tachistoscopic recognition of words and faces. *Neuropsychologia*, 1976, 14, 55–66.

Kimura, D. Dual functional asymmetry of the brain in visual perception. *Neuropsychologia*, 1966, 4, 275–285.

Leehey, S., Carey, S., Diamond, R., & Cahn, A. Upright and inverted faces: The right hemisphere knows the difference. *Cortex*, 1978, 14, 411–419.

Levin, H. S., Grossman, R. G., & Kelly, P. J. Impairment in facial recognition after closed head injuries of varying severity. *Cortex*, 13, 119–130.

Lezak, M. D. *Neuropsychological Assess-ment*, 2nd Edition. New York: Oxford University Press, 1983.

Lhermitte, F., Chain, F., Escourolle, R., Ducarne, B., & Pillon, B. Etude anatomo-clinique d'un cas de prosopagnosie. *Revue Neurologique*, 1972, 126, 329–346.

Lhermitte, F., & Pillon, B. La prosopagnosie: Rôle de l'hémisphere droit dans la perception visuelle. *Revue Neurologique*, 1975, 131, 791–812.

Malone, D. R., Morris, H. M., Kay, M. C., & Levin, H. S. Prosopagnosia: A double dissociation between the recognition of familiar and unfamiliar faces. *Journal of Neurology, Neurosurgery and Psychiatry*, 1982, 45, 820–822.

McGlone, J. Sex differences in human brain asymmetry: A critical survey. *Behavioral and Brain Sciences*, 1980, 3, 215–227.

Meadows, J. C. The anatomical basis of prosopagnosia. *Journal of Neurology, Neurosurgery and Psychiatry*, 1974, 37, 489–501.

Nardelli, E., Buonanno, F., Coccia, G., Fiaschi, A., Terzian, H., & Rizzuto, N. Prosopagnosia: Report of four cases. *European Neurology*, 1982, 21, 289–297.

Oltman, P. K., Ehrlichman, H., & Cox, P. W. Field independence and laterality in the perception of faces. *Perceptual and Motor Skills*, 1977, 45, 255–260.

Pizzamiglio, L., De Pascalis, C., & Vignati, A. Stability of dichotic listening test. *Cortex*, 1974, 10, 203–205.

Pizzamiglio, L., & Zoccolati, P. Sex and cognitive influence on visual hemifield superiority for face and letter recognition. *Cortex*, 1981, 17, 215–226.

Rapacynski, W., & Ehrlichman, H. Opposite hemifield superiorities in face recognition as a function of cognitive style. *Neuropsychologia*, 1979, 17, 645–652.

Rizzolati, G., Umiltà, C., & Berlucchi, G. Opposite superiorities of the right and left hemispheres in discriminative reaction time to physiognomical and alphabetical material. *Brain*, 1971, 94, 431–442.

Rondot, P., & Tzavaras, A. La prosopagnosie après vingt années d'études cliniques et neuropsychologiques. *Journal de Psychologie Normale et Pathologique*, 1969, 66, 133–166.

Rondot, P., Tzavaras, A., & Garcin, R. Sur

un case de prosopagnosie persistant depuis quinze années. *Revue Neurologique*, 1967, 117, 424–428.

Sergent, J., & Bindra, D. Differential hemispheric processing of faces: Methodological considerations and reinterpretation. *Psychological Bulletin*, 1981, 89, 541–554.

Sherman, S. M. Visual fields of cats with cortical and tectal lesions. *Science*, 1974, 185, 355–357.

Smith, A. Nondominant hemispherectomy. *Neurology*, 1969, 19, 442–445.

Sprague, J. M. Interaction of cortex and superior colliculus in visually guided behavior in the cat. *Science*, 1966, 153, 1544–1547.

St. John, R. C. Lateral asymmetry in face perception. *Canadian Journal of Psychology*, 1981, 35, 213–223.

Teuber, H. L. Effects of focal brain injury on human behavior. In T. N. Chase (Ed.), *The Nervous System*, vol, 2, *The Clinical Neurosciences*. New York: Raven Press, 1975.

Tzavaras, A., Hécaen, H., & Le Bras, H. Le problème de la spécificitè du déficit de la reconnaissance du visage humain lors les lésions hemisphériques unilatérales. *Neuropsychologia*, 1970, 8, 403–416.

Tzavaras, A., Merienne, L., & Masure, M. C. Prosopagnosie, amnésie et troubles du langage par lésion temporale gauche chez un sujet gaucher. *Encéphale*, 1973, 62, 383–394.

Turkewitz, G., & Ross, P. Changes in visual field advantage for facial recognition: The development of a general processing strategy. *Cortex*, 1983, 19, 179–185.

Warrington, E. K., & James, M. An experimental investigation of facial recognition in patients with unilateral cerebral lesions. *Cortex*, 1967, 3, 317–320.

Whitely, A. M., & Warrington, E. K. Prosopagnosia: A clinical, psychological and anatomical study of three patients. *Journal of Neurology, Neurosurgery and Psychiatry*, 1977, 40, 395–403.

Young, A. W., & Bion, P. J. Accuracy of naming laterally presented faces by children and adults. *Cortex*, 1981, 17, 97–106.

Zoccolati, P., & Oltman, P. K. Field dependence and lateralization of verbal and configurational processing. *Cortex*, 1978, 14, 155–163.

VIII.
Developmental Neuropsychology

24.

The Concept of Pseudofeeblemindedness*

In recent years, pseudofeeblemindedness, considered as either a clinical condition or a problem of differential diagnosis, has received increasing attention from workers in the field of psychopathology of childhood. Apparently, more frequently than was the case in previous years, the clinician encounters conditions that he is unwilling to designate as "true" mental defect, even though, as the term "pseudofeeblemindedness" implies, these cases exhibit some of the characteristics of mental defect. Obviously, he must have in mind some concept of "true" mental defect which serves as a standard whereby he evaluates the individual case. Within this frame of reference, certain cases are judged to be not mentally defective. Among these cases, a certain proportion are further designated as being "pseudofeebleminded."

When one reflects on the situation, a number of questions raise themselves. One has to do with the exact meaning of

* A. L. Benton, *Archives of Neurology and Psychiatry*, 1956, 75, 379–388. Copyright 1956, American Medical Association.

the diagnosis of pseudofeeblemindedness. And, since the diagnosis depends basically upon the concept of "true" mental defect, one must also ask what is meant by "true" mental defect. The present paper deals with these questions. It attempts to analyze both the concept of pseudofeeblemindedness and that of "true" mental defect. As will be seen, this analysis suggests that the two concepts ought perhaps to be unified into a single broad concept of behavioral defect.

PSEUDOFEEBLEMINDEDNESS AS FALSE DIAGNOSIS

We have first to distinguish between two meanings of "pseudofeeblemindedness." The term has been employed in two senses, which are in essence mutually exclusive and which require explicit differentiation. In one usage of the term, it represents a mistaken diagnosis; i.e., from the data at hand, a child is judged to be behaviorally retarded or deficient when in fact he is not. In its second usage, pseudofeeblemindedness denotes a condition of behavioral retardation or deficiency which is ascribable to factors other than those customarily held to be the essential antecedent conditions of "true" mental defect. In the first sense, pseudofeeble-mindedness means a false inference regarding current behavioral status. In the second sense, it means a true inference which is accompanied, however, with the implication that unusual etiologic factors are responsible for the behavioral deficiency. The simultaneous use of the term in both senses (sometimes by the same author) has led to considerable confusion and misunderstanding.

The inference of mental defect is necessarily made on the basis of observation of a limited sample of behavior. Ordinarily it rests upon the evaluation of the patient's behavior in the interview situation, his performances in the psychological test situation, and the verbal reports of relatives, coupled with the results of physical examination. One measure of the validity of these procedures is the accuracy with which they predict the "true" behavioral status, i.e., the behavioral level generally characteristic of the patient in real life situations. The procedures are "valid" to the degree that a correlation exists between the behavior exhibited under the special conditions of observation provided by the interview or test (or that reported in the case history) and the behavior manifested in daily life. Numerous extraneous factors may operate to affect the observed or reported behavior and thus to attenuate the correlation between these behaviors and actual life behavior. Such an attenuation in relationship results in inferences of less validity than would otherwise be possible.

Extraneous factors which may affect the nature of test or interview behavior are numerous and of a varied character. Temporary physical disability may go unrecognized while adversely affecting a child's behavior in an interview or the quality of his performance on a psychologic examination. Timidity, hostility, or distrust may have a similarly adverse effect upon the performances of adults as well as of children. Successful deliberate simulation of mental incompetence is probably not as rare as is usually assumed. The examiner himself constitutes an important variable. His skill and experience in eliciting optimal performance is often a decisive factor in affecting the validity of the findings, and his personal traits may be a significant determinant of the subject's performances. Those characteristics of the interaction between patient and examiner which are designated as "rapport" play an important role, particularly with younger children and emotionally disturbed patients.

Another source of invalid inference lies in the frequent utilization of inappropriate statistical norms in the interpretation of performance. An even more potent source of error is the employment of inappropriate procedures for the assessment of intelligence, e.g., verbal scales on children with speech or hearing deficits, performance tests on children with visual defects, etc. The information provided by persons concerned with the patient is also subject to distortions which may seriously affect the validity of inferences drawn from it. The retrospective reports of parents provide a type of data which has long been recognized as having only a moderate degree of credibility. The accuracy of descriptions of current behavior by teachers and social workers may be affected by attitudinal and motivational factors, particularly if the child is disturbing the classroom or family structure.

A false diagnosis of mental defect is most frequently made in the case of children who are showing delinquent or antisocial conduct. By definition, these children are behaving incompetently in a social sense. The basic question is, of course, whether a fundamental intellectual inadequacy is responsible for the social incompetence. In the absence of striking evidence to the contrary, the untrained observer is likely to consider that the question is already answered; i.e., he tends to confuse the lack of capacity for social adjustment with intellectual inadequacy. In addition, the conviction on the part of the social or eductional authorities that a child should be institutionalized may play a role in presenting a bleaker picture of the intellectual aspects of his behavior than is actually warranted. On the child's part, hostility and distrust may so constrict his behavior in the interview and test situations that over-all efficiency of performance in these diagnostic situations is that of a mental defective. If he is in difficulty with the law, an element of simulation may enter the picture.

It is not difficult to understand how a false inference of mental defect, i.e., that a child is socially incompetent by reason of intellectual subnormality when in fact he is not, might be made on the basis of observational data and evaluations such as have been described. Acceptance at face value of the verbal reports of informants and an uncritical interpretation of performance in diagnostic situations without consideration of the possible influence of distorting factors might lead, in any given case, to a diagnosis of mental deficiency, when in reality the child's social incompetence is determined by motivational and attitudinal factors rather than by intellectual inadequacy.

If such an erroneous diagnosis is made and if, in later years, the person's behavior and achievements show clearly that he does not suffer from significant intellectual inadequacy, a review of his case may lead to the conclusion that the original inference was false; i.e., he never was

intellectually subnormal. The presumption is, then, that the initial diagnosis was based on inadequate data or on a faulty interpretation of the available data. His behavior suggested mental defect, but fuller or more critical examination would have disclosed the patient's intellectual adequacy. Because the patient gave the impression of being mentally defective, such an erroneous diagnosis is often referred to as pseudofeeblemindedness.

In my opinion it is difficult to justify such a designation for what is essentially an error in diagnosis. Certainly, it would seem better to keep the focus of attention on the responsible clinician rather than to project it, so to speak, on the patient. Errors in diagnosis ought not to be given the status of a clinical entity, and it is reasonable to conclude that in the first sense of the term there is no such thing as "psuedofeeblemindedness."

PSEUDOFEEBLEMINDEDNESS AS MENTAL DEFICIENCY OF ATYPICAL ETIOLOGY

The second sense in which the term "pseudofeeblemindedness" is employed presents a quite different situation. It rests upon the conception that "true" mental defect implies the operation of certain etiologic factors. If it can be assumed that defect or disease of certain critical cerebral areas is at least the proximate cause of "true" mental deficiency, then, in contrast, pseudofeeblemindedness presents a picture of behavioral retardation which is virtually identical with that associated with "true" mental deficiency but which is determined by other factors, most (but not all) of which are extracerebral in nature. Thus, the distinction between "true feeblemindedness" and "pseudofeeblemindedness" depends upon the nature of the responsible etiologic factors. Pseudofeeblemindedness may be said to represent mental deficiency of atypical etiology.

This atypical etiology may be classified into a number of broad classes of determinants: (1) sensory deprivation, such as visual or auditory handicap; (2) motor deficit, as in cerebral palsy; (3) cultural deprivation, as represented by a nonstimulating social or family environment and inadequate schooling; (4) emotional disturbance, which is conceived as exerting an inhibitory effect on intellectual function and, consequently, on the acquisition of basic mental abilities.

It is generally appreciated that each of these classes of factors is capable of exercising a depressing effect of at least a moderate degree on intellectual level, and it is not difficult to construct a theoretical model, illustrating how retardation in the acquisition of the numerous intellectual skills subsumed under the global valuistic concept of "intelligence" can result from the operation of one or another factor. The general tenor of empirical findings which show moderate retardation in intelligence to be characteristic of groups of handicapped children, such as the blind, the deaf, and the culturally underprivileged, also supports this formulation. As a consequence, the experienced examiner, when he evaluates the performances of a handicapped child, tends to take account of the general finding of a moderate retardation being characteristic of the group to which the child belongs. He is also careful to base his evaluation on procedures requiring performances which are well within the behavior repertory of the child, e.g. visual rather than auditory tests to the hard of hearing child, performance rather than verbal tests to the culturally handicapped child, etc. His interpretation of the performances of the child is likely to be rather "liberal," and the finding of a moderate retardation in intellectual development in such a child, e.g., an intelligence quotient of 80–85, is usually interpreted as presumptive evidence that the child's intelligence is within normal limits.

However, the examiner can hardly afford to be too "liberal" in his evaluation. He knows that the typical effect of physical or social handicap is only a relatively slight depression in intelligence level. He also knows that these handicaps tend to be correlated with the occurrence of mental deficiency. Therefore, if a handicapped child's performance is definitely below normal limits, e.g., below an intelligence quotient of 80, the retardation in intellectual development cannot reasonably be ascribed to the typical operation of a physical or social handicap. If, then, the totality of data is consistent in presenting a picture of significant behavioral retardation, the diagnostic inference of mental deficiency must be made.

Theoretically, two distinct sets of factors may be operating to produce the observed behavioral deficiency in such a case. The first possibility is that we are dealing with a "true" mental deficiency; i.e., the cerebral defect or disease which is customarily held to be responsible for states of mental deficiency is present. The physical or social handicap is either an incidental accompaniment of the mental deficiency, or, in the case of physical handicap, it may point to a global developmental disturbance, of which both the behavioral deficiency and the physical deficit are part expressions. In either case, the handicap per se is not a significant determinant of the mental deficiency.

The second possibility is that we are dealing with a case of pseudofeeblemindedness, that is, with an atypically severe effect of the physical or social handicap. The reasons why a handicap should have particularly severe depressive effects on behavioral development in the case of one child and not in the case of another are

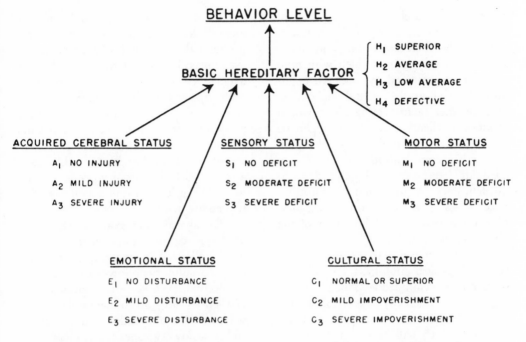

Fig. 12. Theoretical schema illustrating interaction of determinants of mental deficiency and pseudofeeblemindedness.

not well understood. However, clinical experience does suggest that a particularly deleterious effect may occur when a handicap affects a child whose intellectual potentialities are rather limited to start with or when combinations of handicaps are present. One might think in terms of an hereditary core with respect to intellectual potential, varying from individual to individual, through which various factors—cerebral status, sensory status, motor status, emotional status, and cultural status—operate to produce a behavior resultant. This conception is illustrated in Figure 12.

As outlined in Figure 12, "Behavior Level" is conceived to be the resultant of a number of determining factors. A prime determinant is the variable designated as the "Basic Hereditary Factor." This is a continuous variable which, for practical purposes, might be subdivided into four levels, as indicated. The defective level,

H_4, can be assumed to account for mental deficiency of a purely hereditary character. Other factors being held constant, the other levels, viz., H_1, H_2, and H_3 would account for variations in the intelligence quotient within the normal and superior ranges, e.g., 80–150.

This hereditary factor has a double significance. Not only is it a potent determinant in its own right, but it also serves the function of "host," so to speak, for the other factors. That is to say, the other determinants—"Acquired Cerebral Status," "Sensory Status," "Motor Status," etc.——operate through the medium of the nuclear factor of hereditary status, interacting with it to produce their effects.

With respect to the factor of acquired cerebral status, I have in mind the occurrence of brain injury or disease of all degrees of severity. Severe insult suffered in early life (A_3) would account for the category of purely exogenous mental defect. Moreover, a relatively poor, but not defective, hereditary status, as represented by level H_3, combined with mild injury, as represented by level A_2, might produce high-grade mental deficiency, when neither factor acting alone would produce it, leading to what might be called "mixed" mental defect. Thus, we have the combination H_3A_2 as an adequate determinant of high-grade mental deficiency. A good many institutionalized cases seem to fall in this category, perhaps as many as fall in either of the "pure" categories.

Turning to the defect states of presumably atypical etiology, the conditions of pseudofeeblemindedness, the determining factors of sensory status (S), motor status (M), emotional status (E), and cultural status (C) will be noted. Each is a continuous variable, which, for convenience, has been analyzed into three levels: (1) no defect, (2) moderate defect, and (3) severe defect. As has already been mentioned, empirical data on the blind, the deaf, and the culturally underprivileged indicate that, while the handicap involved does lead to some retardation in behavioral development, mental deficiency is not the typical outcome. Since these are group results, it may be assumed that the typical outcome holds for an average hereditary status, i.e., H_2. What these clinical findings can be interpreted to mean is that the interaction of defective sensory or motor function, emotional disturbance, or cultural handicap with an average hereditary status does not lead to mental defect; i.e., such combinations as H_2S_3, H_2M_3, or H_2C_3 are *not* determinants of mental defect. However, if one considers the possibility of an interaction between, for example, defective sensory or motor function with a low-average hereditary status, that is, an H_3S_3 or H_3M_3 combination, it is conceivable that such

an interaction could lead to high-grade mental defect. Indeed, it seems rather probable that it would. In concrete terms, the conception is that while a child with average or superior endowment might, with proper educational guidance, overcome the handicap of deafness or cerebral palsy and attain an intellectual efficiency which is within normal limits, the same sensory or motor handicap would lead to a mental defect state of moderate degree in a child of low- or dull-average intellectual endowment.

To take another example, the factor of severe cultural impoverishment does not usually lead to mental deficiency. The typical resultant is a low- or dull-average intellectual level, i.e., the combination of H_2C_3 does not lead to mental defect. But what of the combination H_3C_3? Can the child of low-average endowment overcome the handicap? It is distinctly possible that he might suffer a sufficiently serious retardation in intellectual growth as to make him a borderline or moron-level mental defective. One suspects that a good many cases of so-called familial mental defect actually belong in this category rather than in the purely hereditary category.

All these situations represent theoretical examples of pseudofeeblemindedness, the general formula being the interaction of a specific handicap with a subnormal (but not defective) hereditary endowment. One speaks of the inability of the child to overcome the deleterious behavioral effects of the sensory, motor cultural, or emotional handicap. This inability might be permanent, or it might be temporary; i.e., over a period of time, the developing person might be able to overcome the more significant effects of the handicap. Under these conditions, one would have the situation of a person who is mentally defective as a child but who, gradually, through the adolescent years gains enough in behavioral efficiency so that he is no longer classifiable as a mental defective.

In addition to the interaction of a specific deficit with a subnormal hereditary endowment as a determinant of mental defect, there is the possibility that combinations of special defects themselves will produce mental defect even in a child of average intellectual potentialities. Deafness combined with cultural impoverishment or blindness combined with motor deficit might constitute sufficiently severe handicaps as to cause a gross retardation in behavioral development.

It must be emphasized that there is nothing false or unreal about these intellectual defect states, even though they may be called "pseudofeeblemindedness." They are true mental defect states from the behavioral standpoint, differing from the more conventional types of mental deficiency only in respect to etiology. Nor is there necessarily an impermanent quality to these conditions. They can continue without alleviation throughout life, in much the same manner as untreated cretinism.

While this conception of physical, psychological, and social handicap causing mental deficiency in a child seems clear enough theoretically, in practice it is not easy to distinguish between such a state of affairs and that represented by the coincidental occurrence of the handicap with so-called "true" mental defect. Limitations in knowledge, as well as lack of precision in psychodiagnostic methods, make it quite difficult to differentiate between the two conditions. At the time of initial examination, the diagnostic inference is more likely to be that one is dealing with a coincidence of the mental defect state and the handicap than with a condition of pseudofeeblemindedness. The first inference often seems to the clinician to be the more "parsimonious" one. Actually, it does not involve fewer

assumptions than does the inference of mental deficiency on the basis of the handicap. However, it does involve more conventional (hence, more acceptable) assumptions and therefore appears easier to make. The diagnosis of pseudofeeblemindedness is more likely to be made only after a period of time has elapsed during which the course of the handicapped patient's development has been such as to show clearly that the diagnosis of mental deficiency is no longer tenable. In short, an impermanent pseudofeeblemindedness is more readily diagnosed than a permanent one. But this cannot be taken to mean that permanent conditions of pseudofeeblemindedness do not exist.

CONCEPT OF "TRUE" MENTAL DEFICIENCY

In order to understand the meaning of pseudofeeblemindedness and to assess its place in clinical thinking, it is necessary to review the notion of mental deficiency itself. It is not at all a simple concept. On the contrary, it is a rather complex one, which possesses behavioral, etiologic, developmental, and prognostic implications. It is also evident that the concept does not mean quite the same thing to different people. With respect to each of these aspects, one finds considerable disagreement among workers in the field.

This is true even with respect to the intellectual aspect. Most students regard the proposition that the cardinal behavioral feature of mental deficiency is intellectual subnormality as virtually axiomatic. Nevertheless, as eminent an authority as Tredgold[1] would not admit this and would insist that the nuclear manifestation of mental deficiency is a defect in behavioral adaptability, which may or may not be accompanied by intellectual subnormality. Similarly, Delay, Pichot and Perse[2] have advanced the notion of "camouflaged mental deficiency," as they call it, i.e., social incompetence camouflaged by a good intelligence quotient.

However, the issues of etiology and prognosis are decidedly more important. With regard to etiology, it is reasonable to state that some concept of defect or disease of critical cerebral areas is what most clinicians have in mind when they think of at least the proximate cause of mental deficiency, whether the defect state be of a hereditary or an acquired nature. Thus, Tredgold writes that "the brain is the organ for the manifestations of mind . . . the material basis of mental deficiency consists in an inadequate development, or persistent imperfection of function, of the neurones of the mantle of the brain . . . primary amentia is the result of an inherent incapacity of these neurones to attain an adequate degree of development and function, while secondary amentia is due to their development having been arrested by some external cause.[1]*

In evaluating this statement by Tredgold, it is useful to consider separately the neuropathologic findings in low-grade deficiency as contrasted with high-grade deficiency, since the general picture seems to be different in these two broad groups. In low-grade deficiency, positive neuropathologic findings, while apparently not demonstrable in every single case, seem to be the rule.[1,3,4,5] However, a somewhat different picture is encountered in high-grade defect. Positive neuropathologic findings are *not* the rule. On the other hand, it would be inaccurate to conclude that negative findings *are* the rule. It appears that the neuropathologic picture is simply unpredictable. In many cases the findings are a normal anatomy and histology. Tredgold, who cannot be accused of being overly skeptical about the assump-

tion of neuropathologic basis for the high-grade defect, summarizes the situation as follows:

In general, the brains of the milder aments are a little less in size and weight than the normal, and their convolutions tend to be wider and simpler; but they rarely present any of the gross abnormalities which characterize those of lower grade. Further, microscopical examinations do not show the marked paucity and imperfection of neurones which occur in idiots and imbeciles, and with our present methods of investigation the brains of many high-grade feebleminded individuals would pass muster as normal.[1]†

Thus, it is probably fair to say that there is a lack of convincing evidence of a consistent neuropathologic basis for high-grade mental deficiency. There are two possible interpretations for this state of affairs. The first is that these negative, or at least inconsistent, findings are a consequence of limitations in our present methods of laboratory investigation. The second interpretation holds that we must accept the facts as they are and that, in any case, it is not necessary to assume that all mental defect necessarily rests on cerebral defect. The idea that neurosis and psychosis are necessarily based on cerebral disease or maldevelopment has long been abandoned. There is no reason to hold to it in the case of high-grade mental defect.

Tredgold's assertion that high-grade mental defect is always based upon cerebral defect or pathology, which is often not demonstrable, is a statement of faith. One may or may not accept this statement of faith. If one does not, one looks to other determinants of the defect state, i.e., determinants other than demonstrable cerebral pathology. When one does this,

* pp. 106–107.   † p. 121.

one moves into the area of pseudofeeble-mindedness.

PROGNOSIS IN MENTAL DEFICIENCY

The question of the ultimate fate of persons who, in childhood, show the behavioral symptom complex of mental deficiency has occupied investigators for half a century. However, before reviewing the findings and discussing the implications of these studies, it is necessary to consider a point of view which, in a sense, "eliminates" the problem of prognosis by establishing a poor prognosis as one of the essential characteristics of this behavioral disorder.

For some workers, the concept of mental deficiency is defined not only by etiologic factors and behavioral manifestations but also by the course and outcome of the disorder. For example, Doll,[6] in his formulation of an "inclusive concept" of mental deficiency, lists as an essential criterion for the diagnosis the condition that the behavioral defect must obtain at maturity. Thus, he states that "the concept of the essential incurability of feeble-mindedness is part of the diagnostic picture. If the prognosis suggests a possibility of amelioration of symptoms amounting to prospects of ultimate normality, then a diagnosis of mental deficiency is not warranted."*

Nevertheless, while it is true that at the present time a poor prognosis is characteristic of virtually all cases of lower-grade defect and of the majority of cases of higher-grade defect, most workers in the field, however conservative their expectations in regard to prognosis may be, probably would not include the idea of a fixed outcome as an essential part of the concept of mental deficiency. Instead, they would prefer to rely on etio-

logic and behavioral criteria to establish the diagnosis and to make the question of outcome a matter for empirical investigation and for possible modification.

There are sound reasons for this refusal to include outcome as an *essential* part of any diagnosis, however important it may be in the *description* of a disease or condition. This holds true even in such instances where an empirical relation has been so securely established that at the present time the diagnosis does in fact predict the terminal state with a high degree of accuracy. The fundamental objection to such a procedure derives from the fact that the course and outcome of a disease are not solely a characteristic of the disease itself but are also a function of the efficiency of medical, psychologic, and educational practice at any given time. In other words, course and outcome depend upon the prevailing level of technologic efficiency. Since this efficiency level changes with time, a diagnostic concept which is based on course and outcome can hardly have a firm foundation.

This idea of poor prognosis as an integral part of the concept of mental deficiency appears to represent an application of the old doctrine of "malignancy," characteristic of a bygone era of medicine, when the physician, lacking a knowledge of pathology and possessing only the most meager therapeutic resources, could claim distinction solely on the basis of his ability to prognosticate. As pathologic anatomy and physiology developed during the nineteenth century, this notion of "malignancy," i.e., of a poor outcome being inherently characteristic of a disease and therefore essential for its diagnosis, was abandoned in most fields of medicine. Apparently, it lingered in psychiatry until at least the early years of the twentieth century. When Kraepelin made his great diagnostic synthesis of catatonia, hebephrenia, and other symp-

---

* p. 423.

tom pictures into the single category of dementia praecox, he included a typical course and outcome as essential features of the disorder. But these were precisely the aspects of his conception that encountered the most significant resistance among his contemporaries, and it was not many years before these elements of the diagnosis succumbed to Bleuler's formulation, which explicitly excluded course and outcome as necessary features of the disease.

The notion of "malignancy" plays little role in current neuropsychiatric thinking. This is not to say, of course, that a diagnosis may not have prognostic implications but says only that such implications do not serve as the essential basis for the diagnosis. They follow, rather than precede, the diagnosis. For example, the diagnosis of schizophrenia depends upon evaluation of a patient's present and past behavior. Once the diagnosis is established, it is not dependent upon the vicissitudes of the course or the response to treatment. Thus, it is not generally held, because a patient responded favorably to insulin, electroshock, frontal leucotomy, or some other treatment, that he was not "really" schizophrenic, that he was a "pseudoschizophrenic," or that his behaviour merely "simulated" schizophrenia.

But this is precisely the type of reasoning tht is often applied to cases of mental deficiency which do not follow the "prescribed" course. Thus, when follow-up study indicates that a patient, diagnosed in earlier years as mentally deficient, is socially competent and shows no more than minimal intellectual retardation, a post hoc judgment is made that the initial diagnosis was false, i.e., the patient was "pseudofeebleminded." This judgment is often accompanied by the suggestion that had a more careful initial examination been done, the original diagnosis would

not have been made. However, the procedures which would have made the examination more careful, or the criteria necessary for a differential diagnosis between "true" and "false" feeblemindedness, are seldom specified.

It is probably fair to state that the majority of workers reject such post hoc reasoning. The diagnosis of mental deficiency cannot depend upon a patient's status 10 years later. His future status is a matter for empirical investigation and analysis.

In considering the ultimate status of persons who in childhood were diagnosed as mentally defective, it is desirable to consider the lower and higher grades separately, for, as in the case with neuropathologic aspects, the two levels present rather different pictures. In the case of low-grade defect, follow-up study may or may not disclose significant changes in the intelligence quotient. However, even if a large change has occurred, it usually has no decisively important implications for the basic issue of social competence. Thus, a change in the intelligence quotient from 35 to 55 or 60 may be recorded, but one finds that the patient is still mentally defective, the only shift being in the category of defect.

Follow-up studies of higher-grade defectives have yielded more interesting results.[7–12] Some of these studies date back many years. All of them are in accord in finding that a significant proportion of persons who, in childhood, were diagnosed as mentally defective and who were treated as such (i.e., were institutionalized or placed in special classes) prove to be socially competent adults. This proportion varies from one-sixth to one-fourth, depending upon the criteria of the investigator and his particular sample of cases. The socioeconomic adjustment of these subjects is found to be variable, ranging from marginal to high-average. Their intelligence test performances vary from borderline to high-average. Their typical socioeconomic adjustment and intelligence test rating can perhaps best be designated as dull-average.

Thus, these studies indicate that some patients appear to show an alleviation of their mental defect state as they reach maturity, their improvement being reflected in a rise in the intelligence quotient and in socioeconomic competence. The reasons for this change in status are unknown, but, whatever be the determinants, the facts are incontestable.

CONCLUSIONS

In summary, we find that in a proportion of cases of high-grade mental deficiency it is not possible to demonstrate a neuropathologic basis. Further, a proportion of cases of mental deficiency prove to be of a temporary nature. Such cases sound suspiciously like those which have been designated as "pseudofeebleminded," in that, by definition, the case of pseudofeeblemindedness lacks the neuropathologic condition responsible for so-called "true" mental defect and, in practice, pseudofeeblemindedness is usually diagnosed when a change in status has occurred, that is, when it exists as a temporary condition. However, we do not know that these cases represent pseudofeeblemindedness in the explicit sense in which I have described the condition, i.e mental defect of atypical etiology. It is possible that we are dealing with erroneous initial diagnoses, i.e., pseudofeeblemindedness in the first sense of the term, as discussed in this paper. But there is no evidence for this supposition, either. It seems clear that there are a not inconsiderable number of cases with a diagnosis of mental deficiency in childhood which do not square with traditional notions about the etiology and prognosis of this group of disorders. On the other hand, the distinction between such cases and those in which the condition might be designated as pseudofeeblemindedness is not at all clear.

The implications of these findings are that traditional concepts of mental deficiency, to the degree that they include a specific etiology, neuropathologic basis, or course as defining terms, should be abandoned. A broader formulation such as that recently proposed by Benda,[3] which calls for a reexamination of the relations between mental "deficiency" and mental "illness" and which reopens the general question of etiology, appears to be more adequate. Since we deal with symptom pictures of multiple etiology, no one specific etiology has any claim to precedence over any other as being the primary antecedent condition of so-called "true" mental deficiency. All cases are examples of "true'" defect, by behavioral criteria. Conditions of "pseudofeeblemindedness" can be conceived as being "true" defect states with certain types of etiologic background. Because of their clinical importance, detailed study of the pathogenesis of these conditions is strongly indicated.

REFERENCES

1. Tredgold, A. F.: A Textbook of Mental Deficiency, Ed. 8, Baltimore, Williams & Wilkins Company, 1952.

2. Delay, J.; Pichot, P., & Perse, J.: La notion de débilité mentale camouflée, Ann. méd-psychol. 110:615–619, 1952.

3. Benda, C. E.: Developmental Disorders of Mentation and Cerebral Palsy, New York, Grune & Stratton, Inc., 1952.

4. Schob, F.: Pathologische Anatomie der Idiotie, in Bumke, O.: Handbuch der Geisteskrankheiten, Berlin, Springer-Verlag, 1930, Vol. 7, pp. 779–995.

5. Weygandt, W.: Der jugendliche

Schwachsinn, Stuttgart, Ferdinand Enke, 1936.

6. Doll, E. A.: Is Mental Deficiency Curable? Am. J. Ment, Deficiency 51:420–428, 1947.

7. Baller, W. R.: A Study of the Present Social Status of a Group of Adults Who, When They Were in Elementary Schools, Were Classified as Mentally Deficient, Genet. Psychol. Monog. 18:165–244, 1936.

8. Charles, D. C.: Ability and Accomplishment of Persons Earlier Judged Mentally Deficient, Genet. Psychol. Monog. 47:3–71, 1953.

9. Fairbank, R.: The Subnormal Child—17 Years after, Ment. Hyg. 17:177–208, 1933.

10. Kennedy, R. J. R.: The Social Adjustment of Morons in a Connecticut City, Hartford, 1948.

11. Muench, G. A.: A Follow-up of Mental Defectives after 18 Years, J. Abnorm. & Social Psychol. 39:407–418, 1944,

12. Schneider, O.: Das Gesetz zur Verhütung erbkranken Nachwuchses und seine Bedeutung für die Hilfsschule, Deutsche Sonderschule 1:401–408, 1934; abstracted, Zentralbl. Neurol. u. Psychiat. 75:228, 1935.

25.

Interactive Determinants of Mental Deficiency*

I should like first to express my appreciation to Dr. Bialer for his presentation. It is comprehensive and stimulating and, at the same time, it offers a sober and thoughtful appraisal. Quite obviously he has given long and careful consideration to the complex issues associated with this problem area of the relationship of mental deficiency to emotional disturbances and physical disability. My discussion will be focused on some of the etiological and diagnostic questions which he has raised.†

His presentation, as do so many of the earlier ones in this Conference, shows what a profound change has taken place during the past 20 years in our thinking about mental deficiency. Earlier it was conceived as an entity; one, to be sure, that could be analyzed in different ways and about which there was room for con-troversy, but nevertheless a "condition" or group of "conditions." Today, in contrast, we think of mental deficiency simply as an end-result which is associated (and not necessarily in an obligatory way) with a variety of conditions or events. These conditions or events are, we say, of a physical, emotional, or social "nature," meaning by this simply that at the present time we find it most useful to describe these particular conditions or events in physical, emotional, or social terms.

One effect of this shift of emphasis from a fixed "condition" to a mere "end-result" has been to introduce a certain degree of fluidity in our thinking and this in turn sometimes has created problems in defining our terms. Dr. Bialer has handled these definitional questions in a forthright and clear way. One may or may not agree with all his definitions but at least one knows what he is talking about.

Dr. Bialer rejects the concept and term "pseudoretardation" as being without substantial foundation and indeed as being a positive hindrance to effective practice and communication. This is a point of view with which most of us now

* A. L. Benton in H. C. Haywood (Ed.) Social-cultural Aspects of Mental Retardation. New York, Appleton-Century-Crofts, 1970, pp. 661–671. Reprinted by permission of Prentice-Hall, Inc., Englewood Cliffs, N.J.

† I. Bialer, "Relationship of mental retardation to emotional disturbance and physical disability," in Haywood, op. cit., pp. 607–660.

agree and one which some of us advanced with considerable vigor a decade or so ago. Yet the battle has not been completely won. The term (if not the concept which it once represented) continues to be used in clinical and educational circles.

What accounts for the persistence of this term which refers to a now generally discredited concept? The prefix "pseudo" means false or not genuine and, of course, pseudoretardation originally meant "not genuine" retardation. No doubt some people still mean this when they use the term but others do not. What they mean is genuine retardation of a particular type or types. We meet an analogous situation in medical classification. There is "bulbar palsy" and "pseudobulbar palsy," "sclerosis" and "pseudosclerosis." Pseudobulbar palsy and pseudosclerosis do not correspond to unreal or spurious conditions; they are quite real indeed. They do correspond to conditions which resemble in some ways the conditions designated as bulbar palsy and sclerosis but which are the product of different mechanisms. Thus the patient with pseudobulbar palsy shows motor disabilities just as does the patient with bulbar palsy but his disabilities are caused by a lesion at a higher level in the central nervous system.

I do not know the precise details about the historical development of these medical conceptualizations, but it is a fairly safe guess that the prefix "pseudo" was used because it served to link a more recently discovered condition (in terms of both similarity and contrast) with an older and more familiar condition. At the same time, it is clear that the prefix was *not* used in this context to imply a condition which is spurious—as it is, for example, in the concept of pseudodementia.

Roughly the same situation would appear to hold for the designation of pseudoretardation or pseudofeeble-mindedness. *If* one thinks in terms of a nuclear type of mental deficiency which is the product of maldevelopment or disease of critical areas of the brain, then one feels impelled to call other types of mental deficiency which are the product of other mechanisms by different names in order to distinguish them from, and at the same time, to associate them with, the nuclear type. However, just as is the case with the medical conceptualizations, the prefix "pseudo" does not imply a spurious or unreal condition.

But this is a rather curious use of the prefix "pseudo." And, while its employment does not seem to pose difficulties for neurologists in the contexts within which they use the term, historical circumstances make it a source of potential confusion in the field of mental deficiency. Certainly there is no place for the term or concept of pseudoretardation in our diagnostic classification. Like Dr. Bialer, I wish that clinicians would abandon it. However, it may persist for a while, in informal communication at least. One reason is that, as the tenor of Dr. Bialer's presentation suggests, there is in fact an atmosphere of doubt surrounding these special types of mental deficiency which were once called "pseudofeeblemindedness." Another possible reason is that these special types of mental deficiency often call for special therapeutic measures which are not particularly indicated in the nuclear types, e.g., psychotherapy or special education focused on a specific sensory defect.

What about this atmosphere of doubt which tends to surround the concept that sensory impairment, motor impairment, and emotional disorder are sufficient determinants of the state of global mental subnormality which defines mental deficiency? Dr. Bialer has expressed these doubts explicitly, pointing out that sensorimotor defect, even when severe, does not typically lead to mental deficiency and that therefore we are scarcely justified in considering them to be important determinants. Similarly, there is no substantial evidence that emotional disorder per se is a causative factor, even though empirically we observe a rather close association between mental deficiency and the presence of emotional disturbances. The complexities of the latter situation and the difficulties in the interpretation of the facts are well described by Dr. Bialer and, in the end, he comes to the conclusion that it is not useful to think of these variables as primary determinants of mental deficiency.

My own point of view is close to that of Dr. Bialer but does differ from it in certain respects. I believe that the importance of sensory impairment, motor impairment, and emotional disturbance as determinants of mental deficiency has been greatly overrated. As Dr. Bialer has pointed out, normative observations on the blind and on the deaf disclose an overall intellectual inferiority of rather small degree in these groups as compared to normal children. Their mean intelligence level is likely to be in the low- or dull-average range. At the same time, each group shows a higher-than-expected proportion of cases of frank mental deficiency. The diagnostic question here is whether we deal with a concurrence of two conditions or with a situation in which the state of mental deficiency is a resultant of the sensory impairment. A frequent background datum is a history of early cerebral disease and in these instances it often seems reasonable to conclude that both the sensory impairment and the global mental defect are concurrent consequences of brain damage. But, while this is a reasonable conclusion, it is not necessarily correct in every case.

In other cases of combined sensory impairment and mental deficiency, one finds no independent evidence of history of brain damage. Dr. Bialer's conceptualization of this problem is rather interesting. He presents the idea that this situation might be interpreted as reflecting "the operation of certain sociocultural variables detrimental to the acquisition of necessary experience" and, more specifically, "as lack of intervention in the form of stimulation from family or other meaningful persons." This, I think, is tantamount to saying that the sensory impairment is in fact a significant determinant of the observed mentally defective state. Perhaps environmental manipulation would alleviate or eradicate the state of mental deficiency and perhaps an "early prosthetic environment" (a happy application of this concept sometimes used by Dr. Bialer) would have prevented it. But these possibilities only reinforce the concept that sensory impairment can be a significant determinant of mental deficiency.

There is a suggestion here that perhaps Dr. Bialer's insistence that sensory impairment is not a significant determinant of mental deficiency has led him astray. For, in this context, he uses the term "functional retardation" with at least the possible implication that this is to be contrasted with mental retardation of a more substantial or enduring nature. But "functional retardation," in this sense, is only a synonym for "pseudoretardation." All types of mental deficiency, whatever their antecedents may be, are of a functional nature. We deal here with a behavioral (that is to say, a functional) concept, and not, as in an earlier era, with one which combines behavior with etiology and pathogenesis. If this type of mental deficiency is preventable by early intervention (as is, for example, phenylketonuria), so much the better. But let us not make the error of incorporating a prognostic or "response-to-treatment" criterion into our basic definition of mental deficiency.

In any case, the issue of the existence of sensorially or emotionally determined types of mental deficiency is not entirely settled. I have already expressed the opinion that the importance of sensori-motor defect and emotional disorder in the production of the clinical picture of mental deficiency has been overrated. This is quite definitely a "quantitative" opinion. I mean by it that the preconceptions of theorists and the unfounded assumptions of clinicians have led to an overestimation of the prevalence of these types of mental deficiency. At the same time, I do not doubt that these types, although they may be relatively uncommon, do exist.

What is the evidence that sensory impairment and emotional disorder are significant determinants of mental deficiency? It must be conceded that we lack anything approaching compelling evidence for the thesis. Uncontrolled clinical observation provides such support as we have for this conviction. To put the case simply, in clinical practice one encounters life histories which are most satisfactorily explained by the principle that sensory impairment or emotional disorder can be significant determinants of a state of mental deficiency. These life histories concern individuals who showed an impermanent state of mental defect which endured over the course of several years but which then showed a remission. However, it would be a mistake to assume that this is always the case. By their very nature, these cases come to light precisely because of the fact that they showed a change in intelligence level. If they had not shown this change, either they would have been considered simply as cases of mental deficiency or they would have posed the diagnostic problems which Dr. Bialer has discussed.

Some examples of this state of affairs, which every experienced clinician has encountered, may be cited.

BLINDNESS COMBINED WITH CEREBRAL PALSY AS A POSSIBLE DETERMINANT OF MENTAL DEFECT

A 6-year-old boy, blind and with cerebral palsy following meningitis at the age of 1 year, was seen for evaluation and found to have an IQ of about 33 (i.e., MA about 2 years). Practically his entire speech consisted in saying radio commercials, either spontaneously or in response to questions. He could articulate long and rather elaborate commercials clearly but evidently had no appreciation of the meaning of his utterances. His behavior was in fact strikingly similar to that of a demented patient who shows repetitive and automatic speech but who can neither understand oral language nor engage in propositional speech.

Inquiry revealed that he had been a tractable infant and child. To get him out of the way, his busy mother was in the habit of sitting him before the radio for hours at a time and she was grateful that he did not object to this. He would listen attentively and obviously enjoyed living in the world of radio.

His fluent articulation, the history of environmental deprivation, and the indications of an autistic personality development suggested that intensive treatment aimed at strengthening his ties to his personal environment and developing his knowledge of the semantic aspects of language should be given a trial. The physical therapist and the speech therapist went to work with a will and his progress during the first month of treatment was gratifying. As one observer put it, he now behaved "more like a child than a radio." For example, he responded appropriately when asked what his favorite programs were, naming one or two. Similarly, when asked to sing, he did so, singing one or two songs that he had heard countless times. However, continued treatment during the second month resulted in no further progress and he seemed to have reached a plateau. He was discharged with the recommendation that he should receive a good deal of personal attention and not be permitted to spend hours at a time before the radio.

Seen 3 years later, he still proved to be defective but he was nevertheless a changed child. His IQ was about 60 (i.e., his MA was about 5.5 years). From a qualitative standpoint, his automatic speech had disappeared and he was obviously functioning on the level of propositional language in both its receptive and expressive aspects. (I lost track of the child after that).

We see here a decided rise in IQ coincident with a change in the handling of the child. He had gained 3.5 years in mental age over the course of 3 years. To be sure, he was still defective, but on a moderate rather than a severe level. The treatment measures that were instituted were not radical or intensive, consisting simply of a changed regime at home and the bringing in of a visiting teacher. I do not know whether or not he would have continued to improve in respect to relative mental level. There is no basis for prediction and it is entirely possible that he had once again reached a plateau. But one wonders what the introduction of a truly prosthetic environment at, for example, the age of 2 might have done for this child.

DEAFNESS AS A POSSIBLE DETERMINANT OF MENTAL DEFECT

A 21-year-old man, who had a mixed nerve and middle ear deafness and who wore a hearing aid which brought his pure tone auditory acuity up to 10 decibels below normal, was seen for vocational counseling. His Full Scale Wechsler IQ was 91 (Verbal Scale IQ = 84; Performance Scale IQ = 100). He was quite anxious and easily upset but friendly and cooperative. Expressive speech and understanding of oral language were normal. He was oriented in all spheres and showed good memory for both recent and remote personal events.

When his history was obtained, it proved to be shocking. He had been institutionalized as a mental defective for 17 years. His mother was incompetent and his father unknown. Soon after his illegitimate birth, he was placed in an orphanage where, at the age of about 1 year, he had an infectious episode involving otitis media, bilateral mastoiditis, and possibly encephalitis. He had developed no effective language by the age of 3 years, appeared to be globally retarded, and was transferred to an institution for mental defectives. Here his IQ was found to be 40, with nonverbal development being slightly better than verbal development. Repeated psychometric determinations between the ages of 3 and 6 years yielded IQ's between 38 and 46. No hearing deficit was noted. Psychometric determinations between the ages of 8 and 16 years yielded IQ's between 56 and 65, indicating a rise of 20 points in IQ coincident with schooling and on-the-job training in this fairly good state school.

It was at this point in his life, at the age of 16 years, that (for reasons which are now unknown) the question of a possible hearing deficit was raised. He was evaluated by an otologist who confirmed that he did in fact have bilateral hearing loss with practically no hearing in the left ear and a mixed type of loss in the right. He was fitted with a hearing aid which, as mentioned, brought his auditory acuity close to normal limits. He immediately began to show further intellectual progress, particularly in language under-standing, and psychometric examin-ations disclosed an additional gain of about 30 points over the course of the next three years. Interestingly, his level on so-called nonverbal tasks, such as the Wechsler Performance subtests, rose even more impressively than did his level on verbal tests.

We see here a rather complex situ-ation involving early emotional depriva-tion and possible brain damage as well as sensory deficit. However, the unrecog-nized hearing loss certainly would appear to have been crucial in producing and maintaining the state of mental deficiency which endured throughout the patient's childhood. When the impairment was recognized and at least partially compen-sated for, a significant rise in intelligence level, "nonverbal" as well as "verbal," occurred. Again one cannot help but speculate whether the introduction of an early "prosthetic" environment would not have completely prevented this state of mental defect.

EMOTIONAL DISORDER AS A POSSIBLE DETERMINANT OF MENTAL DEFECT

A 26-year-old woman, with a diagnosis of paranoid schizophrenia, was seen for evaluation because of assaultive and des-tructive behavior. Psychometric examin-ation indicated a dull- to low-average level of intellectual function. Performance on Information and Vocabulary subtests was low-average, while performance on other subtests was on a dull or borderline level. Because effort and cooperation were marginal, these results were considered to provide a minimal estimate of her intelli-gence.

Her history proved to be most inter-esting. She was born in a family of below average socioeconomic status. Nothing

remarkable is recorded about her infancy or preschool childhood. She started to talk at about the age of 15 months but showed an articulation defect until the age of 10 years. She entered the first grade at the age of 6 years. Her school work is recorded as being barely passing in the first and second grades and as being grossly inadequate in grades 3 to 5. At this time, when she was 11 years old, the ques-tion of institutionalization was raised because her father was an invalid, her mother had to leave the home to work, and the child obviously required more supervision than the parents could give. She was reported to have an adequate memory and to count well but as being poor in arithmetic. Her reading and writ-ing skills were described as "fair." She was able to run simple errands but was untruthful, disobedient, and occasionally destructive. A Vineland Social Maturity Scale given to her at that time indicated overall social competence to be at the 5- to 6-year level. The general impression was that of mental deficiency, as evi-denced by poor scholastic achievement and low social competence.

Upon admission to a state school the clinical and psychometric impression was that of so-called primary mental deficiency, moron level. Her IQ was found to be 66, with an even level of perfor-mance and no undue scatter. It was noted that she "seemed childish for her chrono-logical age." The first two years of her institutionalization were uneventful. The records state that her adjustment to the institution was good and that, although she was inclined to be lazy, her behavior was not unusual. Her school work was up to expectations for her mental age. Psy-chometric reexamination at the age of 13 years yielded an IQ of 60.

At this time she was returned home at her mother's request. At first she pre-sented no adjustment problems but, after her father died some months later, she became destructive and assaultive and was returned to the state school. Here she immediately quieted down. Over the next two years her behavior at the institution was unremarkable. She was noted as being quiet, well-behaved, suggestible, and easily led.

At the age of 16 years, she once again returned home, but within a few months was again a severe behavior problem. This time she was sent to a state psychiatric hospital where a diagnosis of psychosis with mental deficiency was made. During the next few years there was a succession of admissions to the state hospital or the local sanitarium that served the city. Each time that she was institutionalized she would quiet down sufficiently to warrant her return home, and each time that she returned home there would be flareups of destructive behavior of ever-increasing intensity. By the time she was 22 years old, a chronic psychosis was evident and she remained at the state hospital where she became a serious custodial problem. She was suicidal, as well as assaultive, and in time well-developed delusions of persecution came to the fore.

At the age of 25 years, she was transferred to another state hospital. Here a fresh evaluation indicated that the diagnosis of psychosis with mental deficiency was untenable since both clinical and psychometric study disclosed a mental level within normal limits. As I have mentioned, from the psychometric standpoint, she was estimated as being of at least low-average intelligence.

What can we make of this history? A tenable (but admittedly not necessarily correct) interpretation is that this patient always suffered from profound emotional disorder, having to do primarily with her relationship to her parents. This emotional disorder manifested itself first in the form of stupidity, i.e., in a global

intellectual inhibition which perhaps served as a defense against destructive impulses. Later, for reasons unknown (perhaps biological maturation, perhaps her father's death), this inhibition broke down and the behavioral picture changed to that of frank psychosis. But, with this change, intellectual functions were now free to operate (since her stupidity no longer served an adaptive purpose) and her measured intelligence level rose by 25 IQ points—within the setting of a closed ward in a state hospital!

In the three cases that I have cited, socioeconomic background was below average and therefore one can think of cultural deprivation as a factor which was operating in combination with the specific factor of sensory impairment or emotional disorder. It might be argued that, if these patients had come from a better social background, there would have been early therapeutic intervention and the observed mentally defective state might have been prevented. I accept this possibility. However, I would insist that this consideration does not argue against the significance of the specific factors of sensory impairment and emotional disorder as determinants of the mentally defective state which in fact was manifested. Indeed it supports the thesis. For the chances are that, if these specific disabilities had not been present, these patients would not have been defective despite their background of cultural deprivation. Here one can draw an analogy with phenylketonuria. The error of metabolism involved in this type of mental deficiency leads to a behaviorally defective state under one dietary regime (normal diet) but not under another (phenylalanine-free diet). But, of course, the fact that early introduction of the special diet may prevent brain damage and consequent mental deficiency does not eliminate the significance of the metabolic fault as the decisive determinant of the mentally defective state in those cases which did not have the benefit of the special diet.

As Dr. Bialer has indicated, all these factors—biological, interpersonal, and social—act in concert. Whether a single given factor will be a determinant of mental deficiency will depend often upon the status of the other factors. With respect to sensory impairment and emotional disturbance, it seems clear that, by themselves and within the setting of an otherwise normal internal and external milieu, they are not *sufficient* determinants of mental deficiency. But they are *significant* determinants in the sense that under adverse general conditions their presence can be responsible for the appearance of the global state of subnormal intellectual functioning which we call mental deficiency.

Some years ago I developed a graphic model to try to depict this state of affairs in which intelligence level is determined by multiple interacting variables. The current version of this model is presented in Figure 13. As indicated, Intellectual Level is conceived as the product of a number of determining factors of different types—Cerebral Status, Sensory Status, Motor Status, Emotional Status and Cultural Status. Each of these factors, as well as Intellectual Level, is a continuous variable which, for the sake of convenience, is subdivided into three to five levels.

The model clearly postulates that the variable of Cerebral Status is itself determined by endogenous, as well as exogenous, factors. This is no doubt true of other variables such as Sensory Status and Motor Status but it is particularly important to make this explicit for the factor of Cerebral Status. The endogenous determinants may be considered to be of two types: first, the specific genetic anomalies involved in such conditions as phenylketonuria; second, the less specific and more

problematic genetic variables which, in the absence of specific genetic anomalies, form the background of level of general intelligence, as postulated by some human geneticists. It will also be noted that provision is made for a superior level of function with respect to Cerebral Status, as well as Cultural Status.

Applying this model, the "formula" for phenylketonuria would be endogenously determined B_5, with other determining variables being unremarkable. Early therapeutic intervention means in effect the neutralization of the endogenous factor producing B_5. The "formula" which would be applied to cultural-familial mental deficiency depends upon one's convictions (unfortunately, the model cannot compensate for factual ignorance). A popular formula today would be C_3 or C_4, with other determining factors being unremarkable. A generation ago the popular formula would have been endogenously determined B_4, with other determining factors being unremarkable. A distinct possibility, to my way of thinking, is $B_3 \times C_3$, i.e., a combination of relatively poor (but not defective) cerebral status (endogenously or exogenously determined) and substandard cultural background.

Turning to the specific issues under discussion, one might say that S_3, M_3, or E_3, by themselves, do not produce I_4, a state of global mental defect. However, a combination of them ($S_3 \times M_3$ or $S_3 \times E_3$) might produce it. Or the combination of any one of these with C_3 or C_4 might well produce I_4. Thus the formula for the first case I described—the blind child with cerebral palsy—would be $S_3 \times M_2 \times C_4$.

Within the context of this model, the importance of an early prosthetic environment which Dr. Bialer mentions is obvious. It consists essentially of changing cultural status from C_2, C_3, or C_4 to C_1 whenever B_3, S_3, M_3, or E_3, or any combi-

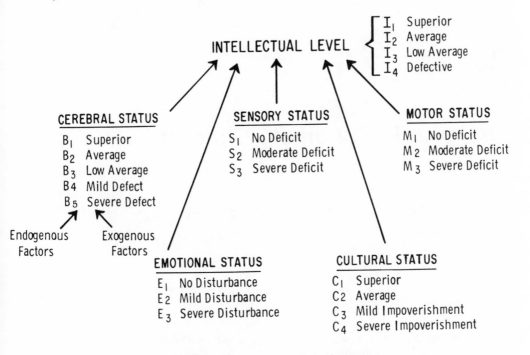

Fig. 13. Determinants of intellectual level.

nation of these, is observed. In the first two cases I described, C_4 was changed to C_2 (at rather late times in life), with a consequent rise in intellectual level.

The interactions among the determinants should not be considered as necessarily being of a simple additive or multiplicative nature. Unusual interactions may occur. In this respect, I would again call attention to the provision in the model for a superior level of cerebral function. As of today, one would think of this as being endogenously determined; however, the future certainly includes the possibility of the operation of exogenous factors. The postulation of a genetically determined superior cerebral endowment may sound hopelessly old-fashioned, but I am convinced that we would do well to overcome our extreme environmentalist bias and retain this possibility. In any

case, given a superior endowment in respect to cerebral status, the interaction between cerebral status and other determinants may be quite different from those occurring within the setting of a more mediocre cerebral status. Thus the combination of $B_1 \times S_3$ or $B_1 \times M_2$ or $B_1 \times E_2$ may result in an enhancement of intellectual level rather than a decline. Similarly, whether endogenous cerebral status is B_2 or B_3 may be a most important determinant of the effects of cultural impoverishment.

Whatever mode of analysis we adopt should serve as a guide for therapeutic intervention of a physical, interpersonal or educational nature. Dr. Bialer has sketched some of the possibilities. These, as well as others, should be given a fair trial within clinical service settings that permit a valid assessment of the results.

26.

Dyslexia: Evolution of a Concept*

It was recognized at a relatively early stage of medical history that injury or disease of the brain in adult patients could cause a loss of a specific cognitive skill such as the ability to name objects or the ability to read. Indeed observations of this type were often employed as an argument in favor of localization of function of the brain. Thus specific anomia or "loss of memory for words" was clearly described in the sixteenth century and the syndrome of alexia without agraphia was identified in the seventeenth century.

But neither physicians nor educators were as quick to recognize that children might also suffer from specific cognitive disabilities as a consequence of congenital or early acquired disease. It was only in 1853 that the Dublin otologist, William Wilde, published his observations on children who were "dumb, but not deaf," i.e., suffering from specific language disability. As we know, developmental dyslexia went unrecognized until the end of the

* A. L. Benton, *Bulletin of the Orton Society*, 1980, 30, 10–26.

nineteenth century when Morgan published his famous case report. As so often happens, once the attention of physicians was called to the condition, they immediately observed it in their practice and a steady stream of papers on dyslexia appeared in the English and German medical literature between 1900 and 1910. Somewhat later, clinical psychologists recognized dyslexia as a distinctive condition and attempted to relate its occurrence to more basic defects in visualization, auditory perception and associational processes. On the other hand, educators were less ready to accept the real existence of "congenital wordblindness" as a clinical entity.

THE EARLY HISTORY

Morgan (1896) described a classic case of dyslexia. His patient was an intelligent 14-year-old boy who was severely disabled in reading and writing despite individual tutoring as well as years of conventional school instruction. The boy knew the phonetic value of most letters and could read short, high frequency words but he could not blend letter sounds and had gained no appreciation of the characteristic spelling patterns of English. Yet he could read three-digit numbers fluently and could solve written problems in algebra. Morgan considered the boy to be "word-blind" but not "letter-blind." Since alexia in adults was known to be related to disease in the territory of the left angular gyrus, he supposed that defective development of this area was responsible for the boy's disability. A very similar case was reported by Bastian (1898) who also ascribed the disability to congenital weakness or early damage of the "visual word centre" in the angular gyrus.

In 1900 James Hinshelwood published the first in what was to be a long series of papers on developmental dyslexia. The two additional cases which he reported added little to what Morgan and Bastian had described. However, Hinshelwood did express the opinion that the condition was "by no means so rare as the absence of recorded cases would lead us to infer. Their rarity is, I think, accounted for by the fact that when they do occur they are not recognized."

There followed a paper by Nettleship (1901) in which he described five cases that he had seen in his practice, two of them dating back to 1882. In addition to confirming the observations of Hinshelwood, Bastian and Pringle Morgan (whom he inexplicably called "Campbell Brown"), Nettleship made a number of new points. He was the first to describe developmental dyslexia in young adults, one of his patients being 23 years old and another 21 years old. He was the first to describe dyslexia in a woman and at the same time also the first to call attention to the preponderance of males with the condition, pointing out that eight of the nine

cases reported up to that time were boys or men. Finally, he made a perceptive sociological observation about reading disability. "The detection of congenital word-blindness is easy in the children of well-educated parents whose young children receive much individual attention. It must be much more difficult, both to recognize and deal with, in the children who crowd our Infant Elementary Schools."

Hinshelwood's second paper in 1902 reported two further cases and addressed the problem of teaching dyslexic children to read. He insisted that they should not be taught in the regular classes along with normal readers but by special methods in a separate setting. Since defective development of the "visual word centre" in the angular and supramarginal gyri of the left hemisphere has impaired their visual memory for words and letters, these children need to be taught by methods that utilize the sense of touch to strengthen sight sound associations. For this he recommended the employment of block letters which the child could learn to identify by touch as well as vision and which he could use in reading and spelling words.

Over the course of the next few years, case reports from Holland, Argentina, France, Germany and the United States appeared in the medical literature, for the most part in ophthalmologic journals (Lechner 1903; Wernicke 1903; Foerster 1905; Brunner 1905; Variot & Lecomte 1906; Claiborne 1906; Jackson 1906; Peters 1908). Although some of these added little to what was already known, they at least demonstrated that dyslexia was not confined to England and Scotland. Claiborne (1906) was the first to raise the question of whether linguistic factors might play a role in the genesis of specific reading disability. Having pointed out the characteristically inconsistent grapheme-phoneme relationships of English, he wrote:

Those who learn to read English always have this difficulty before them, and it would be interesting to know what difference there is in the relative facility with which children learn English, which is filled with such arbitrary pronunciation, and some other language in which each vowel and consonant has a definite value and the same value always under the same circumstances, such as Italian, Spanish, and German. Compare the English words, "tough," "though" and "slough," for example. No such difficulties, I believe, exist in the three other languages mentioned. I believe, and it is reasonable to assume, that word-amblyopia exists more frequently in English-speaking children than in those speaking other languages that have not the difficulties of the English.

The tendency for dyslexia to run in families was noted as early as 1905 by Fisher and by Thomas. Further evidence for a basic hereditary determinant in at least some cases of dyslexia was furnished by the case reports of Stephenson (1907), Hinshelwood (1909) and Plate (1909). Jackson (1906) was the first to suggest that "developmental alexia" would be a more appropriate designation for the condition than "congenital word-blindness."

The 28 papers on dyslexia published between 1896 and 1910 (15 of them by British authors) provided a substantial amount of information about the disability. They established the real existence of the condition and defined its characteristic features. Many more boys than girls were subject to the disability. An hereditary determinant seemed evident in a proportion of the cases. Cerebral damage resulting from birth trauma probably was causative in other cases and perhaps explained the predominance of dyslexic boys. Linguistic factors may affect the relative frequency of the condition in different countries. A striking dissociation between the ability to read numbers as contrasted to letters and words may be shown. Estimates of the frequency of word-blindness in school children ranged from 1 in 2000 (Fisher 1905) to 1 in 100 (Warburg 1911).

However, the growth of empirical knowledge during this period was not accompanied by any basic change in conceptions about the etiology of dyslexia or its underlying mechanisms. The early aphasiologists thought of the territory of the angular gyrus in the dominant hemisphere as being a center in which visual memory images of letters and words were deposited. Injury or faulty development of that center entailed a partial or complete loss of these memory images with consequent impairment in the ability to read. Hinshelwood, the leading theorist of the time, adopted this simplistic conception to "explain" specific dyslexia. The dyslexic child suffered from maldevelopment of the left angular gyrus area with consequent inability to retain the visual memories of letters and words. Hence, he had to use the homologous area in the right hemisphere to learn to read and, since this area was not well adapted for the purpose, his progress was defective. The fact that many dyslexic children could read numbers with greater facility than words was interpreted as meaning that there were separate centers for the visual memories of numbers and words. Hinshelwood contended that the auditory memory of dyslexic children was invariably good, a notion which fits in with his concept of localized pathology and defective visual-verbal imagery.

It was agreed that a child could overcome his disability, at least in part, but special educational arrangements and methods were required to accomplish this. Among other procedures, Fisher (1905) recommended that the "look and say" method calling for global word recognition be employed with these children who experienced so much difficulty with phonemic analysis. Another recommendation was that, since the right hemisphere was subserving the learning of reading by these children with defective left hemispheres, it would be logical to teach them to write with the left hand.

THE PSYCHOLOGICAL PERIOD (1912–1926)

As psycho-educational clinics and child guidance centers were established in the second decade of the twentieth century, educational and clinical psychologists became concerned with dyslexia. Their approach to the problem posed by non-reading children was quite different from that of the ophthalmologists and school doctors who had first described the condition. They were primarily interested in a functional analysis of the dyslexic child with the aim of identifying those basic disabilities that might underlie his failure to learn to read. The psychologists appreciated that reading was more than a matter of simple sight-sound associations, as had been assumed by most of the early workers in the field, and that it involved "perception, interpretation of symbols, memory, comprehension, motor processes, emotions and complex associations" (Bronner 1917, p. 77). They were, therefore, prepared to investigate all aspects of mentation and cognition in their effort to understand the determinants of reading failure. An early example is the application of the free association test to a dyslexic boy by Voss (1914) who found that his responses deviated markedly from normative values and who therefore suggested that the basic defect in dyslexia extended beyond visuoverbal processes to encompass oral language as well.

The major studies of this period presented detailed analyses of the performances of disabled readers on diverse perceptual, associational and learning tasks with the aim of identifying the basic disabilities underlying their failure to learn to read. Bronner (1917), for example, found different performance patterns in individual dyslexics. One might be poor in auditory memory and motor speech expression, another might fail nonverbal visual memory tests. From her observation of successful approaches to the remediation of reading disability, Schmitt (1918) concluded that dyslexics were deficient in developing the complex of meanings connected with both oral and written symbols and hence their recognition of these symbols was uncertain and unstable. In essence, she conceived of the basic disability in reading failure as being one of the association rather than perception and memory. Bronner had expressed the same idea in a rather vague way when she wondered "whether in reading there is not involved some subtle synthetic process which, at the present time, we have no means of studying but defects of which, nevertheless are of extreme significance." Similarly, Wallin (1920) wrote:

Although the source of the difficulty has been considered to be a defect in visual word imagery, it is possible that the seat of the trouble may be in the connections between the centers for the images of spoken words and for the images of written words. We suggest this as an important topic for investigation.

In consonance with this conclusion, Wallin reported that his dyslexic children did not show defects in visual imagery or memory, as measured by their performances on the ball-and-field and memory for designs subtests of the Binet. Nor did they show impairment in auditory memory, as measured by auditory-vocal digit span.

Further studies in the 1920s reinforced the concept that dyslexia could not be construed as a purely visuoverbal disability. Fildes (1922) found that many disabled readers showed defects either in visual form discrimination and memory or in auditory memory for numbers and sentences. She therefore concluded that reading disability is partly an expression of a more general impairment involving vision, hearing and their interrelations. Similarly, Hincks (1926) reported that her dyslexic subjects showed a variety of perceptual defects, most notably in visual form perception and pitch discrimination. On the other hand, a dissenting note was sounded by Gates (1922) who found no evidence of defective visual or auditory perception and memory in children who were relatively poor readers (but not necessarily dyslexics). He severely criticized such concepts as faulty "visualization" or "ability to associate auditory and visual symbols" as too poorly defined and too global to be meaningful. Instead, he ascribed poor reading achievement to environmental factors such as inadequate instruction and poor habit training.

Another line of thought that emerged during this period deserves to be mentioned. An association between hand preference, and particularly forced change in preference, with stammering had been noted as early as 1912 by Ballard. Dearborn (1925) extended the association to reading disability, noting that at least one third of the non-readers whom he had seen were left-handed. His student, Hincks (1926), who made the same observation, commented:

Many non-readers are left-handed, and many who are not actually so, show traits that we might call "left-minded." They often begin to read a word at the right instead of the left end.

The words "saw" and "was" are apt to be bugbears for all non-readers. Their confusion of letters, numbers and forms alike except for orientation is another characteristic of "left-mindedness." One is inclined to wonder whether some early transfer of handedness may not have caused a disturbance similar to that of stammering, but resulting in reading difficulty. Statistics on a large number of non-readers might prove very enlightening.

Clearly the state of knowledge about dyslexia in the mid-1920s was far more differentiated than it had been in 1910. Attention had shifted from the description of surface characteristics to the analysis of underlying mechanisms. Two schools of thought had emerged. One school postulated diverse perceptual and cognitive disabilities as the basis for the observed failure in learning to read. The other school emphasized environmental and characterological variables, such as faulty instruction, inadequate nurture and poor habits. There was no great interest in identifying a neurological basis for the disorder. However, the theory put forth by Morgan and Hinshelwood that dyslexia arises from focal maldevelopment of the posterior parietal territory of the dominant hemisphere was generally regarded as inadequate.

THE WORK AND INFLUENCE OF S. T. ORTON

A new and highly original neurological theory of dyslexia was advanced by Orton in a series of papers published between 1925 and 1929 (see Orton 1966). Starting from the observation that dyslexic children tended to show reversals in right-left orientation in the reading of letters and words, he related this disturbance in directionality to a defective interhemispheric organization of cerebral function. Proposing the term "strephosymbolia" (twisted symbols) as a designation for developmental dyslexia, he identified two types of reversals in reading; the reversed reading of letters was designated as static reversals, the reversed reading of words as kinetic reversals.

At the same time, Orton was equally strongly impressed by the high frequency of left-handedness, lack of established hand preference and mixed hand and eye preference in disabled readers as well as in children with speech defects. Calling attention to the well-known association between mirror writing and left-handedness, he reported that many of his dyslexics read mirror image text as well as they read conventional text. He saw these perceptual and motor deviations as reflecting a specific fault in cerebral development, namely, a failure to establish hemispheric specialization for the visual perception of symbolic stimuli. He pointed out that, while the occipito-parietal areas of the two hemispheres are functionally equivalent at the levels of simple visual perception and object recognition, the occipito-parietal cortex of the dominant hemisphere alone mediates reading, i.e., the recognition of visual symbolic material. This concentration of function in a single hemisphere is necessary for fluent reading in order to effect the suppression of antidromic or mirror image information in the subordinate hemisphere that would compete with correctly orientated information in the dominant hemisphere. Specific reading disability results from a failure to establish this specialization of function in a single hemisphere.

This suggests that the process of learning to read entails the elision from the focus of attention of the confusing memory images of the nondominant hemisphere which are in reversed form and order, and the selection of those which are correctly oriented and in correct sequence. . . .

The frequency in these cases of reading disability, of reversals of letter pairs, of whole syllables . . . or of the major parts of words strongly suggests that there has been an incomplete elision of the memory patterns in the nondominant hemisphere, and that therefore either right or left sequence may be followed in attempting to compare presented stimuli with memory images, and that this leads to confusion or delay in selection. . . .

The term "congenital word-blindness" because of its association with the acquired condition and the implications therefrom, does not seem to be properly descriptive of this disability and I would therefore like to offer the term "strephosymbolia" . . . as a descriptive name for the whole group of children who show unusual difficulty in learning to read (Orton 1925, pp. 607–609).

Orton's theoretical formulation decisively influenced the direction of subsequent research on dyslexia. Over the past 50 years no topic in the field has been so thoroughly investigated as has the question of whether specific reading disability is systematically related to incomplete or anomalous hemispheric dominance. As everyone knows, the outcome of this vast amount of research has not led to any firm conclusions. Again and again evidence for an association between reading disability and deviant laterality (e.g., left-handedness, ambidexterity, inconsistent hand-eye preference) has been obtained. On the other hand, many studies have reported negative results. Even discounting this inconsistency, the positive findings do not permit a simple interpretation. For example, a paper may report that indications of left-handedness or ambidexterity were found in 35 percent of a sample of dyslexic children as compared to a 15 percent frequency in an age-matched sample of normal readers. The between-groups difference is real enough. But, before inferring any causal relationship, one has to account for the 65 percent of dyslexics who are purely right-handed ind the 15 percent of adequate readers who show deviant laterality.

The development of techniques such as dichotic listening and tachistoscopic stimulation of the left and right visual fields has made it possible to investigate the auditory and visual information processing capacities of each cerebral hemisphere and thus has provided measures of hemispheric dominance that are more directly related to the Orton theory. As is well known, a right ear (i.e., left hemisphere) superiority in the recognition and recall of verbal stimuli (digits, words) is shown by a majority of normal right-handed adults and older children in the dichotic listening situation. Similarly a right visual field superiority in the recognition and recall of verbal stimuli (words, nonsense syllables) is shown by a majority of normal right-handed adults and older children under the condition of tachistoscopic stimulation of either or both visual fields.

That these measures have serious limitations as indicators of hemispheric specialization for language function must be acknowledged. It is generally accepted that left hemisphere dominance for language is true of almost all right-handed persons. Right hemisphere dominance for language, as reflected in the occurrence of aphasia from a right hemisphere lesion in a right-handed patient is a very uncommon event, occurring in not more than six percent of cases (Conrad 1949; Russell & Espir 1961). Similarly, application of Wada's intracarotid sodium amytal test indicates that at least 92 percent of right-handed subjects are left hemisphere dominant for language (Milner 1973).

But the experimental auditory and visual tasks have not generated comparable results, for one finds the proportion of normal subjects making performances indicative of left hemisphere dominance for language to be almost always less than 90 percent and often less than 80 percent (Kimura 1964, 1967; Bryden 1965; Fontenot & Benton 1972; Hilliard 1973; McGlone & Davidson 1973). Thus, if the clinical findings in aphasic patients with unilateral brain disease and the Wada test results are taken as criterion measures, it is evident that ear advantage and visual field differences are quite imperfect indicators of hemispheric dominance for language.

In any case, studies comparing these measures in normal and dyslexic children have produced the same blend of negative and mildly positive findings as have the studies on handedness (cf. Bryden 1970; Zurif & Carson 1970; Witelson & Rabinovitch 1972; McKeever & Van Deventer 1975; Yeni-Komshian, Isenberg & Goldberg 1975; Leong 1976; Thomson 1976). Nevertheless, while some workers in the field have dismissed laterality as a significant factor in reading failure, others still believe that anomalous or incomplete hemispheric cerebral dominance is characteristic of a specific subgroup of developmental dyslexics (e.g., Zangwill 1960, 1962). It is possible that the dyslexic cases identified by means of computerized tomography as having a pattern of structural asymmetry opposite of that seen in normal right-handers belong to this subgroup. In a sample of 24 dyslexics, Hier and his co-workers (1978) found 10 who showed a wider parieto-occipital region in the right hemisphere than in the left while the usual finding is a wider region in the left hemisphere (Geschwind & Levitsky 1968; LeMay 1976). These dyslexics differed from the other subjects in the sample in their lower WAIS or WISC Verbal Scale IQ and in their more frequent histories of delayed development of oral speech, two characteristics which Zangwill postulated as being part of a specific dyslexic syndrome.

The next development in thought

about dyslexia took a rather different direction. In the 1930s, some clinicians and educational psychologists became impressed with the high frequency of behavioral maladjustment and personality disorder in dyslexic children. The impression was perhaps inevitable given the fact that very often these children were brought to clinical attention because of conduct problems and not specific reading failure. Systematic study of the question indicated that an excessively high proportion of cases did in fact show evidence of emotional disturbance (Monroe 1932; Robinson 1946). A reasonable interpretation was that the learning disability created stresses and failure experiences which led to the child's emotional disturbances. This was acknowledged but some clinicians viewed the personality disorder as primary and the reading disability as only one expression of it. The practical implication of this view was that psychotherapy was a necessary element in treatment and one which had to precede tutoring or be carried out in conjunction with it (Blanchard 1935).

DYSLEXIA SINCE WORLD WAR II

After World War II, there was an enormous growth of interest in dyslexia or at least in the failure of children to acquire fully adequate reading skills. Estimates of the prevalence of reading disability ranged from 10 percent to a hardly credible 30 percent (Benton 1975). One reason for this wide variation was that educators and researchers often failed to distinguish between dyslexia, or specific reading disability, and what has come to be called "reading backwardness," i.e., reading failure due to low intelligence, sensory defects or lack of educational opportunity (Benton 1975; Rutter 1978). A tremendous expansion of investigative work

paralleled this increased interest in reading failure.

Investigation proceeded along various lines. Early themes such as the relationship of deficiencies in visual and auditory perception to dyslexia were taken up again (Benton 1962; Nielsen & Ringe 1969; Vellutino, Steger & Kandel 1972; Vellutino 1978). As already mentioned, Orton's theory continued to be evaluated through the application of newer experimental methods. There were also fresh approaches to the question of the neurological basis of dyslexia. Electroencephalography provided a measure of brain function which could be utilized to assess the presence of diverse types of functional abnormality (Hughes 1978). Possible structural anomalies have been investigated, as in the CT study of Hier et al. (1978) and the autopsy report of Galaburda and Kemper (1979). Methods of clinical evaluation developed for the assessment of brain injury and anomalous development in children were applied to dyslexics (Denckla 1977). The confusing results from studies of perceptual functions in dyslexic children led researchers to probe other cognitive processes such as intersensory integration, sequential perception and defects of language function (Birch & Belmont 1964; Bakker 1972; Shankweiler & Liberman 1972, 1976; Vellutino 1978). Finally, proceeding from the assumption that dyslexia is not the single disorder which it was once thought to be but instead consists of a number of syndromes, each with its own cognitive characteristics and antecedent conditions, attempts have been made to establish valid and clinically useful classifications of the disorder (Mattis, French & Rapin 1975; Doehring & Hoshko 1977).

The impressive magnitude of this research effort is indicated by the fact that a recent book summarizing the current state of knowledge about dyslexia lists more than 900 monographs, papers and reports published between 1960 and 1977 (Benton & Pearl 1978). The studies described in these publications investigate dyslexic children from every standpoint—genetic, neurologic, psychologic, educational and social. As a consequence, we now possess a large body of information about every aspect of dyslexia. But somehow this mass of information has not proved to be as useful as one would have anticipated.

This is not to say that advances in knowledge and practice have not been achieved. Thanks to recent work on the prediction of reading disability, the preschool child at risk for later reading failure can be identified with fair accuracy (Benton 1976; Jansky 1978; Satz, Taylor, Friel & Fletcher 1978). This means that remediation can be instituted before the child begins the learning of reading and it offers the possibility that the experience of reading failure can at least be mitigated, if not avoided. This is a first step toward prevention but is not equivalent to prevention which depends upon an understanding of the causes and basic nature of dyslexia. As yet we do not possess this understanding.

Similarly, the dedicated efforts of reading specialists have made a variety of remediation methods available to the teacher who can select those which appear to be most appropriate for an individual child (Johnson 1978). Yet there is considerable doubt about the effectiveness of many remedial instruction programs since all too often a specific therapeutic effect cannot be demonstrated. The reasons for this are obscure. It may be that the remedial techniques have not been applied skillfully or that their duration and intensity have been inadequate. Whatever the reason, the fact remains that remediation proceeds without knowledge of causation and often seems to be without proven value.

Clinical and experimental observations during the past 20 years have taught us a great deal about the disorder in terms of its genetic, neurologic, behavioral and social correlates. Yet it is very difficult to integrate these observations into a coherent body of knowledge, particularly since there are so many instances of contradictory empirical findings in the literature. As a consequence, the concept of dyslexia has become quiite complex and seems to mean different things to different people. Indeed, the very definition of the disorder is considered to be a serious problem (Eisenberg 1978; Benton 1978).

We have yet to find our way out of this impasse. The point is often made that one reason for our failure to find stable correlates of reading failure is that we are dealing with not one but a number of different conditions. Hence the identification of more homogeneous dyslexic syndromes would seem to be a necessary task. Different approaches to the problem of classification have been employed and systems based on the characteristics of reading performance (Boder 1973; Doehring & Hoshko 1977), on associated cognitive disabilities (Mattis, French, & Rapin 1975), on the presence or absence of cerebral electrophysiologic abnormality (Hughes 1978) or of clinical signs of neurologic abnormality (Rutter, Graham, & Yule 1970; Denckla 1977) have been investigated. However, for the most part, these classifications have been developed in isolation from each other and their interrelations have not been determined. For example, it has not been established whether or not dyslexic children who show different profiles of reading performance also show different associated cognitive disabilities, although it would seem likely that this is the case. Similarly, neurologic and cerebral electrophysiologic studies of dyslexic children generally have treated them as a homogeneous group without regard to characteristics of their reading performances or the associated cognitive disabilities which they may show. Consequently, it is not known whether neurologic or electrophysiologic abnormality is characteristic of certain types of dyslexic children and not of others. The discordant results of studies on the frequency of neurologic and EEG abnormality in dyslexic children suggest that this may well be the case.

In the 1930s the idea that dyslexia was an expression of a more pervasive personality disorder was advanced. More recent study has shown that, whether the idea is valid or not, emotional disturbance and conduct disorders are indeed frequent correlates of dyslexia (Rutter, Graham & Yule 1970; Rutter, Tizard & Whitmore 1970; Wender 1971). However, the meaning of this association and, specifically, the possible role it plays in the genesis of developmental dyslexia remains obscure.

There is another approach to dyslexia that deserves to be considered. At the beginning of this paper I mentioned that, while physicians quickly recognized congenital word-blindness as a distinctive condition once it had been described, teachers were less ready to accept it as a defined entity. Certainly this was not because they did not see children who had failed to learn to read. It was a question of a difference in attitude. Where the physicians saw disease the teachers saw a challenge. As Zigmond (1978) phrased it " . . . failure of the 'dyslexic' to learn is the result of failure of teachers to teach." She pointed out that learning by its very nature is an interactive process.

Learning is an interactive process. Whatever learning occurs is a complex product of what the learner brings to the situation and what the situation brings to the learner . . . In this con-

text, failure to learn to read can be seen as the result of something being wrong with the person, *or* the result of something being wrong with the environment (teaching) *or* an interaction of both. While the preponderance of literature on reading disabilities attributes the problem to the person, we must not use the concept of dyslexia as an excuse to condone poor teaching. Teaching which disregards the significant differences among students in motivation, developmental levels, and rate and style of learning in planning instruction is poor teaching. We believe that it produces disabled learners. If "dyslexic" children are placed in educational environments which acknowledge individual differences and which provide for alternative teaching strategies related to these differences, then a significant number of "disabled" learners will begin to learn effectively. These learners could then no longer be viewed as having some "intrinsic specific disorders," leaving only a small minority who continue to have problems to be labelled "dyslexic," i.e., unable to profit from reading instruction as we currently know how to deliver it (Zigmond 1978, pp. 437–438).

Similarly, Adelman (1970) speaks of "the not so specific learning disability population" and points out how extremely heterogeneous it is with regard to etiology and appropriate remedial strategies.

A number of comments may be made about this point of view. First to the extent that it encourages more vigorous and imaginative teaching, it is of heuristic value. Secondly, support for this interactionist position comes from other sources. We know, for example, that the prevalence of specific reading failure is related to a variety of social and cultural factors, such as size of family and neighborhood. A reasonable interpretation is that the observed educational disability is a product of the interaction of some endogenous defect with environmental forces. Finally, in emphasizing the heterogeneous nature of the problems posed by children diagnosed as dyslexic it is in harmony with current thinking.

Thus we see that the evolution of the concept of dyslexia has been in the direction of a progressively greater degree of differentiation. It is a multifaceted concept which includes genetic, neurologic, cognitive, emotional, educational, and social components. But there is little agreement among experts about which components are primary and which are secondary or, stated in another way, which components define dyslexia and which do not. We hope and expect that in the 1980s investigative work will be sufficiently comprehensive to take account of this complexity and thus generate findings which will advance our understanding of dyslexic children and enable us to help them more effectively.

REFERENCES

Adelman, H. S. 1970. Learning problems: An interactional view of causality. *Academic Therapy* 6:117–123.

Bakker, D. 1972. *Temporal Order in Disturbed Reading*. Rotterdam: Rotterdam University Press.

Ballard, P. B. 1912. Sinistrality and speech. *Journal of Experimental Pedagogy* 1:298–310.

Bastian, H. C. 1898. *A Treatise on Aphasia and Other Speech Defects*. London: H. K. Lewis; New York: Appleton and Company.

Benton, A. L. 1962. Dyslexia in relation to form perception and directional sense. *In* J. Money (ed.). *Reading Disability: Progress and Research Needs in Dyslexia*. Baltimore: Johns Hopkins University Press.

Benton, A. L. 1975. Developmental dyslexia: Neurological aspects. *In* W. J. Friedlander (ed.). *Advances in Neurology* (Vol. 7). New York: Raven Press.

Benton, A. L. 1976. Developmental dyslexia. *J. Ped. Psychol.* 1:28–31.

Benton, A. L. 1978. Some conclusions about dyslexia. *In* A. L. Benton & D. Pearl (eds.). *Dyslexia: An Appraisal of Current Knowledge*. New York: Oxford University Press.

Benton, A. L. & Pearl, D. (eds.). 1978. *Dyslexia: An Appraisal of Current Knowledge*. New York: Oxford University Press.

Birch, H. G. & Belmont, L. 1964. Auditory-visual integration in normal and retarded readers. *Amer. J. of Orthopsychiat.* 34:852–861.

Blanchard, P. 1935. Psychogenic factors in some cases of reading disability. *Amer. J. of Orthopsychiat.* 5:361–374.

Boder, E. 1973. Developmental dyslexia: A diagnostic screening procedure based on three characteristic patterns of reading and spelling. *In* B. Bateman (ed.). *Learning Disorders*. Seattle: Special Child Publications.

Bronner, A. F. 1917. *The Psychology of Special Abilities and Disabilities*. Boston: Little, Brown.

Brunner, W. E. 1905. Congenital word-blindness. *Ophthalmology*. 1:189–195.

Bryden, M. P. 1965. Tachistoscopic recognition, handedness, and cerebral dominance. *Neuropsychologia* 3:1–8.

Bryden, M. P. 1970. Laterality effects in dichotic listening: Relations with handedness and reading ability in children. *Neuropsychologia* 8:443–450.

Claiborne, J. H. 1906. Types of congenital amblyopia. *J. Amer. Med. Assoc.* 47:1813–1816.

Conrad, K. 1949. Ueber aphasische Sprachstörungen bei hirnverletzten Linkshändern. *Nervenarzt* 20:148–154.

Dearborn, W. F. 1925. The etiology of congenital word blindness. *Harvard Monogr. Educ. Ser.*1, Vol.1, No.1, 50–76.

Denckla, M. B. 1977. Minimal brain dysfunction and dyslexia: Beyond diagnosis by exclusion. *In* M. E. Blaw, I. Rapin, & M. Kinsbourne (eds.). *Topics in Child Neurology*. New York: Spectrum Publications.

Doehring, D. & Hoshko, I. M. 1977. Classification of reading problems by the Q-technique of factor analysis. *Cortex* 13:281–294.

Eisenberg, L. 1978. Definitions of dyslexia: Their consequences for research and policy. *In* A. L. Benton & D. Pearl (eds.). *Dyslexia: An Appraisal of Current Knowledge*. New York: Oxford University Press.

Fildes, L. G. 1922. A psychological inquiry into the nature of the condition known as congenital word-blindness. *Brain* 4:286–307.

Fisher, J. H. 1905. Case of congenital word-blindness (inability to learn to read). *Ophthalmic Rev.* 24:315–318.

Foerster, R. 1905. Beiträge zur Pathologie des Lesens und Schreibens (congenitale Wortblindheit bei einem Schwachsinnigen). *Neurol. Centralbl.* 24:235–236.

Fontenot, D. J., & Benton, A. L. 1972. Perception of direction in the right and left visual fields. *Neuropsychologia* 10:447–452.

Galaburda, A. M., & Kemper, T. L. 1979. Cytoarchitectronic abnormalities in developmental dyslexia: A case study. *Ann. Neurol.* 6:94–100.

Gates, A. I. 1922. *The Psychology of Reading and Spelling with Special Reference to Disability.* Teachers College Contr. Educ. No. 129.

Geschwind, N. & Levitsky, W. 1968. Human brain: Left-right asymmetries in temporal speech region. *Science* 161:186–187.

Hier, D. B., LeMay, M., Rosenberger, P. B. & Perlo, V. P. 1978. Developmental dyslexia: Evidence for a subgroup with a reversal of cerebral asymmetry. *Arch. Neurol.* 35:90–92.

Hilliard, R. D., 1973. Hemispheric laterality effects on a facial recognition task in normal subjects. *Cortex* 9:246–258.

Hincks, E. M. 1926. Disability in reading in relation to personality. *Harvard Monogr. Educ.* Ser.1, Vol. 1, No. 1, 1–92.

Hinshelwood, J. 1900. Congenital word-blindness. *Lancet* 1:1506–1508.

Hinshelwood, J. 1902. Congenital word-blindness, with reports of two cases. *Ophthalmic Rev.* 21:91–99.

Hinshelwood, J. 1909. Four cases of congenital word-blindness occurring in the same family. *Brit. Med. J.* 2:1229–1232.

Hughes, J. R. 1978. Electroencephalographic and neurophysiological studies in dyslexia. *In* A. L. Benton & D. Pearl (eds.). *Dyslexia: An Appraisal of Current Knowledge.* New York: Oxford University Press.

Jackson, E. 1906. Developmental alexia (congenital word-blindness). *Amer. J. Med. Sci.* 131:843–849.

Jansky, J. J. 1978. A critical review of

"some developmental and predictive precursors of reading disabilities." *In* A. L. Benton & D. Pearl (eds.). *Dyslexia: An Appraisal of Current Knowledge.* New York: Oxford University Press.

Johnson, D. J. 1978. Remedial approaches to dyslexia. *In* A. L. Benton & D. Pearl (eds.). *Dyslexia: An Appraisal of Current Knowledge.* New York: Oxford University Press.

Kimura, D. 1964. Left-right differences in the perception of melodies. *Quart. J. Exp. Psychol.* 16:355–358.

Kimura, D. 1967. Functional asymmetry of the brain in dichotic listening. *Cortex* 3:163–178.

Lechner, C. S. 1903. Aangeboren woordblindheid. *Ned. Tijdschr. Geneeskunde.* 39:235–244.

LeMay, M. 1976. Morphological cerebral asymmetries of modern man, fossil man, and non-human primates. *Ann. N. Y. Acad. Sci.* 280:349–366.

Leong, C. K. 1976. Lateralization in severely disabled readers in relation to functional cerebral development and synthesis of information. *In* R. M. Knights & D. J. Bakker (eds.). *The Neuropsychology of Learning Disorders.* Baltimore: University Park Press.

Mattis, S., French, J. H., & Rapin, I. 1975. Dyslexia in children and young adults: Three independent neuropsychological syndromes. *Develop. Med. Child Neurol.* 17:150–163.

McGlone, J. & Davidson, W. 1973. The relationship between cerebral speech laterality and spatial ability with special reference to sex hand preference. *Neuropsychologia* 11:105–113.

McKeever, W. F., & Van Deventer, A. D. 1975. Dyslexic adolescents: Evidence of impaired visual and auditory language processing associated with normal lateralization and visual responsivity. *Cortex* 11:361–378.

Milner, B. 1973. Hemispheric specialization: Scope and limits. *The Neurosciences: Third Study Program.* Cambridge, Massachusetts: MIT Press.

Monroe, M. 1932. *Children Who Cannot Read.* Chicago: University of Chicago Press.

Morgan, W. P. 1896. A case of congenital word-blindness. *Brit. Med. J.* 2:1378.

Nettleship, E. 1901. Cases of congenital

word-blindness (inability to learn to read). *Ophthalmic Rev.* 20:61–67.

Nielson, H. H., & Ringe, K. 1969. Visuoperceptive and visuo-motor performance of children with reading disability. *Scand. J. Psychol.* 10:225–231.

Orton, S. T. 1925. "Word-blindness" in school children. *Arch. Neurol. Psychiat.* 14:581–615.

Orton, S. T. 1966. *"Word-blindness" in School Children and Other Papers on Strephosymbolia (Specific Language Disability–Dyslexia) 1925–1946.* Towson, Maryland: Orton Society.

Peters, A. 1908. Ueber kongenitale Wortblindheit. *Münchener Med. Wschr.* 55:1116–1119.

Plate, E. 1909. 4 Fälle von kongenitale Wortblindheit in einer Familie. *Münchener Med. Wschr.* 56:1793–1796.

Robinson, H. M. 1946. *Why Pupils Fail in Reading.* Chicago: University of Chicago Press.

Russell, W. R. & Espir, M. L. E. 1961. *Traumatic Aphasia.* London: Oxford University Press.

Rutter, M. 1978. Prevalence and types of dyslexia. *In* A. L. Benton & D. Pearl (eds.). *Dyslexia: An Appraisal of Current Knowledge.* New York: Oxford University Press.

Rutter, M., Graham, P., & Yule, W. 1970. *A Neuropsychiatric Study in Childhood.* London: Heinemann.

Rutter, M., Tizard, J. & Whitmore, K. 1970. *Education, Health and Behavior.* London: Longman.

Satz, P., Taylor, H. G., Friel, J., & Fletcher, J. 1978. Some developmental and predictive precursors of reading disabilities: A six year follow-up. *In* A. L. Benton & D. Pearl (eds.). *Dyslexia: An Appraisal of Current Knowledge.* New York: Oxford University Press.

Schmitt, C. 1918. Developmental alexia. *Elem. School J.* 18:680–700, 757–769.

Shankweiler, D. & Liberman, I. Y. 1972. Misreading: A search for causes. *In* J. F. Kavanaugh & I. G. Mattingly (eds.). *Language by Ear and by Eye.* Cambridge, Massachusetts: MIT Press.

Shankweiler, D. & Liberman, I. Y. 1976.

Exploring the relations between reading and speech. *In* R. M. Knights & D. J. Bakker (eds.). *The Neuropsychology of Learning Disorders.* Baltimore: University Park Press.

Stephenson, S. 1907. Six cases of congenital word-blindness affecting three generations of one family. *Ophthalmoscope* 5:482–484.

Thomas, C. J. 1905. Congenital "word-blindness" and its treatment. *Ophthalmoscope* 3:380–385.

Thomson, M. E. 1976. A comparison of laterality effects in dyslexics and controls using verbal dichotic listening tasks. *Neuropsychologia.* 14:243–246.

Variot, G. & Lecomte. 1906. Un cas de typholexie congénitale (cécité congénitale verbale). *Bulletins et Memoires de la Société-Medicale des Hôpitaux de Paris* 23:995–1001.

Vellutino, F. F. 1978. Toward an understanding of dyslexia: Psychological factors in specific reading disability. *In* A. L. Benton & D. Pearl (eds.). *Dyslexia: An Appraisal of Current Knowledge.* New York: Oxford University Press.

Vellutino, F. F., Steger, J. A. & Kandel, G. 1972. Reading disability: An investigation of the perceptual deficit hypothesis. *Cortex* 8:106–118.

Voss, G. 1914. Ueber die Assoziationsprüfung bei Kindern nebst einem Beitrag zur Frage der "Wortblindheit." *Z. Neurol.* 26:340–351.

Wallin, J. E. W. 1920. Congenital word blindness—some analyses. *Training School Bulletin* 17:76–84; 93–99.

Warburg, F. 1911. Ueber die angeborene Wortblindheit und die Bedeutung ihrer Kenntnis für den Unterricht. *Z. Kinderforschung* 16:97–113.

Wender, P. 1971. *Minimal Brain Dysfunction in Children.* New York: Wiley-Interscience.

Wernicke, O. 1903. Ceguera verbal congenita. *Rev. Soc. Med. Argentina* 11:477–485.

Wilde, W. 1853. *Practical Observations on Aural Surgery.* London: J. Churchill; Philadelphia: Blanchard and Lea.

Witelson, S. F., & Rabinovitch, M. S. 1972. Hemispheric speech lateralization in children with auditory-linguistic deficits. *Cortex* 8:412–426.

Yeni-Komshian, G. H., Isenberg, D., &

Goldberg, H. 1975. Cerebral dominance and reading disability: Left visual field deficit in poor readers. *Neuropsychologia* 13:83–94.

Zangwill, O. L. 1960. *Cerebral Dominance and Its Relationship to Psychological Function.* Edinburgh: Oliver and Boyd.

Zangwill, O. L. 1962. Dyslexia in relation to cerebral dominance. *In* J. Money (ed.). *Reading Disability: Progress and Research Needs in Dyslexia.* Baltimore: Johns Hopkins University Press.

Zigmond, N. 1978. Remediation of dyslexia: A discussion. *In* A. L. Benton & D. Pearl (eds.). *Dyslexia: An Appraisal of Current Knowledge.* New York: Oxford University Press.

Zurif, E. B., & Carson, G. 1970. Dyslexia in relation to cerebral dominance and temporal analysis. *Neuropsychologia* 8:351–361.

27.

Child Neuropsychology: Retrospect and Prospect*

Child neuropsychology seeks to elucidate the relationship between brain and behavior in the developing human being. As compared to adult neuropsychology, the discipline has its own distinctive problems. From a functional standpoint, the central nervous system of the child is different from that of the adult. Moreover, it is in a state of rapid evolution while the changes of the nervous system of the adult are not only much slower, but also in the opposite direction of devolution. Cerebral dysfunction in the child tends to be expressed in a failure to acquire new cognitive skills and behavioral capacities while the adult with brain disease more often shows impairment in abilities that were learned in earlier years. The nature of the problems that impel clinical and theoretical study of brain-behavior relationships also differs in the fields of child and adult neuropsychology. In the case of children, diverse types of behavioral disability such as mental retardation, specific learning disabilities, and conduct disorders provide the primary impetus for investigating the role of brain dysfunction in the production of these problems. In contrast, it is more often the case in adult neuropsychology that brain disease itself is the presenting problem and one's task is to define the behavioral correlates of the disease.

Child neuropsychology has both theoretical and applied aspects but these are so intimately intertwined that it is difficult to specify where one leaves off and the other begins. As our basic knowledge of the role of the brain in mediating children's behavior grows, the more effective our efforts to help deviant children overcome their disabilities become. Conversely, the deviant children who are brought to us for help provide the parameters and variability that are indispensable for gaining that basic knowledge.

THE HISTORICAL BACKGROUND

The dictum that the brain is the "organ of mind" and that injury to it can cause dis-

* A. L. Benton in J. de Wit and A. L. Benton (Eds.), *Perspectives in Child Study*. Lisse, Swets, and Zeitlinger, 1982, pp. 41–61.

turbances in mentation and behavior was widely accepted by physicians and philosophers as early as 400 B.C., when the Hippocratic school of medicine flourished. Localization of specific mental functions is an almost equally ancient concept, dating back to A.D. 200. Moreover, specific deficits such as sudden loss of the ability to read and inability to recall the names of objects and persons were considered to be the consequence of brain disease as well as the more or less general decline in mental function that was called "dementia."

However, before the second half of the nineteenth century, knowledge of the structure of the brain and the interactions among its parts was too fragmentary and concepts of the nature of behavior were too vague to permit the formulation of any cogent theory of the nature of the relation between brain and behavior. This state of affairs changed radically after Broca established the association between aphasia and left-hemisphere disease and Fritsch and Hitzig demonstrated the existence of the excitable motor cortex. These landmark discoveries provided the impetus for the systematic study of the neurological foundations of behavior that began in the 1870s and continues to the present day. In adult psychology it is now possible to make reliable, although not precise, correlations between neurological events and behavioral events, and this body of information provides the basis for a progressively increasing understanding of how the central nervous system operates to support cognitive processes and affective reactions.

The development of child neuropsychology followed a parallel course but at a slower pace. So far as one can see, there was no interest in the topic of brain-relationships in children until the beginning of the nineteenth century when the more severe forms of mental retardation were

related to congenital or early acquired structural malformation of the brain. This point of view steadily gained ground throughout the nineteenth century and in time the concept that all mental retardation, mild as well as severe, had a neurological basis was widely accepted. But, apart from mental retardation, little attention was paid to the neurological correlates of other behavior disorders of children.

As was the case with adult neuropsychology, two landmark events transformed child neuropsychology into a major field of scientific endeavor. The first was the description by Pringle Morgan in 1896 of developmental dyslexia. Like the correlation which Broca had made, Morgan's brief note represented a true discovery. For, as soon as he published his case report, other physicians immediately encountered dyslexic patients in their practice. By 1910 no less than 28 papers on dyslexia had been published, among them the first contribution from Holland in 1903 by the Leiden opthalmologist, C. S. Lechner. The dominant concept was that dyslexia (or, as it was called, congenital wordblindness) was a true neuropsychological disorder resulting from maldevelopment of the posterior parietal area of the left hemisphere.

The other landmark event, some 20 years later, was the pandemic of encephalitis which swept through Europe and North America between 1916 and 1924. This dreadful disease left in its wake thousands of surviving children with severe personality disturbances, conduct disorders, and intellectual impairments that were obviously ascribable to postencephalitic brain disease. The finding that many of these children were not mentally retarded, although they did suffer from specific defects in intellect and impulse control, gave rise to the concept of the nondefective brain-injured child.

THE CONTEMPORARY PICTURE

We turn now to a review of the present situation and a consideration of future prospects. Let us first address the topic of specific reading disability.

Developmental dyslexia

The amount of investigative work on this disorder has been truly prodigious. Inspection of abstract journals and reference lists shows that during the last decade over 1,000 monographs and papers have been published on the topic. Although all aspects of the condition have been studied, the main concern of recent research has been with two questions, namely, the neurological basis of the disability and the nature of the basic cognitive defects which may give rise to it.

Turning to the question of a neurological basis for reading disability, we have seen that the early workers in the field assumed that congenital wordblindness was due to defective development of the territory of the angular gyrus which was regarded as being a "center for the visual memory of words and letters." Stated in another way, congenital wordblindness was viewed as the infantile counterpart of acquired pure alexia in adult patients. However, this formulation appeared to be less tenable as it became apparent that many dyslexic children had other types of cognitive defects, for example, impaired auditory (rather than visual) verbal memory and that the left hemisphere did not have quite the same dominating influence on language function in young children as it did in adults. Moreover, the simplistic notion that the angular gyrus was the repository of visual memory images of letters and words was rejected. Nevertheless, "parietal theory," to give it a name, is still very much alive as a research topic. The clearest formulation of it has been offered by Geschwind

(1965) who considers the inferior parietal lobule (i.e., the angular and supramarginal gyri) to be an association area where visual, auditory, and tactile information is integrated, this information coming from modality-specific association areas such as Wernicke's area for audition and the peristriate occipital cortex for vision. Thus, in Geschwind's view, this area can provide a cerebral mechanism for the establishment of those crossmodal or intersensory associations which may be the basis for the development of and maintenance of skill in reading. Of course, this is consonant with the hypothesis advanced by Herbert Birch (Birch & Belmont, 1964, 1965; Birch & Lefford, 1963) that defective capacity for intersensory integration is a potent cause of dyslexia in children.

Does the posterior parietal association area in fact function as a mechanism for effecting intersensory integrations? There have been a number of approaches to the question. The posterior parietal region shows only a rudimentary development in infrahuman primates and at the same time it has been demonstrated that the capacity of chimpanzees, orangutans, and monkeys to form stable intersensory associations is quite limited (Davenport & Rogers, 1970; Drewe, Ettlinger, Milner, & Passingham, 1970; Ettlinger, 1967). The combination of findings is consistent with the theory but it scarcely provides cogent evidence in favor of it. The relative failure of infrahuman primates to learn intersensory associations may be due to lack of development of frontal association cortex, to experiential deprivation, or to their lack of language as a mediating instrument rather than to their relatively undeveloped posterior parietal region (cf. Ettlinger, 1967; Geschwind, 1965).

Another approach has been through study of patients with focal brain disease, the experimental question being whether or not those with posterior parietal lesions show poorer performance on crossmodal matching tests than do those with lesions in other parts of the brain. Butters and Brody (1968) and Butters, Barton, and Brody (1970) reported that patients with lesions involving (but not confined to) the posterior parietal area showed poorer performance on both crossmodal and ipsimodal matching tasks than did patients with lesions sparing the parietal territory, but the serious methodological weaknesses of their studies prevent accepting the results at face value.

The only direct approach to the question, i.e., through study of dyslexic children, has utilized the visual evoked response as a measure of parieto-occipital function. Several investigators (e.g., Bakker, Licht, Kok, & Bouma, 1980; Conners, 1971; Hughes, 1971; Preston et al., 1974, 1977) have found that dyslexics show deviant temporo-parieto-occipital responsiveness to visual stimulation, particularly in the territory of the left angular gyrus and particularly to verbal-visual stimulation. Although there is some disagreement about the specific nature of the abnormal activity, a difference between disabled and normal readers seems evident.

On balance, one can say that the "parietal" theory of developmental dyslexia has some, but not very substantial, empirical support. It remains a tenable hypothesis, its current weakness stemming from insufficient empirical testing rather than from an array of negative findings that would tend to disprove it.

The other major neurological theory of dyslexia implicates defective interhemispheric organization of cerebral function as being responsible for the disability. Since its original formulation by Orton in the 1920s, no hypothesis has been so thoroughly investigated as has the question of whether dyslexia is explicable in terms of incomplete or anomalous hemispheric cerebral dominance.

In advancing his theory, Orton had in mind abnormalities of hemispheric cerebral dominance as they relate to visuoverbal information processing. For decades the quesion was addressed indirectly through study of the lateral aspects of motor activity, such as hand, eye, and foot preference and the interrelations among them, on the assumption that these characteristics provided an index of hemispheric specialization for linguistic functions. Evidence for an association of modest degree between reading failure and deviant motor laterality (e.g., lefthandedness, ambidexterity, and inconsistent lateral preferences) has been obtained repeatedly but many studies have also reported negative results (cf. Balow, 1963; Balow & Balow, 1964; Belmont & Birch, 1965; Bettman, Stern, Whitsell, & Gufman, 1967; Shankweiler, 1963; Sparrow & Satz, 1970; Zangwill, 1962). This inconsistency in the empirical findings, as well as the fact that even the positive studies report only rather weak relationships between deviant laterality and reading disability, have led some specialists to discount this factor completely as a significant correlate of the educational disability. However, it is probably the case that the majority of workers in the field still believe that, despite the inconclusiveness of the results, deviant motor laterality plays some role in the genesis of dyslexia.

The development of the techniques of dichotic listening and tachistoscopic stimulation of the left and right visual fields made it possible to investigate the auditory and visual information processing capacities of each cerebral hemisphere and thus provided measures of hemisphere cerebral dominance and interhemispheric integration that are more directly related to the theory. The outcome of the substantial amount of research on dichotic listening response patterns and visual field relationships in disabled and normal readers has been mixed. Investigative work in this area has produced the same blend of negative and moderately positive findings as have the studies of lateralized motor function (cf. Bakker, Teunissen, & Bosch, 1976; Bryden, 1970; Leong, 1976; McKeever & Van Deventer, 1975; Thomson, 1976; Witelson, 1976; Witelson & Rabinovitch, 1972; Yeni-Komshian, Isenberg, & Goldberg, 1975; Zurif & Carson, 1970).

There are a number of possible reasons for this disappointing state of affairs. One is the thoughtless way in which some otherwise careful researchers go about selecting subjects for their investigations. All types of poor readers, including the mentally subnormal, the culturally deprived, and those with conduct problems, are often included for study if they satisfy the single criterion of being poor readers. It is at least highly probable that, under this circumstance, the neurological background of the reading disorder differs from group to group and to search for a common factor is a fruitless exercise. Another possible reason for discrepant findings is that two rather different types of studies have contributed considerable amounts of data in the field. One group of studies deals with children in the regular grades who are relatively poor readers. The other group deals with more severely disabled children who often have other handicaps and whose difficulties are severe enough to warrant their referral to a clinical facility or a special school. There is suggestive evidence that the latter category of child is far more likely to show signs and characteristics supportive of one or another neurological theory of dyslexia.

Still another possible basis for confusion is the implicit assumption underlying most of the work in the field that dyslexia is a single entity. If, in fact, dyslexia is not a single entity but instead only the common outcome of a number of different syndromes, each with its own distinctive defining characteristics and antecedent conditions, then the search for a single neurological basis for the disorder is probably misdirected. Finally, the predilection for the utilization of parametric statistics, with its emphasis on mean scores and variability, instead of individual case analysis, may be a factor that has hindered our efforts to achieve insight into the neurological bases of specific reading disability.

We turn now to the behavioral correlates of dyslexia. The aim of the vast amount of research on this question has been to identify those basic disabilities which may be responsible for the failure in reading. The main trends of thought, which are considered in detail in a number of recent reviews (Benton, 1975; Benton & Pearl, 1978; Knights & Bakker, 1976; Vellutino, 1980) may be listed as follows:

(1) Visuoperceptive and Visuomotor Defects. The concept that dyslexia is the outcome of a more basic perceptual and perceptuomotor disability was very popular 20 years ago. However, subsequent research has failed to confirm its importance as a correlate of dyslexia except for the identification by Mattis, French, and Rapin (1975) of a small group of reading-disabled children who show a constellation of deficits in visual perception and short-term visual memory.

(2) Disturbances of the Body Schema. The observations that some dyslexic children show disturbances in the right-left orientation and in finger localization led some medical specialists (e.g., Hermann, 1959, 1964; Hermann & Norrie, 1958; Kinsbourne & Warrington, 1963) to formulate a theory that dyslexia is a by-product

of a disturbance of the body schema, a sort of "developmental Gerstmann syndrome." The empirical evidence on the issue is conflicting (Benton, 1975). To the degree that there are concurrent associations between reading achievement and such body schema performances as right-left orientation and finger recognition, they are likely to be stronger among younger children in the early school grades than among older children (Benton, 1962; Fletcher, Taylor, Morris, & Satz, 1982; Sparrow & Satz, 1970). There are also indications that lateral differences in the capacity to identify the fingers may be related to reading achievement (Fletcher et al., 1982; Reed, 1967).

However, there is now fairly substantial evidence that performance on finger localization tests in kindergarten children is a significant *predictor* of subsequent reading achievement, particularly in the beginning school grades (Fletcher et al., 1982; Lindgren, 1978; Satz & Friel, 1973, 1974). Why finger recognition should possess this predictive significance and whether it is the body schema component of performance that is important is not clear (Benton, 1979). Finger localization does not represent a single task but rather a series of tasks, each of which may make distinctive demands on different perceptual or cognitive abilities such as intrasensory discrimination, intersensory integration, perceptual-representational processes and verbal coding. The recent analysis of Fletcher et al. (1982) indicates that the different task performances load on different factors and that each may make a specific contribution to the prediction of reading achievement at different grade levels.

(3) Defects in Intersensory Integration. The concept that impaired capacity to transfer information across sensory modalities is responsible for failure in at least a subgroup of cases has been a topic of investigation ever since its formulation by Birch (1962) and Birch and Belmont (1964, 1965). The hypothesis appears to be a reasonable one, both because it coincides with the commonsense view that the formation of sight-sound association underlies the acquisition of beginning reading skills and because, as we have seen, it fits in so well with the "parietal" theory of the neurological basis of dyslexia. The empirical facts upon which Birch developed his hypothesis have been confirmed repeatedly; a sizable number of reading-disabled children, especially the younger ones, do show deficiencies in auditory-visual matching (Benton, 1975; Benton & Pearl, 1978; Vellutino, 1980). However, the findings of subsequent research have engendered considerable doubt that a specific deficiency in the capacity for intersensory integration is primarily responsible for poor performance on these intersensory matching tasks. Instead, a variety of other factors such as limitations in short-term memory, deficiency in ipsimodal associative capacity, incapacity to attend to multiple stimuli, impairment in the perception of temporal sequences and deficiencies in verbal mediation, have been invoked as possible explanations.

(4) Defects in Sequential Perception. The accuracy of perception of the temporal order of sequentially presented stimuli, of both an ispimodal and crossmodal nature, has been intensively investigated (Allen, 1975; Bakker, 1967, 1970(a), 1972; Corkin 1974; Groenendaal & Bakker, 1971; Senf, 1969; Weiner, Barnsley, & Rabinovitch, 1970). With one or two exceptions, the empirical results clearly indicate that poor readers tend to be inferior to normal readers in recalling the serial order of visual, auditory, and tactile stimuli of a verbal and nonverbal nature. The infer-

ence from these findings that a specific deficiency in sequential perception is an important determinant of reading failure has been criticized on various grounds (Vellutino, 1980) but the hypothesis is not only tenable but also of considerable heuristic value.

(5) Limitations in Language Development. The view that specific reading disability is the most obvious expression of a more general language retardation has become increasingly prominent in recent years. There is much clinical evidence to support the application of the concept to at least a subgroup of dyslexic children. A history of delayed oral speech development is often elicited. An association between such a history and a particularly low WISC Verbal Scale IQ in dyslexics has been demonstrated (Warrington, 1967). The oral speech productions of poor readers are often impoverished, both quantitatively and qualitatively (Fry, Johnson, & Muehl, 1970). Their performance on naming tests may be slower and less accurate than even those of less intelligent nondyslexic children with a diagnosis of minimal brain dysfunction (Denckla & Rudel, 1976a, 1976b). The capacity to analyze the spoken word into its phonemic units has been found to be closely correlated with reading ability in young school children (Liberman & Shankweiler, 1978; Shankweiler & Liberman, 1976). Thus an impressive case for the existence of a specific "language disorder" syndrome of dyslexia, as described by Mattis et al. (1975), Denckla (1977), and Petrauskas and Rourke (1979) can be made.

Minimal brain dysfunction

Both as a term and as a concept, "minimal brain dysfunction" (MBD) is still a somewhat controversial topic. Probably by now the majority of neurologists and neuropsychologists consider the concept to be valid and see it as a significant advance in the evaluation and treatment of deviant children. However, other clinicians (e.g., Ingram, 1973; Schmitt, 1975) condemn MBD as a myth that has retarded progress in understanding and helping children with behavioral and educational problems.

Even those who find the MBD concept to be useful concede that it is amorphous and lacking in precision. It is not a diagnosis not does it refer to a specific syndrome. It is only a label that is applied to a number of diverse abnormalities of behavior shown by children.

The behavioral disorders covered by the MBD label are indeed extremely diverse. There is almost no type of intellectual, psychomotor or emotional disability of childhood that has not been classified by some author under the rubric of MBD. The only exceptions are mental retardation and cerebral palsy and these are excluded only because they are major disabilities with demonstrable brain pathology. Some of the disorders that have been considered to be expressions of MBD are:

1. The hyperkinetic syndrome, characterized by overactivity, distractability, and impulsive behavior, is surely the most prominent type of behavior disorder covered by the MBD label. In fact it is responsible for the development of the concept.

2. Academic difficulties that cannot be ascribed to subnormal intelligence or extraneous factors, are interpreted as an expression of MBD.

3. It is well known that children with cerebral palsy may show defective perceptual capacity, as reflected in their inability to discriminate between complex figures, to differentiate figure from ground and to

analyze a visual configuration into its basic elements. When this disability is seen in a child who does not suffer from cerebral palsy, it is often interpreted as a sign of MBD.

4. The child of adequate intelligence who is motorically awkward and slow in developing fine motor skills, the so-called "clumsy child" (Dare & Gordon, 1970; Gubbay, 1975; Reuben & Bakwin, 1968; Walton, Ellis, & Court, 1962) is often placed in the MBD category.

5. Anxiety and disorders of mood in children have been interpreted as a behavioral expression of MBD (Wender, 1971).

Each of these presumed MBD syndromes has its own diagnostic problems. Let us take the hyperkinetic syndrome as an example. As we saw, hyperactivity, impulsivity, and aggressiveness were noted to be prominent features of the postencephalitic state in children after the pandemic of encephalitis which had run its course by the middle of the 1920s. It seemed clear that this hyperkinetic syndrome was the result of brain disease. Later the importance which Strauss and Lehtinen (1947) placed on hyperactivity and distractibility as characteristic features of the behavior of high-grade mental retardates who were assumed to have exogenous brain damage reinforced this belief. Consequently, it was natural to assume that hyperactivity and distractibility in a child of adequate intelligence and without a history of clear evidence of brain disease also implied brain disease. Since there was no firm evidence of brain disease and since the behavior disorder manifested by the child, although important, was not comparable in severity to mental retardation or cerebral palsy, the inferred dysfunction was regarded as "minimal."

The first observation that may be made about the hyperkinetic syndrome is that, as described by present-day writers, it is only a pale imitation of the hyperactivity, destructiveness, and aggressiveness characteristic of the postencephalitic state. Today a child exhibiting these symptoms would be classified as psychotic and not be placed in the MBD category. Moreover, observations on children who have been diagnosed as "hyperkinetic" indicate that, in fact, many of them are not motorically hyperactive but instead lack the capacity for sustained attention. Nor is it clear how much hyperactivity (or distractibility) a child must show in order to be considered pathologically "hyperactive." Normative studies have shown that a substantial proportion of school-age boys are characterized by their parents and teachers as hyperactive, distractible, and having a short attention span (cf. Tuddenham, Brooks, & Milkovich, 1974; Werry & Quay, 1971). That clinicians have differing concepts of what constitutes the hyperkinetic syndrome is indicated by the wide variation in the estimates of the prevalence of the condition. At least there is general agreement that the syndrome is more frequently encountered in boys than in girls.

These and other considerations have led some clinicians to question the reality of the association between the hyperkinetic syndrome and cerebral abnormality. On the one hand, it has been noted that most children with demonstrable brain disease do not manifest the syndrome. On the other hand, hyperkinesis, distractibility, and restlessness are seen in children who are judged to have psychogenic disorders. It has also been pointed out that behavioral descriptions of the hyperkinetic child and of the autistic child show a high degree of communality with overactivity, distractibility, and impaired interpersonal relationships being prominent features of both clinical pictures.

Despite these questions and despite the fact that overactivity and distractibility may have a psychogenic basis, there is much evidence to suggest that in many instances the hyperkinetic syndrome is related to cerebral abnormality. The observation that most children with frank brain disease are not hyperkinetic is not a compelling argument against this conclusion; it may mean only that the hyperkinetic syndrome results from a particular form of cerebral dysfunction. Although the nature of this dysfunction is unknown, the significant response of hyperkinetic children to amphetamine, methylphenidate, and antidepressant drugs suggests the presence of neurochemical abnormalities and involvement of neurotransmitter systems in the limbic region and basal ganglia. In this connection it may be noted that the hyperkinetic syndrome in children with convulsive disorders is specifically associated with temporal lobe epilepsy (Ounsted, Lindsay, & Norman, 1966). Nor does the alleged similarity of symptoms in the hyperkinetic syndrome and autism raise a major problem in view of the mounting evidence that the latter condition has an organic basis (A. R. Damasio & Maurer, 1978; H. Damasio, Maurer, Damasio, & Chui, 1980; Rutter, 1974).

Still another point is that, although by definition the intelligence of hyperkinetic children is within the normal range, the condition tends to be associated with a lowered level of intellectual function (Miller, Palkes, & Stewart, 1973; Palkes & Stewart, 1972), and this finding in itself raises the question of cerebral dysfunction.

These considerations apply with equal force to the other MBD syndromes. What then is the answer to the problem posed by this multi-faceted, amorphous con-

cept? We have seen that one answer is to reject it altogether. But there is another approach to the problem which recognizes that the MBD concept arose out of sound observation and filled a need to identify a variety of conditions that do not fit into established diagnostic categories. Denckla (1977) has outlined this position quite clearly. She recognizes that the MBD concept is lacking in precision and that it is not a diagnosis. But she points out that it can be a "first step in clinical diagnosis," i.e., a working hypothesis that one is dealing with an organically based behavioral disorder. Comparing the MBD concept to the equally broad and vague notion of "convulsive disorder," she has described how the hypothesis can be tested and the diagnosis can be refined through information gained by the history, clinical examination, neuropsychological evaluation, and laboratory procedures. Given this information, one should be able to identify specific MBD syndromes defined by distinctive etiological factors, presenting features and indications for therapy.

Normative and comparative neuropsychology

Perhaps the most interesting facet of the contemporary picture is the emergence of a neuropsychological approach to the developmental study of normal and deviant children. The data are still relatively sparse but a beginning has been made. Much of the research in this area has been focused on the changing status of hemispheric cerebral dominance as a function of age and sex. Another topic of interest has been the course of development of body schema performances, visuoconstructive abilities, motor skills, and other performances that have long been utilized as measures of cerebral status in the adult subject.

Hemispheric cerebral dominance

That hemispheric specialization of function in children differs from that of adults has been known ever since Cotard (1868) demonstrated that congenital and early acquired disease of the left hemisphere does not lead to the obvious and specific loss of linguistic capacity that follows the occurrence of such lesions in later life. However, until recently our knowledge of interhemispheric relationships in children was based on fragmentary and often ambiguous clinical data. Now, with the aid of newer techniques of investigation, it is possible to undertake systematic studies of the many questions associated with hemispheric cerebral dominance in the normal child.

Audition. One such technique is, of course, dichotic listening. A right-ear superiority in the recall of speech sounds has been demonstrated in children as young as 4–5 years, indicating that hemispheric asymmetry in respect to speech and language has been established by that age (Bakker, Hoefkens, & Van der Vlugt 1979; Geffner & Hochberg, 1971; Kimura, 1963; Knox & Kimura, 1970; Nagafuchi, 1970; Rosenblum & Dorman, 1978; Satz, Bakker, Teunissen, Goebel & Van der Vlugt, 1975). The same asymmetry in the recall of speech sounds in school children can be demonstrated by monaural, as well as dichotic, stimulation (Bakker, 1967, 1969, 1970b). Indeed, findings obtained through other methods of investigation, e.g., auditory evoked responses to speech sounds, suggest that there is already hemispheric lateralization of function in infants less than one year of age (Molfese, Freeman, & Palermo, 1975).

Some studies of acquired aphasia in children have led to the conclusion that an increasing degree of left-hemisphere specialization for speech and language develops until about the age of 11–12 years (Collignon, Hécaen, & Angerlergues, 1968; Lenneberg, 1967). However, for the most part, the dichotic listening results with normal children have not shown a developmental curve of increasing right-ear superiority that would be consistent with this conclusion which, in any case, is by no means securely established. More often than not, the right-ear superiority at the age of 5 or 6 years has been found to be as great as that at the age of 10 or 11 years. In passing it may be noted that dichotic listening study of younger and older adults also shows no changes as a function of age (Borod & Goodglass, 1980). A sex difference in degree of right-ear superiority, which might be expected in view of the more rapid development of verbal abilities in young girls as compared to boys, also has not been demonstrated. An association between social class and the age of onset of right-ear superiority has been reported by Geffner and Hochberg (1971) who found it at the age of 4 years in middle-class children but only at the age of 7 years in children of lower socio-economic background.

The left-ear superiority in the auditory processing of nonspeech sounds that is found in adult subjects has also been demonstrated in children (Bakker, 1967, 1970b; Knox & Kimura, 1970). Again, direct relationships between degree of ear superiority and increasing age are not apparent.

The failure of so many studies to find a simple growth curve of increasing right- or left-ear superiority after the age at which it has become evident has been the subject of discussion in which diverse factors, such as limitations in experimental design, the type of stimulus employed, task requirements, handedness, and lateral awareness, have been invoked as possible determinants of the phenomenon

(Porter & Berlin, 1975; Satz et al., 1975). The question is quite complicated and it remains unresolved.

Vision. Hemispheric asymmetry in the processing of visual information by children has been demonstrated by means of lateral monoptic and dichoptic stimulation of the visual fields. There is a right visual field superiority for the recognition of verbal material, which may be apparent as early as 5–7 years (Buffery, 1971; Forgays, 1953; Marcel, Katz, & Smith,1974). Evidence of a left visual field superiority for the recognition of faces in 5–11-year-old children has also been adduced (Marcel & Rajan, 1975; Young & Ellis, 1976). Whether or not there is a progressive development of increasing lateral asymmetry with age remains obscure. Observations on facial recognition in normal adults indicate that visual field differences are generally small and that there is considerable inter-individual variation (Benton, 1980). Thus it seems doubtful that a straightforward association between age and degree of hemispheric asymmetry will be found for this performance.

Somesthesis. Both single and simultaneous double presentations have been used to determine whether there are hand differences in the processing of somesthetic information. A superiority of the left hand in the reading of Braille sentences by blind children and in learning Braille letters by sighted children has been demonstrated (Hermelin & O'Connor, 1971; Rudel, Denckla, & Spalten, 1974). The tactile matching of Braille letters by sighted children who do not know this alphabet is also accomplished better with the left hand (Rudel, Denckla, & Hirsch, 1977). In this study, the Braille letters functioned as a stimulus that was devoid of verbal significance. Studies involving other nonverbal tasks, such as matching palpated meaningless shapes and judging the direction of lines traced with the fingers, have found the same left-hand superiority in righthanded children (Lindgren, 1977; Witelson, 1974, 1976).

An interesting aspect of the Braille studies is their indication of right-hemisphere superiority for a task with verbal content. In this respect somesthetic information processing appears to differ from processing in the auditory and visual modalities. There is suggestive evidence that boys show this left-hand advantage at a younger age than girls and that it may be present as early as the age of 6 years.

Diverse performances

Considerable attention has been given to the course of development of various abilities in school-age children, as indexed by relevant test performances. The impetus for these normative studies came from clinical observations that these abilities frequently appear to be impaired in brain-damaged adults and children. It was, therefore, felt necessary to establish normative standards in relation to age and sex as a basis for clinical judgment. The measurement of perceptual and motor capacities has been a prominent part of this endeavor, no doubt because of the assumption that the nondefective child with brain damage is likely to show impairment in these areas. Among the performances for which age-sex norms have been established are: finger recognition (Benton, 1959; Lefford, Birch & Green, 1974), right-left orientation (Benton, 1959, 1968; Spreen and Gaddes, 1969), motor impersistence (Garfield, 1964; Rutter, Graham, & Yule, 1970), tactile form perception (Spreen & Gaddes, 1969); three-dimensional block construction (Spreen & Gaddes, 1969); facial recognition (Benton, Van Allen, Hamsher, & Levin, 1978). In addition to serving the standard purpose of providing a guide for clinical investigation, these normative studies have disclosed interesting features in the growth curves of some abilities. For example, there is an apparent plateau in the development of accuracy in facial recognition at ages 9–10, a phenomenon that may be related to the shift from "piecemeal" to a "configurational" approach to facial perception postulated by Carey and Diamond (1977).

PROSPECTS FOR THE FUTURE

Of necessity this review has been selective in nature. It has not been possible to consider a number of important topics in the field such as, for example, developmental aphasia (Wyke, 1978), the neuropsychological aspects of mental retardation (Benton, 1970; Matthews, 1974), advances in clinical neuropsychological assessment (Lezak, 1976) and the genetics of dyslexia (McLearn, 1978; Childs, Finucci, & Preston, 1978). Yet, in spite of its limitations, I think that the review provides ample evidence of the significant gains in knowledge that have been achieved during the last 25 years. With respect to developmental dyslexia, we now know something about the conditions under which it develops, the settings in which it occurs and the cognitive disabilities associated with it. The concept of minimal brain dysfunction has been clarified to some degree. Methods of neuropsychological assessment now rest on a firmer basis and a beginning has been made toward developing neuropsychologically oriented programs of remediation and management.

Yet so much remains to be done. To take developmental dyslexia as an example, we possess an enormous amount of information about the antecedents and correlates of reading disability in children. However, the findings that have come from the application of diverse neurological and behavioral approaches to the problem have not been correlated with each other. As a consequence, we do not have a truly coherent body of knowledge about the disorder (or group of disorders). We do not know whether the EEG abnormalities that are so often found in dyslexic children are more closely associated with defects in intersensory integration than they are with the presence of oral language disabilities. We do not know whether distinctive qualitative features of the reading performances of dyslexics are differentially related to any of the diverse cognitive defects that have been described. Nor do we know whether deviant hemispheric dominance relationships are characteristic of one of the dyslexic syndromes that have been described but not of others. These and many other lacunae in our knowledge pose research questions that now need to be addressed. There are no significant conceptual or technical difficulties that prevent us from answering these questions. However, there are logistic problems. It is doubtful that a single research unit, with its inevitable limitations in subject population, resources, and scientific expertise, has the capability of answering these questions which require a multidisciplinary approach for their solution. What is needed is a coordinated effort on the part of a number of reseach units so that we have the tools to undertake this complicated research task.

Another aspect of the present situation and its continuing development that deserves comment is the neurological side of brain-behavior relationships, that is to say, the "neuro" component of "neuropsychology." Much of the research and clinical and educational service that we categorize as neuropsychological is, in fact, purely behavioral in nature. Thus, if I assess finger localization in dyslexic children, I may say that I have done a neuropsychological study. But, strictly speaking, it is a purely psychological study in which two behavioral variables, reading ability and finger recognition, are being correlated without any *necessary* reference to the central nervous system. It is neuropsychological only because of my assumption, which is derived from observations of adult patients *with* demonstrable brain disease, that finger localization capacity reflects the integrity of brain function in children *without* demonstrable brain disease. My assumption may or may not be correct.

A neuropsychological study in the strict sense is one in which *both* the nervous system *and* behavior are investigated. EEG studies of dyslexic and MBD children satisfy this criterion, as do the evoked potential studies of Conners (1971), Preston et al. (1974) and Bakker et al., (1980). Other examples are the CT (computerized tomography) studies of developmental dyslexia in adults by Hier, Le May, Rosenberger, & Perlo (1978) and of autistic children by H. Damasio et al. (1980). In view of the continuing rapid development of non-invasive electrophysiological and neuroradiological techniques, it may be anticipated that neurobehavioral studies utilizing them will be an important component of future research. It is likely that evoked potential and EEG studies with special reference to regional differences in the electrical activity of the brain will be a prominent feature of this effort (Duffy, Denckla, Bartels, & Sandini, 1979). Although Hier et al. (1978) were able to demonstrate structural anomalies of the brain in a subgroup of dyslexics by means of computerized tomography, this technique has not been very informative. However, computerized tomography is still in a developing stage and it may yet prove to be a valuable research tool. The interesting findings of the cytoarchitectonic autopsy study of a dyslexic by Galaburda and Kemper

(1978) suggest that the current effort of the Orton Society to collect additional autopsy data is a promising approach. It is also possible that modified techniques of cerebral blood flow measurement and positron emission tomography (PET) that make these procedures non-invasive will enable the neuropsychologist to employ them as measures of brain function. Finally, the development of new techniques may enable us to test the still speculative theory that some aspects of MBD symptomatology are the product of disturbed neurochemical mechanisms in the brain (Wender, 1976). On the practical level, the claim of Feingold (1975) that artificial dyes and other food additives are responsible for MBD, which was at first not taken seriously, has now received enough empirical support (Swanson & Kinsbourne, 1980; Weiss et al., 1980) to warrant more comprehensive investigation.

This is not to say, of course, that purely behavioral studies are lacking in neuropsychological significance. Indeed, much of what we know about brain-behavior relationships in children has come from such studies. Nevertheless, I believe that the time has come to incorporate independent measures of cerebral function and structure into neuropsychological research if we are to get to the heart of the matter.

At the other end of the spectrum, we have to note that much of the behavior of interest to the child neuropsychologist is correlated with, if not influenced by, environmental and interpersonal factors associated with socio-economic status. This is particularly true of reading skill but it applies to other performances as well. For example, as we have seen, Geffner and Hochberg (1971) found that the age of onset of right-ear superiority in the verbal dichotic listening situation was associated with the socio-economic background of children. With respect to dyslexia, Rutter (1978) has pointed to its correlation with size of family, the educational standards of the community, the area in which a child lives, and the characteristics of the school which he attends. In their studies of kindergarten children, Satz and his coworkers found that socio-economic status was a more potent predictor of subsequent reading failure than any behavioral measure (Satz, Taylor, Friel & Fletcher, 1978). The early students of dyslexia, such as Hinshelwood (1917), drew a sharp distinction between congenital wordblindness and reading failure due to low intelligence or lack of educational opportunity. At the time the distinction served a useful purpose in helping to define a condition, the real existence of which some educators tended to deny. The distinction is still valid but the implication that dyslexia is independent of social factors, which is so often derived from it, is not valid.

There is also substantial evidence that MBD symptoms, such as hyperactivity and attentional deficit, are influenced by socio-familial factors. From her review of the literature on the determinants of the behavior of children with MBD symptoms or at risk for the development of these symptoms, Werner (1980) concluded that the most powerful predictor was "social status and family characteristics of the caretaking environment." In her own follow-up studies (Werner, Bierman, & French, 1971), she found a significant interaction between socio-economic status and the effects of perinatal complications with socio-economically handicapped children showing more severe behavioral disturbances. Similarly, the detailed investigations of Paternite and Loney (1980) and Paternite, Loney, and Langhorne (1976) have demonstrated that the symptomatology of MBD, most notably aggressive behavior, is specifically

correlated with diverse aspects of the child's environment. These include more general factors such as socio-economic status, family size and crowding, as well as factors that would appear to affect parent-child relationships more directly, such as marital harmony and whether or not the father or mother is rated as being "too busy," "too strict," or "too short-tempered." Paternite and Loney hesitate to ascribe particular importance to any specific environmental factor as a determining variable before their findings are confirmed by independent studies. However, they feel confident in concluding that "home environmental influences are related to the development and expression of symptomatology of hyperactive-MBD boys, not only when they are young, but also when they reach adolescence."

The implications of these observations for clinical neuropsychological investigations are, I think, fairly clear. They tell us that the behavioral changes following brain dysfunction in children are, or at least are likely to be, the product of an interaction between that dysfunction and environmental variables, and not a direct invariant effect of neurological status. It follows that we shall have to identify the specific nature of these interactions and take them into account if our research efforts and clinical evaluations are to yield meaningful and useful information.

Finally, the question of the practical applications of child neuropsychology needs to be addressed. From a practical standpoint, neuropsychology has been largely a diagnostic speciality that attempts to identify basic cognitive disabilities of personality deviations in children with educational problems or conduct disorders. The assumptions underlying the assessment are, on the one hand, that the disabilities which are disclosed are related to disturbed cerebral function and, on the other hand, that these disabilities are responsible for a child's educational or interpersonal difficulties. Having made the assessment, the neuropsychologist has been content to report the findings and make recommendations for remediation and management with the expectation that the teacher, special educator, or school psychologist will be able to use these to advantage in their efforts to help the child. However, this expectation is not always fulfilled. The educator may not find a report that a child has a specific cognitive or perceptual disability, deviant hemispheric dominance relationships or a weakness in attention or concentration to be particularly useful. It may not be clear to him how he can proceed to alleviate these supposedly basic "brain-dependent" impairments and sometimes his own observation of the child in school and at play leads him to doubt that the impairments disclosed by the neuropsychological examination are in fact responsible for the child's difficulties.

Perhaps it is this failure of the two specialties to communicate effectively with each other that is responsible for the trend, particularly noticeable during the past decade, for neuropsychologists to assume a more active role in the remediation and management of children with learning disabilities and conduct disorders (cf. Gaddes, 1980; Knights & Bakker, 1980). This development, so aptly described by Douglas (1976) as a shift of emphasis from "neurologizing to the problem of finding ways to help the very large number of children who are being diagnosed as learning disabled, MBD or hyperactive," is an important one.

The tasks to be addressed involve the development of remediation and training programs based on the inferences derived from neuropsychological evaluation and the determination of whether or not these programs are in fact effective. It is a fairly safe prediction that the programs will prove to be less than optimally effective. This outcome will necessitate a revision of our inferences, the formulation of new evaluation procedures and the development of new methods of remediation and training. This effort should lead to more successful treatment of neurologically handicapped children. It may lead to significant advances in our understanding of brain-behavior relationships, which at present is so limited.

Thus I think that child neuropsychology is likely to follow new directions in the coming decades. Comprehensive interdisciplinary studies involving parallel measurement of both neurological and behavioral variables will be prominent. More sophisticated research designs will take account of the modifying influence of environmental factors on the behavior of children with cerebral dysfunction. Clinical practice will expand beyond neuropsychological assessment to encompass the development and validation of remedial programs. There is every reason to expect that this expansion of our investigative and clinical acitivities will yield rich rewards.

REFERENCES

Allen, T. W. Patterns of attention to temporal stimulus sequences and their relationship to reading achievement. *Child Development,* 1975, 46, 1035–1038.

Bakker, D. J. Temporal order, meaningfulness, and reading ability. *Perceptual and Motor Skills,* 1967, 24, 1027–1030.

Bakker, D. J. Ear asymmetry with monaural stimulation: task influences. *Cortex,* 1969, 5, 36–42.

Bakker, D. J. Temporal order perception and reading retardation. In D. J. Bakker & P. Satz (Eds.), *Specific reading disability: advances in theory and method.* Rotterdam: Rotterdam University Press, 1970 (a).

Bakker, D. J. Ear asymmetry with

monaural stimulation: relations to lateral dominance and lateral awareness. *Neuropsychologia*, 1970, *8*, 103–117 (b).

Bakker, D. J. *Temporal order in disturbed reading.* Rotterdam: Rotterdam University Press, 1972.

Bakker, D. J., Hoefkens, M., & Van der Vlugt, H. Hemispheric specialization in children as reflected in the longitudinal development of ear asymmetry. *Cortex*, 1979, *15*, 619–626.

Bakker, D. J., Licht, R., Kok, A., & Bouma, A. Cortical responses to word reading by right- and left-eared normal and reading-disturbed children. *Journal of Clinical Neuropsychology*, 1980, *2*, 1–12.

Bakker, D. J., Teunissen, J., & Bosch, J.: Development of laterality-reading patterns. In R. M. Knights & D. J. Bakker (Eds.), *The Neuropsychology of learning disorders.* Baltimore: University Park Press, 1976.

Balow, I. H. Lateral dominance characteristics and reading achievement in the first grade. *Journal of Psychology*, 1963, *55*, 323–328.

Balow, I. H., & Balow, B. Lateral dominance and reading achievement in the second grade. *American Educational Research Journal*, 1964, *1*, 139–143.

Belmont, I. L., & Birch, H. G. Lateral dominance, lateral awareness and reading disability. *Child Development* 1965, *36*, 57–72.

Benton, A. L. *Right-left discrimination and finger localization. Development and pathology.* New York: Hoeber-Harper, 1959.

Benton, A. L. Dyslexia in relation to form perception and directional sense. In J. Money (Ed.), *Reading disability: progress and research needs in dyslexia.* Baltimore: Johns Hopkins University Press, 1962.

Benton, A. L. Right-left discrimination. *Pediatric Clinics of North America*, 1968, *15*, 747–758.

Benton, A. L. Neuropsychological aspects of mental retardation. *Journal of Special Education*, 1970, *4*, 3–11.

Benton, A. L. Developmental dyslexia: neurological aspects. In W. J. Friedlander (Ed.), *Advances in Neurology* (Vol. 7). New York: Raven Press, 1975.

Benton, A. L. Some conclusions about dys-

lexia. In A. L. Benton & D. Pearl (Eds.), *Dyslexia: An appraisal of current knowledge.* New York: Oxford University Press, 1978.

Benton, A. L. The neuropsychological significance of finger recognition. In M. Bortner (Ed.), *Cognitive growth and development.* New York: Brunner/Mazel, 1979.

Benton, A. L. The neuropsychology of facial recognition. *American Psychologist*, 1980, *35*, 176–186.

Benton, A. L., & Pearl, D. (Eds.) *Dyslexia: an appraisal of current knowledge.* New York: Oxford University Press, 1978.

Benton, A. L., Van Allen, M. W., Hamsher, K., & Levin, H. S. *Test of facial recognition.* Iowa City: University of Iowa Hospitals, 1978.

Bettman, J. W., Stern, E. L., Whitsell, L. J., & Gofman, H. F. Cerebral dominance in developmental dyslexia. *Archives of Ophthalmology*, 1967, *78*, 722–729.

Birch, H. G. Dyslexia and the maturation of visual function. In J. Money (Ed.), *Reading disability: progress and research needs in dyslexia.* Baltimore: Johns Hopkins University Press, 1962.

Birch, H. G., & Belmont, L. Auditory-visual integration in normal and retarded readers. *American Journal of Orthopsychiatry*, 1964, *34*, 825–861.

Birch, H. G., & Belmont, L. Auditory-visual integration, intelligence, and reading ability in school children. *Perceptual and Motor Skills*, 1965, *20*, 295–305.

Birch, H. G., & Lefford, A. Intersensory development in children. *Monographs of the Society for Research in Child Development*, 1963, *28*: 5 (Whole No. 89).

Borod, J. C., & Goodglass, H. Lateralization of linguistic and melodic processing with age. *Neuropsychologia*, 1980, *18*, 79–84.

Bryden, M. P. Laterality effects in dichotic listening: relations with handedness and reading ability in children. *Neuropsychologia*, 1970, *8*, 443–450.

Buffery, A. W. H. Sex differences in the development of hemispheric asymmetry of function in the human brain. *Brain*, 1971, *31*, 364–365.

Butters, N., Barton, M., & Brody, B. A. Role of the right parietal lobe in the mediation of cross-modal associations and reversible operations in space. *Cortex*, 1970, *6*, 174–190.

Butters, N., & Brody, B. A. The role of the left parietal lobe in the mediation of intra- and cross-modal associations. *Cortex*, 1968, *4*, 328–343.

Carey, S., & Diamond, R. From piecemeal to configurational representation of faces. *Science*, 1977, *195*, 312–314.

Childs, B., Finucci, J. M., & Preston, M. S.: A medical genetics approach to the study of reading disability. In A. L. Benton & D. Pearl (Eds.), *Dyslexia: an appraisal of current knowledge*. New York: Oxford University Press, 1978.

Collignon, R., Hécaen, H., & Angerlergues, R. A propos de 12 cas d'aphasie acquise de l'enfant. *Acta Neurologica et Psychiatrica Belgica*. 1968, *68*, 245–277.

Connors, C. K. Cortical visual evoked response in children with learning disorders. *Psychophysiology*, 1971, *7*, 418–428.

Corkin, S. Serial-ordering deficits in inferior readers. *Neuropsychologia*, 1974, *12*, 347–354.

Cotard, J. *Etude sur l'atrophie cérébrale*. Thèse, Paris, 1868.

Damasio, A. R., & Maurer, R. G. A neurological model for childhood autism. *Archives of Neurology*, 1978, *25*, 777–786.

Damasia, H., Maurer, R. G., Damasio, A. R., & Chui, H. C. Computerized tomographic scan findings in patients with autistic behavior. *Archives of Neurology*, 1980, *37*, 504–510.

Dare, M. T., & Gordon, N. Clumsy children: A disorder of perception and motor organization. *Developmental Medicine & Child Neurology*, 1970, *12*, 178–185.

Davenport, R. K., & Rogers, C. M. Intermodal equivalence of stimuli in apes. *Science*, 1970, *168*, 279–280.

Denckla, M. B. Minimal brain dysfunction and dyslexia: beyond diagnosis by exclusion. In M. E. Blau, I. Rapin, & M. Kinsbourne (Eds.), *Child neurology*. New York: Spectrum Publications, 1977.

Denckla, M. B., & Rudel, R. Naming of pictured objects by dyslexic and other learning disabled children. *Brain and Language*, 1976, *3*, 1–15 (a).

Denckla, M. B., & Rudel, R. Rapid "automatized" naming (R.A.N.): dyslexia differentiated from other learning disabilities. *Neuropsychologia*, 1976, *14*, 471–497 (b).

Douglas, V. I. Perceptual and cognitive factors as determinants of learning disabilities. In R. M. Knights & D. J. Bakker (Eds.), *The neuropsychology of learning disorders*. Baltimore: University Park Press, 1976.

Drewe, E. A., Ettlinger, J., Milner, A. D., & Passingham, R. E.: A comparative review of the results of neuropsychological research on man and monkey. *Cortex*, 1970, *6*, 129–163.

Duffy, F. H., Denckla, M. B., Bartels, P. H., & Sandini, G. Dyslexia: Regional differences in brain electrical activity by topographic mapping. *Annals of Neurology*, 1979, *7*, 412–420.

Ettlinger, G. Analysis of cross-modal effects and their relationship to language. In C. H. Millikan & F. L. Darley (Eds.), *Brain mechanisms underlying speech and language*. New York: Grune & Stratten, 1967.

Feingold, B. F. *Introduction to clinical allergy*. Springfield, Ill.: Charles C. Thomas, 1975.

Fletcher, J. M., Taylor, H. G., Morris, R., & Satz, P. Finger recognition skills and reading achievement: A developmental neuropsychological perspective. *Developmental Psychology* 1982, *18*, 124–132.

Forgays, D. G. The development of differential word recognition. *Journal of Experimental Psychology*, 1953, *45*, 165–168.

Fry, M. A., Johnson, C. S., & Muehl, S. Oral language production in relation to reading achievement among select second graders. In D. J. Bakker & P. Satz (Eds.), *Specific reading disability: advances in theory and method*. Rotterdam: Rotterdam University Press, 1970.

Gaddes, W. H. *Learning disabilities and brain function: a neuropsychological approach*. New York: Springer-Verlag, 1980.

Galaburda, A. M., & Kemper, T. L. Cytoarchitectonic abnormalities in developmental dyslexia: a case study. *Annals of Neurology*, 1978, *6*, 94–100.

Garfield, J. C. Motor impersistence in normal and brain-damaged children. *Neurology*, 1964, *14*, 623–630.

Geffner, D. S., & Hochberg, I. Ear laterality performance of children from low and middle socioeconomic levels on a verbal dichotic listening task. *Cortex*, 1971, *7*, 193–203.

Geschwind, N. Disconnexion syndromes in animal and man. *Brain*, 1965, *88*, 237–294.

Groenendaal, H. A., & Bakker, D. J. The part played by mediational processes in the retention of temporal sequences by two reading groups. *Human Development* 1971, *14*, 62–70.

Gubbay, S. S. *The clumsy child*. Philadelphia: W. B. Saunders, 1975.

Hermann, K. *Reading disability*. Copenhagen: Munksgaard, 1959.

Hermann, K. Specific reading disability with special reference to complicated word blindness. *Danish Medical Bulletin*, 1964, *11*, 34–40.

Hermann, K., & Norrie, E. Is congenital word-blindness a hereditary type of Gerstmann's syndrome? *Psychiatria et Neurologia (Basel)* 1958, *136*, 59–73.

Hermelin, B., & O'Connor, N. Functional asymmetry in the reading of Braille. *Neuropsychologia*, 1971, *9*, 431–435.

Hier, D., Lemay, M., Rosenberger, P. B., & Perlo, V. Developmental dyslexia: evidence for a subgroup with reversal of cerebral asymmetry. *Archives of Neurology*, 1978, *35*, 90–92.

Hinshelwood, J. *Congenital word-blindness*. London: H. K. Lewis, 1917.

Hughes, J. R. Electroencephalography and learning disabilities. In H. R. Myklebust (Ed.), *Progress in learning disabilities*. New York: Grune & Stratton, 1971.

Ingram, T. T. S. Soft signs. *Developmental Medicine and Child Neurology*, 1973, *15*, 527–530.

Kimura, B. Speech lateralization in young children as determined by an auditory test. *Journal of Comparative and Physiological Psychology*, 1963, *56*, 899–902.

Kinsbourne, M., & Warrington, E. The developmental Gerstmann syndrome. *Archives of Neurology*, 1963, *8*, 490–501.

Knights, R. M., & Bakker, D. J. (Eds.) *The neuropsychology of learning disorders*. Baltimore: University Park Press, 1976.

Knights, R. M., & Bakker, D. J. (Eds.) *Treatment of hyperactive and learning disordered children*. Baltimore: University Park Press, 1980.

Knox, C., & Kimura, D. Cerebral processing of nonverbal sounds in boys and girls. *Neuropsychologia*, 1970, *8*, 227–237.

Lechner, C. S. Aangeboren woordblindheid. *Nederlandsch Tijdschrift voor Geneeskunde*, 1903, *39*, 235–244.

Lefford, A., Birch, H. G., & Green, G. The perceptual and cognitive bases for finger localization and selective finger movement in preschool children. *Child Development*, 1974, *45*, 335–343.

Lenneberg, E. H. *Biological foundations of language*. New York: Wiley, 1967.

Leong, C. K. Lateralization in severely disabled readers in relation to functional cerebral development and synthesis of information. In R. M. Knights & D. J. Bakker (Eds.), *The neuropsychology of learning disorders*. Baltimore: University Park Press, 1976.

Lezak, M. D. *Neuropsychological assessment*. New York: Oxford University Press, 1976.

Liberman, I. Y., & Shankweiler, D. Speech, the alphabet and teaching to read. In L. Resnick & P. Weaver (Eds.), *Theory and practice of early reading*. New York: Wiley, 1978.

Lindgren, S. D. *Spatial perception in children: supramodal spatial ability and hemispheric specialization for spatial processing*. Ph. D. Dissertation, University of Iowa, 1977.

Lindgren, S. D. Finger localization and the prediction of reading disability. *Cortex*, 1978, *14*, 87–101.

Marcel, T., Katz, L., & Smith, M. Laterality and reading proficiency. *Neuropsychologia*, 1974, *12*, 131–139.

Marcel, T., & Rajan, P. Lateral specialization for recognition of words and faces in good and poor readers. *Neuropsychologia*, 1975, *13*, 489–497.

Matthews, C. G. Application of neuropsychological test methods in mentally retarded subjects. In R. M. Reitan & L. A. Davison (Eds.), *Clinical neuropsychology*. Washington, D.C.: Winston, 1974.

Mattis, S., French, J. H., & Rapin, I. Dyslexia in children and young adults: three independent neuropsychological syndromes. *Development Medicine and Child Neurology*, 1975, *17*, 150–163.

McKeever, W. F., & Van Deventer, A. D. Dyslexic adolescents: evidence of impaired visual and auditory language processing associated with normal lateralization and visual responsitivy. *Cortex*, 1975, *11*, 361–378.

McLearn, G. E. Dyslexia: Genetic aspects. In A. L. Benton & D. Pearl (Eds.), *Dyslexia: an appraisal of current knowledge*. New York: Oxford University Press, 1978.

Miller, R. G., Palkes, H. S., & Stewart, M. A. Hyperactive children in suburban elementary schools. *Child Psychiatry and Human Development*, 1973, *4*, 121–127.

Molfese, D. L., Freeman, R. B., & Palermo, D. S. The ontogency of brain lateralization for speech and nonspeech stimuli. *Brain and Language*, 1975, *2*, 356–368.

Morgan, W. P. A case of congenital word-blindness. *British Medical Journal*, 1896. *2*, 1378.

Nagafuchi, M. Development of dichotic and monaural hearing abilities in young children. *Acta Otolaryngologica*, 1970, *69*, 409–415.

Orton, S. T. "Wordblindness" in school children. *Archives of Neurology and Psychiatry*, 1925, *14*, 581–615.

Orton, S. T. Reading disability. *Genetic Psychology Monographs*, 1926, *14*, 335–343.

Orton, S. T. Specific reading disability—strephosymbolia. *Journal of the American Medical Association*, 1928, *90*, 1095–1099.

Ousted, C., Lindsay, J., & Norman, R. Biological factors in temporal lobe epilepsy. *Clinics in Developmental Medicine* Nr. 22. London: Heinemann, 1966.

Palkes, H., & Stewart, M. Intellectual ability and performance of hyperactive children. *American Journal of Orthopsychiatry*, 1972, *42*, 35–39.

Paternite, C. E., & Loney, J. Childhood hyperkinesis: relationships between symptomatology and home environment. In C. K. Whalen & B. Henker (Eds.), *Hyperactive children*. New York: Academic Press, 1980.

Paternite, C., Loney, J., & Langhorne, J. E. Relationships between symptomatology and

SES-related factors in hyperactive/MBD boys. *American Journal of Orthopsychiatry*, 1976, *46*, 291–301.

Petrauskas, R., & Rouke, B. P. Identification of subgroups of retarded readers: A neuropsychological, multivariate approach. *Journal of Clinical Neuropsychology*, 1979, *1*, 17–37.

Porter, R. J., & Berlin, C. I. On interpreting developmental changes in the dichotic right-ear advantage. *Brain and Language*, 1975, *2*, 186–200.

Preston, M. S., Guthrie, J. T., & Childs, B. Visual evoked responses (VERs) in normal and disabled readers. *Psychophysiology*, 1974, *11*, 452–457.

Preston, M. S., Guthrie, J. T., Kirsch, I., Gertman, D., & Childs. B. VERs in normal and disabled readers. *Psychophysiology*, 1977, *14*, 8–14.

Reed, J. C. Lateralized finger agnosia and reading achievements at ages 6 and 10. *Child Development*, 1967, *38*, 213–220.

Reuben, R. N., & Bakwin, H. Developmental clumsiness. *Pediatric Clinics of North America*, 1968, *15*, 601–610.

Rosenblum, D. R., & Dorman, M. F. Hemispheric specialization for speech perception in language deficient kindergarten children. *Brain and Language*, 1978, *6*, 378–389.

Rudel, R. G., Denckla, M. B., & Hirsch, S. The development of left hand superiority for discriminating Braille configurations. *Neurology*, 1977, *27*, 160–164.

Rudel, R. G., Denckla, M. B., & Spalten, E. The functional asymmetry of Braille letter learning in normal, sighted children. *Neurology*, 1974, *24*, 733–738.

Rutter, M. The development of infantile autism. *Psychological Medicine*, 1974, *4*, 147–163.

Rutter, M. Prevalence and types of dyslexia. In A. L. Benton & D. Pearl (Eds.), *Dyslexia: an appraisal of current knowledge*. New York: Oxford University Press, 1978.

Rutter, M., Graham, P., & Yule, W. *A neuropsychiatric study in childhood*. London: Heinemann, 1970.

Satz, P., Bakker, D. J., Teunissen, J., Goebel, R., & Van der Vlugt, H. Developmental parameters of the ear asymmetry: A multi-variate approach. *Brain and Language*, 1975, 2, 171–185.

Satz, P., & Friel, J. Some predictive antecedents of specific learning disability: a preliminary one year follow-up. In P. Satz and J. Ross (Eds.), *The disabled learner*. Rotterdam: Rotterdam University Press, 1973.

Satz, P., & Friel, J. Some predictive antecedents of specific learning disability: a preliminary two-year follow-up. *Journal of Learning Disabilities*, 1974, 7, 437–444.

Satz, P., Taylor, H. G., Friel, J., & Fletcher J. Some developmental and predictive precursors of reading disabilities: A six-year follow-up. In A. L. Benton & D. Pearl (Eds.), *Dyslexia: an appraisal of current knowledge*. New York: Oxford University Press, 1978.

Schmitt, B. D. The minimal brain dysfunction myth. *American Journal of Diseases of Children*, 1975, 129, 1313–1318.

Senf, G. M.: Development of immediate memory for bisensory stimuli in normal children and children with learning disorders. *Development Psychology 6*: Part 2, 1969.

Shankweiler, D. P. A study of developmental dyslexia. *Neuropsychologia*, 1963, 267–286.

Shankweiler, D., & Liberman, I. Y. Exploring the relations between reading and speech. In R. M. Knights & D. J. Bakker (Eds.), *The neuropsychology of learning disorders*. Baltimore: University Park Press, 1976.

Sparrow, S., & Satz, P. Dyslexia, laterality and neuropsychological development. In D. J. Bakker and P. Satz (Eds.), *Specific reading disability: Advances in theory and method*. Rotterdam: Rotterdam University Press, 1970.

Spreen, O., & Gaddes, W. H. Developmental norms for 15 neuropsychological tests age 6 to 15. *Cortex*, 1969, 5, 170–191.

Strauss, A., & Lehtinen, L. *Psychopathology and education of the brain-injured child*. New York: Grune & Stratton, 1947.

Swanson, J. M., & Kinsbourne, M. Food dyes impair performance of hyperactive children on a laboratory learning test. *Science*, 1980, 207, 1485–1486.

Thomson, M. E. A comparison of laterality effects in dyslexics and controls using verbal dichotic listening tasks. *Neuropsychologia*, 1976, 14, 243–246.

Tuddenham, R. D., Brooks, J., & Milkovich, L. Mothers' reports of behavior of ten-year-olds. *Developmental Psychology*, 1974, 10, 959–965.

Vellutino, F. R. *Dyslexia*. Cambridge, Mass.: MIT Press, 1980.

Walton, J. N., Ellis, E., & Court, S. D. M. Clumsy children: developmental apraxia and agnosia. *Brain*, 1962, 603–612.

Warrington, E. K. The incidence of verbal disability associated with reading retardation. *Neuropsychologia*, 1967, 5, 175–179.

Weiner, J., Barnsley, R. H., & Rabinovitch, M. S. Serial order ability in good and poor readers. *Canadian Journal of Behavioral Science*, 1970, 2, 116–123.

Weiss, B., et al. Behavioral responses to artificial food colors. *Science*, 1980, 207, 1487–1489.

Wender, P. H. *Minimal brain dysfunction in children*. New York: Wiley-Interscience, 1971.

Wender, P. H. Hypothesis for a possible biochemical basis of minimal brain dysfunction. In R. M. Knights & D. J. Bakker (Eds.), *The neuropsychology of learning disorders*. Baltimore: University Park Press, 1976.

Werner, E. E. Environmental interaction in minimal brain dysfunctions. in H. E. Rie & E. D. Rie (Eds.), *Handbook of minimal brain dysfunctions*. New York: Wiley, 1980.

Werner, E. E., Bierman, J. M., & French, F. F. *The children of Kauai* Honolulu: University Press of Hawaii, 1971.

Werry, J. S., & Quay, H. C. The prevalence of behavior symptoms in younger elementary school children. *American Journal of Orthopsychiatry*, 1971, 41, 136–143.

Witelson, S. F. Hemispheric specialization for linguistic and nonlinguistic tactual perception using a dichotomous stimulation technique. *Cortex*, 1974, 10, 3–17.

Witelson, S. F. Abnormal right hemisphere specialization in developmental dyslexia. In R. M. Knights & D. J. Bakker (Eds.), *The neuropsychology of learning disorders*. Baltimore: University Park Press, 1976.

Witelson, S. F., & Rabinovitch, M. S. Hemispheric speech lateralization in children with auditory-linguistic deficits. *Cortex*, 1972, 8, 412–426.

Wyke, M. A. (Ed.) *Developmental dysphasia*. London: Academic Press, 1978.

Yeni-Komshian, G. H., Isenberg, D., & Goldberg, H. Cerebral dominance and reading disability: left visual field deficit in poor readers. *Neuropsychologia*, 1975, *13*, 83–94.

Young, A. W. & Ellis, H. D. An experimental investigation of developmental differences in ability to recognize faces presented to the left and right cerebral hemispheres. *Neuropsychologia*, 1976, *14*, 495–498.

Zangwill, O. L. Dyslexia in relation to cerebral dominance. In J. Money (Ed.), *Reading disability: Progress and research needs in dyslexia*. Baltimore: Johns Hopkins University Press, 1962.

Zurif, E. B., & Carson, G. Dyslexia in relation to cerebral dominance and temporal analysis. *Neuropsychologia*, 1970, *8*, 351–361.

IX.
Approaches to Clinical Methodology

28.

Problems of Test Construction in the Field of Aphasia*

I. GENERAL CONSIDERATIONS

I should like to open this discussion of problems of test construction in the field of aphasia by considering first an analogous problem, namely, intelligence test construction. There are many similarities between intelligence and language. Both are extremely complex concepts which are difficult to define in such a way as to secure the agreement of any large number of experts. Both are variables of great clinical and educational importance; therefore, whether he possesses a satisfactory definition or not, the clinician is forced to deal with these concepts as best he can. The potential development of both intelligence and language, as well as their actual level of function at any given time, are strictly determined by central nervous system factors. Yet, at the same time, both are cultural products, the social environment being an indispensable precondition for the development of each. Finally, both intelligence and language are frequently impaired, either in combination or separ-

ately, in adults with acquired cerebral disease and in children with congenital cerebral abnormalities. Given these basic similarities, it may be instructive to review briefly the development of test construction in the area of intelligence since, on the whole, it seems that we have been somewhat more successful here than in the area of aphasia.

The clinical application of tests of mental abilities has a history going back about 90 years. The impetus for their development appears to have come from a desire to probe for the presence of mental impairment in patients who were not obviously demented and also in aphasic patients. Of course, the concept of dementia goes back many centuries. But it was only during the latter half of the nineteenth century that physicians felt the need for defined procedures that would elicit, and also perhaps provide a quantitative measure of, behavioural expressions of dementia. Undoubtedly the controversial question of whether aphasia necessarily involved a deficit in intelligence stimulated the development of

* A. L. Benton, *Cortex*, 1967, 3, 32–58.

special test methods. The definitive description of sensory aphasia by Wernicke in 1874 must also have made it seem imperative to distinguish between specific loss of language comprehension and more general impairment in understanding.

However, the procedures and test methods that were developed were rarely standardized in the modern sense. Starting with a subjective criterion of what constituted normal performance, the clinician defined pathological inferiority as any performance below that level without giving systematic consideration to the limits of normal variability or to the effects of such factors as age, sex and cultural level (although, of course, common sense and clinical experience must certainly have played a corrective role in many instances). Various clinics developed their own favored batteries of tests for memory, reasoning, practical judgment, calculation, reading and other abilities and utilized these tests for making judgments about their patients' mental status. No doubt this was useful within the context of any single clinic but the results usually meant little to other workers who used other tests. Criteria of normality varied from one place to another. In one clinic, failure to repeat seven digits might be considered to indicate defective immediate memory while in another clinic the criterion was failure to repeat five digits. Perhaps each was a valid criterion in the respective clinic, the difference in norms being due to a difference in test administration or scoring performance or perhaps in the type of patient seen in the two clinics. But obviously the test results were not comparable. The unsatisfactory nature of this situation was realized and it was not long before standard mental status examinations or test batteries, designed to be used by all clinics, were proposed.

One such battery was proposed by the Würzburg psychiatrist, Rieger, who outlined an extensive battery of tests (which took about 100 hours to give) and who recommended its general use. Neither Rieger's battery (which was, of course, quite impracticable) nor other proposed test batteries were generally adopted. There were a number of reasons for this. Chief among them was that the assembling of a battery of tests such as this was essentially an armchair exercise. No explicit empirical standardization and no clear demonstration of clinical utility supported the tests. Consequently, there was no convincing evidence that a proposed battery was significantly superior to one's own battery. Thus, while it was readily conceded that the adoption of the same battery by a large number of clinics would be desirable, there seemed to be no compelling reason for adopting any particular battery of tests.

This was the state of affairs in intelligence testing and intelligence test construction when Alfred Binet entered the scene at the beginning of the twentieth century. As we know, Binet was presented with a practical problem by the educational authorities of Paris, namely how can one identify those children who were destined to fail in school because of lack of intelligence and who required special instruction.

Binet undertook to answer the question by developing a battery of mental tests to measure the hypothetical quality of intelligence in children. His tests were *objective*, that is to say, not only was the task explicitly outlined but the procedure for presenting it was exactly described and precise criteria for evaluating whether or not a subject's performance was satisfactory were listed. Moreover, his tests were *standardized*, that is to say, they were given to samples of boys and girls of different ages; those tests which did not show a progressive rise in performance level with increasing age and those which showed a significant sex difference were eliminated. The result was, as we know, a series of tests appropriate to children of different ages ranging from age 3 years to the adult level.

We also know, of course, that the Binet scale enjoyed a phenomenal success. Bobertag in Germany, Burt in England and Terman in the United States standardized the tests for use in these countries and developed equivalent versions. In some countries the scale was merely translated and the French or American standardization was adopted without revision. This was certainly a mistake and must have led to many errors of interpretation. The scale enjoyed this unparalleled success because it was objective, because it was standardized and because its clinical utility was demonstrated. For whatever its limitations were (and it had many), clinical workers in different places at least could now obtain directly comparable results. In short, it established the possibility of meaningful communication among them.

One serious limitation of the Binet scale was that it had been standardized on children and therefore its application to adults sometimes produced results of questionable validity. Another limitation was that most of the tests of the scale were of a verbal nature and therefore were likely to underestimate the true intelligence of individuals who, for one reason or another, suffered a specific weakness of verbal skills.

Both of these limitations were overcome to some degree by the Wechsler scales, which were standardized on adults with due allowance for the effects of age on performance and which provided separate scales for "verbal" and "non-verbal" abilities. The Wechsler scales have many serious defects; it is not necessary to go into these here. The point to be made is that, despite these defects, the scales have enjoyed immense popularity. The reasons for their popularity are the same as those underlying the popularity of the Binet. The scales were objective, they were standardized and they had demonstrable clinical utility.

With this perspective in mind, let us turn to the problem of test construction and application in the field of aphasia. I think it is not inaccurate to say that we are today where intelligence testing was in 1900, i.e., in the pre-Binet stage. Many test batteries, some of them of excellent quality, have been devised and are used in the clinics in which they were developed. A few, such as the battery of Schuell (1965), have been adopted by other clinics but none has been so widely adopted as to make it generally recognized as a standard battery. In recent years important developmental work has been going on in a number of neurological centers, e.g., Berlin, Bucharest, Düsseldorf, Milano, Iowa City (cf. De Renzi, 1960; Kreindler & Fradis, 1961; Bay, 1964; Weigl, 1966; Spreen, Benton, & Van Allen, 1966). It is not surprising that each of these centers is represented at this conference, for these are the centers which have been most keenly aware of the critical nature of the problem facing us and each has made intensive efforts to remedy the situation. Each has reported brief descriptions of a comprehensive series of tests which is used in that particular center and which *could* be used more widely. But none has been generally adopted. The history of clinical intelligence testing perhaps tells us why. Excellent as these batteries are, none of them has been published in *usable form*. None of them presents standardization information, explicitly describes testing procedures, presents exact criteria for scoring or offers detailed guides for the interpretation of performance. Moreover, none of them presents convincing evidence that the battery possesses a degree of clinical utility which is significantly greater than any other series of aphasia tests which might be assembled.

I hope I am not misunderstood. I do not mean to say that the batteries of tests developed in many clinics are not well standardized and objective or do not possess great clinical utility. The point which must be made (and it is a simple one) is that there is little evidence in *published form* that they are well standardized, objective and useful. In brief, the batteries which each of us has developed falls short of accomplishing what the Binet scale or the Wechsler scales have accomplished.

The Binet scale and the Wechsler scales certainly are not the last word in intellectual testing. All of us are aware of their many deficiencies. But, at the same time, it seems to me undeniable that, if the field of aphasia testing could attain at least the Binet-Wechsler stage, a significant advance would be gained. However limited such a "universal" aphasia battery might be, at least it would establish the possibility of effective communication among us.

Let us consider some of the formidable problems involved in developing such an examination.

The first problem which we encounter is of a conceptual nature, for our conception of language will determine what tests we employ to assess language disturbance. How should we conceptualize language? Should we analyze it in terms of different types of stimulus response sequences, establish a classification on this basis and devise tests to assess each type of performance? Should we follow Jacksonian principles and conceive of language in terms of levels of performance which are defined not by specific modalities or specific modes of response but in terms of the complexity of the proposition? If we do, we should adopt a very different set of tests. Do we believe, following the tradition of Marie and Head, that there is only one basic language function and that the different

clinical pictures we see represent essentially adventitious admixtures of a disturbance in the single basic function and various non-linguistic sensory or motor disabilities? Or do we believe, following the tradition of Wernicke, that there are different primary types of aphasic disorder—receptive and expressive, auditory and visual, central and conductive? Or, following the lead of some linguists, should we conceive of language in terms of basic grammatical categories? In each case, our fundamental preconception will determine the nature of our examination and of the specific tasks included in it.

Now, of course, quite the same conceptual problem arises in the field of intelligence test construction. What is the nature of intelligence? What is its structure? Is the nucleus of intelligence a single general ability, which enters into all intellectual performances, as Spearman believed? Or is intelligence "multidimensional" in nature, consisting of a relatively small number of primary mental abilities, as Thurstone stated? Or is it simply the sum total of a large number of specific intellectual skills that the individual has developed during the course of his life as a function of his hereditary predisposition, his formal education and accidental circumstances? Obviously our fundamental conception of the structure of intelligence will determine our choice of test methods. If we believe that intelligence consists essentially of a single general ability, then theoretically the best measure is a single test (e.g., the Progressive Matrices of Raven) which assesses this ability most directly. If we adopt Thurstone's concept of multiple primary abilities, we would develop tests for each of 5, 6 or 8 abilities which have been derived from factorial analysis. If we accept the doctrine of specificity, our test battery will consist of many tests covering as broad a range of diverse abilities as possible.

How did Binet solve this conceptual problem? Very simply . . . he avoided it. At first, he offered some simple armchair definitions, such as anyone might come up with ("intelligence is the capacity to adapt to novel situations," etc.). However, when pressed to defend his scale as a measure of these hypothetical abilities, he retreated to a pragmatic (and circular) definition: "intelligence" is what the tests measure. In short, Binet was prepared to concede that the scale was of no theoretical significance and to defend it on the sole basis of clinical utility. The Wechsler scales are a similar mélange of tasks employed previously in clinical work and with no underlying conceptual basis. This is a grave deficiency of these scales which imposes severe limitations on their usefulness in clinical investigation. As we have seen, their popularity has been due to other factors.

Now we must face the difficult problem of whether it is possible to go beyond the pragmatic level in constructing a standard test battery for aphasia. Given the diversity of conceptual approaches to the problem of aphasia, it may not be possible to do so at the present time. This is a question which we must discuss today. If our answer is negative (i.e., if we see no possibility of achieving a single conceptual framework which is satisfactory to all schools of thought), then perhaps a standardized basic examination can be assembled on pragmatic grounds. For example, it is likely that all students of aphasia would agree that a test of visual object-naming is a necessary part of any aphasia examination, even though there are different conceptions about what information the test provides. On the other hand, probably only some students would consider that a test of tactile object-naming is a necessary part of an aphasia examination. No doubt all would agree that a test of oral language comprehension belongs

in the examination. However, there would be considerable disagreement about the selection of items in such a test, depending upon how one defines "difficulty" or "complexity" (e.g., grammatical form, length of question, number of "bits of information" in the question, etc.) The status of tests of repetition of digits, words or sentences might well be controversial, valued by some but considered by others to be essentially irrelevant to the problem of aphasia.

I do not know the answer to this question. But obviously, it is one which cannot be "wished away". Some kind of solution (or, at least, understanding) of the question must be achieved before a broadly acceptable standard examination for aphasia can be constructed.

The other problems involved in the construction of an aphasia examination are of a technical nature. They are not nearly as difficult as the conceptual problem in the sense that their solution is actually well within our capabilities while the conceptual problem may not be at the present time. However, these technical problems are quite formidable in the sense that their solution demands a great deal of labor. The construction of a technically adequate test battery to evaluate the status of language functions involves a number of tedious, time-consuming tasks: careful selection of items for each test in the battery; pilot testing to determine reliability, validity and level of difficulty; collection of normative data for performance on each test of appropriate groups of subjects, including assessment of the influence of such factors as age, sex and cultural status on performance level; determining the effects of practice or prior experience with the tests; considering whether two or more equivalent forms of the battery should be constructed in order to permit unbiassed repeated examination of the same patient; correcting scores for the influence of age and educational level, when this is necessary; finally, transforming raw scores into standard scores or ranks so that one obtains a valid picture of an individual patient's strengths and weaknesses.

All these steps are necessary components in the development of an aphasia test battery designed for use within a single language community. The development of a standard examination designed for use in two or more language communities raises additional problems. The test battery must be standardized separately for each language community for it will be found that the same item does not necessarily have the same meaning or the same difficulty level in every community. Therefore the task is not one of simple translation of a test from one language to another but the more complicated one of constructing an essentially equivalent test in the second language.

Let me illustrate this problem by some specific examples. In standardizing a test of visual object-naming in our laboratory, we decided to select items on the basis of the age at which young children could name the object under the artificial condition of the psychometric testing situation. This we called the "acquisition age" of the name of the object. Thus we found that (at least in the case of children living in the midwestern section of the U.S.) the acquisition age for the word "key" was 4.1 years; for the word "jar," it was 4.6 years; for the word "shoe-lace," it was 5.2 years, etc. At the same time, Prof. De Renzi and Dr. Vignolo have been developing an Italian version of this visual naming test and, in the course of this, they have been standardizing the same items on Milanese children. Many of the items prove to have approximately the same acquisition age in the American and the Italian standardizations. However, other items prove to have lower or higher ages

in one or the other language community. It is, of course, easy to understand why this should be so. For example, the age at which children in a given language community will learn the name of a safety razor will depend upon the relative prevalence of use by their fathers of safety razors as compared to straight razors or electric shavers. One of the items in our visual naming test is a toy rotary egg-beater representing the instrument which American housewives typically use to whip up various mixtures of eggs, cream, butter, etc. But this is generally a much less familiar object to Italian children since *their* mothers typically use the Continental egg-whisk (*fouet*; *frullino*; *Schneebesen*). Conversely, the Continental egg-whisk is not known by name to most American children.

These considerations may seem at first glance to be an academic exercise without clinical significance. I can assure you that they are not. Rochford and Williams (1962) have demonstrated that the naming of different objects and their parts shows a highly consistent order of difficulty in patients with nominal aphasia and in normal children. Recently we completed a similar study of the relationship between the errors made by aphasic patients in naming various objects and the "acquisition ages" of the names of these objects as determined in young children. The results disclosed extremely high correlation coefficients between the number of errors made by the patients and the age at which children learned the names of the objects. This held for both visual and tactile naming. It was as clear a demonstration of the "law of regression" as one could hope to make and fully confirmed the findings of Rochford and Williams.

What is true of visual object naming will hold, of course, for all the tasks in an aphasia examination. The difficulty of a specific test of language understanding will be determined by factors peculiar to each language such as the relative frequency in each language of the words in the proposition presented to the patient, the relative ease or difficulty of pronouncing the words in each language, and the grammatical form in which the proposition is stated.

It is evident, then, that a valid international aphasia examination will *not* consist of identical tests but rather of *essentially equivalent* tests, each of which has been standardized on the language population to which it is to be applied. It is equally evident that the development of such an examination is a task of considerable magnitude. However, the task can be done. I personally believe that the fruits would be worth the great effort which is required. If we should be successful, we would possess for the first time the means for a direct comparison of our individual findings. This, I think we would all agree, is a prerequisite for truly scientific intercourse among us and this has been lamentably lacking in the field of aphasia. Moreover, in the course of developing such an examination, we may well learn important new facts about aphasia. Finally, it may be anticipated that the very existence of an examination based on rigorous scientific criteria would have the effect of raising the quality of aphasia research throughout the world. This too, we would all agree, is a prerequisite for advancing our knowledge of this group of disorders of ever-increasing medical importance.

II. DESCRIPTION OF AN APHASIA EXAMINATION IN COURSE OF DEVELOPMENT

The construction of this battery of tests to evaluate language disorders was initiated at the Neurosensory Center of the College of Medicine, University of Iowa, in 1962 by Dr. Otfried Spreen and myself. In 1965, Prof. Ennio De Renzi and Dr. L. A. Vignolo of the University Clinic for Nervous and Mental Diseases in Milano began the development of an Italian language version of the battery.

The impetus for undertaking this major project was derived from several considerations: (1) to provide a fairly comprehensive examination that would include assessment of most of the areas of language function which are of clinical interest; (2) to provide sufficiently detailed tests for each area of language function so that a relatively exact measure of performance level can be obtained; (3) to include specific tests in the battery which could be employed to investigate current questions in the field of aphasia (e.g., the reality of the clinical pictures of conduction aphasia, central aphasia and transcortical aphasia; the nature of the pattern of recovery from aphasia; the nature of the pattern of loss in developing aphasia; the question of modality-specific aphasia); (4) to standardize and score test performances in such a way as to introduce necessary corrections for the effects of age, education and sex on performance and to make possible a direct and valid comparison of performances within the individual patient as well as among patients; (5) to include a series of non-linguistic control tests in the battery in order to insure valid interpretation of performance on the language tests; (6) to include a series of non-linguistic supplementary tests assessing various abilities in order to permit investigation of some of the non-linguistic intellectual deficits associated with aphasic disorders.

Selection of tests

The selection of tests was based on theoretical and practical considerations. From the theoretical standpoint, it was believed that the traditional associationist

Table 24. Tests of language function in the aphasia battery

1.	VN	Visual Naming
2.	DU	Description of Use
3.	TNR	Tactile Naming, Right Hand
4.	TNL	Tactile Naming, Left Hand
5.	SRP[a]	Sentence Repetition
6.	DRF[a]	Repetition of Digits
7.	DRR[a]	Reversal of Digits
8.	WF	Word Fluency
9.	SC	Sentence Construction (Masselon Test)
10.	IN	Identification by Name
11.	IS	Identification by Sentence (De Renzi-Vignolo Token Test)
12.	RNO	Reading Names Orally
13.	RSO	Reading Sentences Orally
14.	RNP	Reading Names for Meaning
15.	RSP	Reading Sentences for Meaning (De Renzi-Vignolo Token Test)
16.	VGN	Visual-Graphic Naming
17.	WN	Writing Names
18.	WD	Writing to Dictation
19.	WC	Writing from Copy
20.	ART[a]	Articulation (Oral Repetition)

[a] Presented on tape.

approach still possessed sufficient validity to warrant formulation of certain test procedures along these lines. Thus, tests of tactile object-naming with the right and with the left hand were included as well as the more conventional test of visual object-naming. Analogous tests of reading and writing were included both in order to effect systematic variation in type of stimulus and mode of response and because of their importance for clinical purposes. Tests of language understanding were included for obvious reasons. Tests of repetition of sentences and digits were included with particular reference to the question of the concepts of conduction aphasia and transcortical aphasia. Verbal associative fluency and sentence construction were included with the hope that they might provide assessments of the status of "inner language" in aphasic patients.

The 20 tests of language function that comprise the nucleus of the battery are listed in Table 24. A brief description of each test follows:

1. *Visual Naming (VN)*. The patient is instructed to name 10–40 objects (not pictures); the actual number of objects

presented depends upon the purpose of the test (clinical evaluation or specific research problem) and the level of the patient's performance.

2. *Description of Use (DU)*. The patient is instructed to tell the use of 10–20 objects from the basic set of 40 objects.

3. *Tactile Naming, Right Hand (TNR)*. The patient is instructed to feel the object with his right hand (without the aid of vision) and name it; 10–20 objects from the basic set of 40 are used; in case of failure, stereognostic capacity is evaluated by Control Test 1 (TMR).

4. *Tactile Naming, Left Hand (TNL)*. Same procedure as TNR.

5. *Sentence Repetition (SRP)*. The patient is instructed to repeat tape-recorded sentences ranging from 1 to 26 syllables in length.

6. *Repetition of Digits (DRF)*. The patient is instructed to repeat tape-recorded series of digits ranging from three to nine digits in length.

7. *Reversal of Digits (DRR)*. The patient is instructed to repeat in reverse

order tape-recorded series of digits ranging from two to seven digits in length.

8. *Word Fluency (WF)*. The patient is instructed to say all the words which he can think of that begin with a specific letter of the alphabet (e.g., "F," "A," "S,"); three one-minute trials with three different letters are given.

9. *Sentence Construction (SC)*. Sets of two or three words are presented to the patient who is instructed to make up a sentence with these words; five sets of words are given.

10. *Identification by Name (IN)*. The patient is instructed to point to objects (from the basic set of 40 objects) named by the examiner; the actual number of objects named depends upon the specific purpose of the test and the level of the patient's performance.

11. *Identification by Sentence (IS)*. This test, which is a slight modification of the Token Test of De Renzi and Vignolo, consists of 39 commands of progressively increasing complexity which assess the patient's capacity to understand oral language.

12. *Reading Names Orally (RNO)*. The patient is instructed to read aloud names of objects from the basic set of 40 objects.

13. *Reading Sentences Orally (RSO)*. The patient is instructed to read aloud 12 commands from the De Renzi-Vignolo Token Test.

14. *Reading Names for Meaning (RNP)*. The patient is presented with the written name of an object and instructed to point to it in a display of 10 objects.

15. *Reading Sentences for Meaning (RSP)*. The patient is presented with 12 written commands from the De Renzi-Vignolo Token Test and instructed to carry them out.

16. *Visual-Graphic Naming (VGN)*. The patient is instructed to write the names of 10 visually presented objects

from the basic set of 40 objects; performance is scored in terms of accuracy of naming and not for graphic characteristics.

17. *Writing Names (WN)*. The patient's performance on Test 16 is scored for spelling but not for accuracy of naming; if the patient was not able to write the name of the visually presented object, the name is presented to him orally (i.e., writing to dictation).

18. *Writing to Dictation (WD)*. The patient is instructed to write two short sentences to dictation; performance is scored for spelling, punctuation, omissions and reduplications.

19. *Writing from Copy (WC)*. The patient is instructed to write two short sentences from copy; performance is scored as in Test 18.

20. *Articulation (ART)*. The patient is instructed to repeat clearly 30 meaningful and 8 nonsense words presented by tape; performance is scored in terms of the number of correctly articulated consonant or consonant blends.

Control tests

These control tests are given to certain patients in order to determine whether their failure on certain language tests may be due to sensory or perceptual defect rather than to impairment in language. A brief description of these four tests follows:

C1. *Tactile-Visual Matching, Right Hand (TMR)*. This test is given if the patient has made any errors in the test of tactile naming with the right hand (TNR), its purpose being to determine whether failure in the naming task may have been due to stereognostic defect. A series of objects is presented to the patient for tactile recognition with the right hand without the aid of vision; he is instructed to identify the object in a visual display set before him. The arrangement is illustrated in Figure 14.

C2. *Tactile-Visual Matching, Left Hand (TML)*. This test, which is the same as Test C1, assesses tactile recognition in the left hand and is given to any patient who has made one or more errors in the test of tactile naming with the left hand (TNL).

C3. *Visual-Visual Matching (VVM)*. This test is given if the patient has made any errors in the tests of visual naming (VN) or identification by name (IN); two trays, each containing the same 10 objects, are set before the patient; one tray is in the standard position while the other is in the reversed position so that the locations of the objects are different on the two trays; pointing to an object on one tray, the examiner instructs the patient to point to the same object on the other tray. The purpose of the test is to determine whether the patient's failure on the language tests may have been due to impairment in visual recognition.

C4. *Visual Form Perception (FP)*. This test is given if the patient has made any errors on any reading test (RNO, RSO, RNP, RSP); a visual display of 21 letters is set before the patient (Figure 15); 8 letters are then presented one at a time and the patient is instructed to identify the presented letter on the display; if he makes any errors, a second test is given to obtain a more precise estimate of his visuoperceptive impairment.

Supplementary tests

As their name implies, these tests do not form an essential part of the language battery in the strict sense. They evaluate various aspects of praxis, perception, memory and reasoning and their purpose is to provide a fuller picture of the setting within which a patient's language disturbances appear. As such, they are considered to be

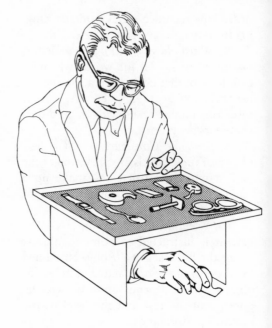

Fig. 14. Arrangement for test of tactile-visual matching, right hand.

useful both for the clinical evaluation and for investigative purposes. The 10 tests are as follows:

S1. *Utilization Praxis, Right Hand (APR)*. The patient is instructed to demonstrate with his right hand the use of each of 10 objects from the basic set of 40 objects. If he does not understand the verbal instructions, the use of other objects in the basic set is demonstrated in an effort to communicate the nature of the task to him. His performance on each task is analyzed in terms of the component actions, e.g., his demonstration of the use of a knife is analyzed in terms of whether he grasps the handle, orientates the knife so that the blade is away from him and makes a cutting or spreading movement.

S2. *Utilization Praxis, Left Hand (APL)*. This test, which is the same as Test S1, employs other objects to assess demonstration of use with the *left* hand.

S3. *Handedness Inventory (H)*. This test consists of a series of questions about

Q W E R T Y U I O P

A W S D F G H J K L Z

Fig. 15. Visual display for test of visual form perception; individual letters are presented singly to the patient who is instructed to identify it on the display; actual height of letters is 5 mm.

hand preference in various activities and is presented orally to the patient or, when this is not possible, to a reliable informant; if doubt exists about the patient's understanding of the concepts of "right" and "left", he is asked to show how he would perform the activity mentioned, e.g., throw a ball or use a screwdriver. The supplementary questions about hand preference among members of the family are presented to the patient or a relative whenever it seems likely that reliable information on this point can be secured. The Inventory is shown in Table 25.

S4. Sound Recognition (SRC). This test consists of 13 tape-recorded familiar sounds which are presented to the patient with the instruction that he name the source of the sound. If performance on this sound-naming task is below the normal level, the test is repeated in the form of a non-verbal multiple-choice task in

Table 25. Handedness questionnaire

A. Are you right-handed or left-handed?	Right	Left	Mixed
B. Do you consider yourself *strongly* or *moderately* right-handed (or left-handed)?	Strongly	Moderately	
C. 1 With which hand do you write?	Right	Left	Both
2 With which hand do you use a scissors?	Right	Left	Both
3 With which hand do you use a screwdriver?	Right	Left	Both
4 With which hand do you throw a ball?	Right	Left	Both
5 In baseball, do you bat right-handed or left-handed?	Right	Left	Both
6 With which hand do you use a hammer?	Right	Left	Both
7 With which hand do you use a needle in sewing?	Right	Left	Both
8 With which hand do you usually carry books?	Right	Left	Both
9 With which hand do you usually carry a suitcase?	Right	Left	Both
10 With which hand do you hold the toothbrush when you brush your teeth?	Right	Left	Both

Hand preferences of members of family

Father:
Mother:
Siblings:
Brother 1 —   Sister 1 —
Brother 2 —   Sister 2 —
Brother 3 —   Sister 3 —
Brother 4 —   Sister 4 —
Husband/wife:
Children (6 years and over):
Son 1 —   Daughter 1 —
Son 2 —   Daughter 2 —
Son 3 —   Daughter 3 —
Son 4 —   Daughter 4 —

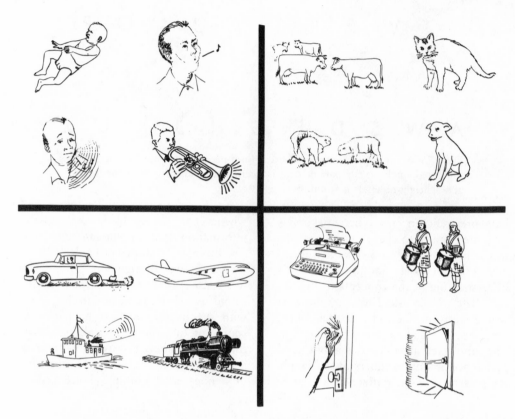

Fig. 16. Examples of multiple-choice items on sound recognition test; patient hears tape-recorded sound (e.g., baby crying, boat whistle, drums) and is instructed to point to the source of the sound on the four-choice card.

which the patient must identify the source of the heard sound among four alternatives presented in visual form to him. Examples of this multiple choice task are presented in Figure 16.

S5. *Three-dimensional Block Construction (BC).* This test of three-dimensional block construction involves the successive presentation of each of three block models to the patient with the instruction that he construct a replica which is exactly like the model (cf. Critchley, 1953; Benton & Fogel, 1962).

S6. *Stereognosis, Right Hand (STR).* In this test the patient is required to identify abtract figures made of sandpaper haptically with *right* hand and without the aid

of vision, identification being accomplished by matching the haptically perceived form with the same form visually presented in a display (Figure 17).

S7. *Stereognosis, Left Hand (STL).* Application of Test S6 to the *left* hand.

S8. *WAIS Block Designs (BD).* This subtest of the Wechsler battery is employed to assess higher-level two-dimensional constructional praxis.

S9. *WAIS Picture Arrangement (PA).* This subtest of the Wechsler battery is employed to assess the patient's ability to organize pictorial information into a meaningful temporal sequence.

S10. *Visual Retention Test, Multiple Choice Form (VRT).* This test of short-

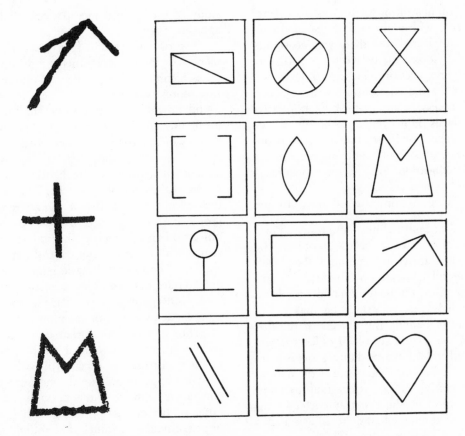

Fig. 17. (*A*) Examples of sandpaper figures used in supplementary tests of stereognosis (STR, STL); actual height of figures is 5 cm. (*B*) Visual display presented to the patient for identification of haptically perceived sandpaper figures; actual size of figures is the same as the sandpaper figures.

term visual memory involves the presentation of each of 15 abstract designs to the patient; after the design has been removed, the patient must identify it among four alternatives presented to him.

Standardization procedures

The steps taken in standardizing [a] test of visual object-naming (VN) may be described to illustrate the standardization procedures utilized in developing the tests in the battery. A total of 60 objects were presented for visual and tactile naming to a group of aphasic patients, a group of control patients and to children of various ages. On the basis of the findings, 40 objects were selected to form the test on the basis of the following criteria: (1) number of failures in visual naming of the item so that there would be a fairly wide range of difficulty; the actual percentage of failure ranged from 3.6 per cent to 35.5 per cent; (2) items that were appropriate for both visual and tactile naming; (3) ease of scoring responses as correct or incorrect. This 40-item test was then divided into four subsets of 10 objects, each subset being of approximately equal difficulty level.

Administration of the test to control patients within the age range of 16–64 years indicated that there was no significant association between performance level and age or educational level and hence that no correction for these factors was necessary in establishing normative standards. However, on other tests (e.g., digit repetition, word fluency) corrections in score to control for the influence of age and education on performance were found to be necessary.

The test is administered in two forms:

1. For most clinical and research purpose, one or two trays (10–20 objects) are presented for visual naming. If the patient names all 10 objects on the first tray correctly, the test is terminated and he is assigned score of 40. If he makes 1–9 errors in naming the objects of the first tray, the second set of 10 objects is presented and the assigned total score is twice the number of objects correctly named. Conversely, if the patient fails to name any object on the first tray correctly, the test is terminated and he is assigned a score of 0.

2. For certain specific research purposes, all four trays (40 objects) are presented (e.g., in studies of visual and tactile naming or of the relationship between frequency of errors in aphasic patients and the age of acquisition of the name of the object in children).

Development of profile sheets

A distribution of the raw scores of the control patients on each test was tabulated and appropriate corrections made for the influence of age and educational level on performance. Each distribution of corrected scores was then converted into a percentile rank distribution. Bay employed an essentially similar procedure of converting raw scores into ranks in his study of the performance patterns of 80 aphasic patients.

A profile sheet based on the performances of the control patients indicating the percentile rank equivalent of different raw scores was then constructed. It was found, however, that this profile sheet was unsuitable for evaluating the performances of aphasic patients because most of the scores of the "typical" aphasic patient fell below the entire distribution of scores of the control group. For example, the typical aphasic patient in our reference group correctly named 32 out of 40 objects on visual naming while the lowest score on this test for any control patient was 37. The typical aphasic patient was able to repeat 14 sentences correctly in the Sentence Repetition Test (SR); the lowest score made by a control patient was 16.

Thus it was evident that this profile sheet, which was developed on the basis of the performances of control patients, was not appropriate for the purpose of comparing aphasic patients with each other or for evaluating differential level of performance within the individual patient. However, it has proved to be useful for investigating the language performances of clinically non-aphasic patients, e.g., in comparing patients with lesions of the left and right hemispheres and in studying the decline of language functions in normal old age and in senile dementia.

In order to study language function in aphasia more precisely, we developed another profile sheet based upon the performances of what we designated as our "reference group" of aphasic patients. Within certain restrictions, this group consisted of all patients with a clinical diagnosis of aphasia who were referred to the Laboratory of Neuropsychology for evaluation. The restrictions consisted in excluding from the group any patient who was uncooperative or confused, whose disability was clearly limited to disturbances in articulation or whose concomitant dysarthria was so severe that his speech was not understandable.

The distribution of the raw scores of the patients on each test was plotted, the appropriate corrections for the influence of age and educational level were made and the corrected scores were converted into percentile rank scores, as in the first profile sheet. This new profile sheet was used as a basis for plotting the scores of individual aphasic patients (Figure 18). The individual profile gives an immediate indication of the overall severity of the aphasic disorder (as compared to our reference group of aphasic patients) and also of the pattern of performance of the patient on this battery of language tests.

Illustrative profiles

Figure 19 shows the profiles of a young woman who presented with a relatively mild aphasic disturbance following a cerebrovascular accident and who recovered virtually completely from a clinical standpoint. "Anomia" was noted on the referral sheet as being the most prominent disability; actually, as the lower profile shows, her poorest performances were on the repetition and reversal of digits. On retest, she showed no aphasic deficits except inferior performances on the repetition tasks.

Figure 18 shows the profile of a patient clinically diagnosed as a case of "expressive aphasia." It will be noted that all oral expressive performances, including the "inner language" performances involved in Word Fluency (WF) and Sentence Construction (SC), are severely impaired. Writing is also severely impaired. On the other hand, both oral and visual verbal understanding are less severely compromised but are nevertheless clearly defective. The profile fits the classic description of "motor aphasia."

Figure 20 shows the profile of a patient with the diagnosis of "jargon aphasia." It will be seen that, with the curious exception of Reading Names for Meaning (RNP), all performances are grossly defective. The profile fits the classic description of "Wernicke's aphasia."

Figure 21 shows the profile of a patient clinically classified as "anomia." However, the pattern of performance indicates that this is scarcely the picture of "pure anomia" or "amnesic aphasia." One notes that Description of Use (DU) is as severely impaired as Visual Naming (VN). In addition, all performances involving reading (i.e., visual discrimination) are severely impaired. It is also to be noted that Writing from Dictation (WD), i.e., via the auditory channel, is not impaired while Writing from Copy (WC), i.e., via the visual channel, is grossly defective. However, control test performances provided no evidence of gross visuosensory or visuoperceptive deficit. Visual-Visual Matching (VVM), Tactile-Visual Matching (TMR, TML) and Visual Form Perception were all performed perfectly. Nevertheless, the possibility of an interaction between a more subtle visual deficit and language performance, as postulated by Kok (1964) and by Bisiach (1966), should not be excluded.

Figure 22 presents the profile of a patient who was referred as having a relatively "pure" Gerstmann syndrome. She did in fact show severe finger agnosia, right-left disorientation, acalculia and agraphia. In addition, she manifested severe constructional apraxia and marked topographic disorientation As would be anticipated, the profile shows that her writing is impaired, particularly writing to dictation and writing from copy. She also shows poor repetition of digits, which is not unexpected. She was considered on an

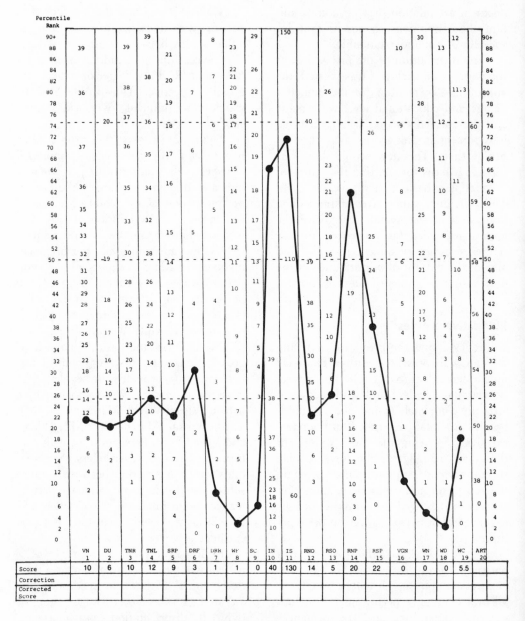

Fig. 18. Profile of patient with clinical diagnosis of "expressive aphasia."

impressionistic-clinical basis to be free from aphasia. The profile suggests why this impression was gained. Her naming performances, description of use of objects and identification of objects when the name is supplied by the examiner are fairly adequate. However, we also note that Reading for Meaning (RSP) is significantly impaired and that the "inner language" tests (Word Fluency and Sentence Construction) are performed quite poorly. Thus there would seem to be a sig-

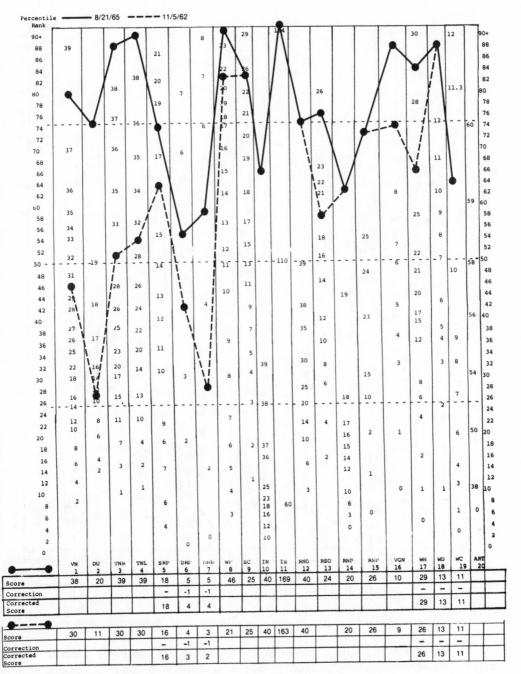

Fig. 19. Profiles of aphasic patient initially referred with notation of "anomia" who showed virtually complete recovery from clinical standpoint.

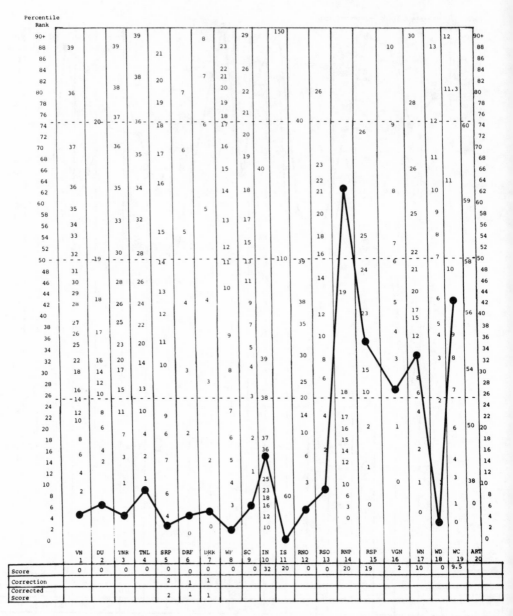

Fig. 20. Profile of patient with referral diagnosis of "jargon aphasia."

nificant impairment of language functions in this ostensibly non-aphasic patient.

Figure 23 shows the test and retest profiles of a patient who initially showed a global aphasia. On the first test, all performances were severely impaired; he could do almost nothing. He could ident-

ify 12 objects out of 40 when the name was supplied to him by the examiner, but that was about all. The impaired naming and reading could not be explained in terms of sensory deficit. He was examined again five months later and showed great improvement in naming, oral understand-

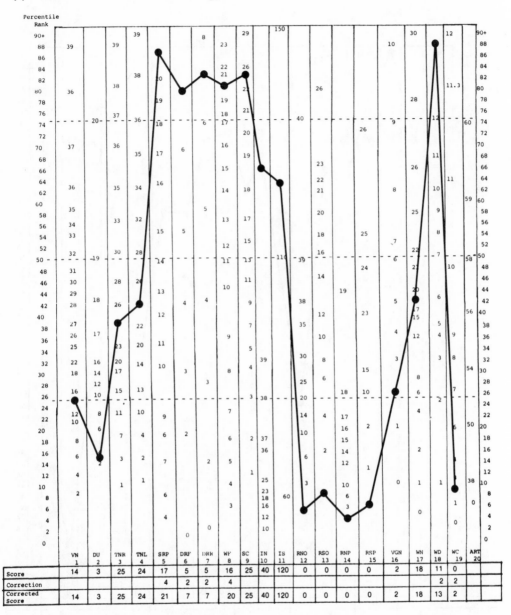

	VN 1	DU 2	TNR 3	TNL 4	SRP 5	DRF 6	DRR 7	WF 8	SC 9	IN 10	IS 11	RNO 12	RSO 13	RNP 14	RSP 15	VGN 16	WN 17	WD 18	WC 19	ART 20
Score	14	3	25	24	17	5	5	16	25	40	120	0	0	0	0	2	18	11	0	
Correction					4	2	2	4										2	2	
Corrected Score	14	3	25	24	21	7	7	20	25	40	120	0	0	0	0	2	18	13	2	

Fig. 21. Profile of patient with referral diagnosis of "anomia"; note that all language performances involving vision are impaired.

ing, reading and writing. But some performances did not improve, e.g., repetition of sentences and digits and reading sentences aloud (RSO). We note also that tactile naming is somewhat better than visual naming. Furthermore, we see that "Des-cription of Use" of visually presented objects is relatively poor. This raises the question, as in a case previously presented, of whether a subtle disturbance in visual recognition may not be a residual deficit. The extreme impoverishment of

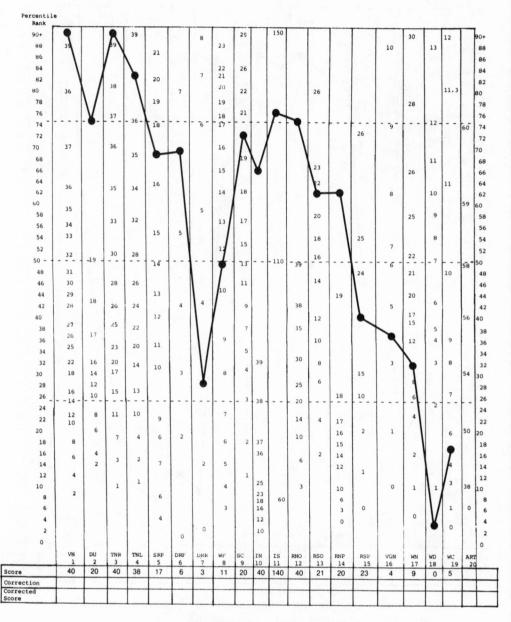

Fig. 22. Profile of patient with referral diagnosis of "Gerstmann syndrome."

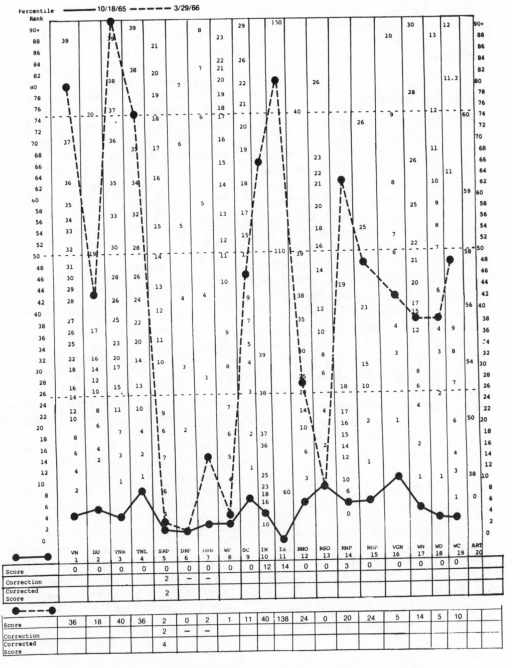

Fig. 23. Profiles of patient with initial global aphasia who showed significant improvement over a period of five months.

his "inner language" processes (despite his remarkable improvement in expression and understanding) is indicated by his absolute failure on the word fluency test.

Concluding comments

This is an outline of the test battery which is in course of development in Iowa City and Milan. We hope that, when perfected, it will provide both a useful instrument for clinical evaluation and a valid research technique. It would seem possible that it, or a similarly standardized battery of tests, could serve as the starting point for the development of a basic multilingual instrument for the investigation of aphasia. Of course, the application of such an international battery would not be restrictive in any way. Certainly it would not preclude the utilization of special tests and approaches by an investigator or in any clinic. On the other hand, the uniform application of a standard examination such as this would go far towards establishing that level of *operational* understanding among workers which is a prerequisite for scientific communication in the field of aphasia.

REFERENCES

Bay, E. (1964) *Principles of classification and their influence on our concepts of language,* in Disorders of Language, ed. by A. V. S. de Reuck & M. O'Connor. Little, Brown and Co., Boston.

Benton, A. L., & Fogel, M. L. (1962) *Three-dimensional constructional praxis: a clinical test.* "Arch. Neurol.," 7, 347–354.

———, Meyers, R. & Polder, G. J. (1962) *Some aspects of handedness,* "Psychiat. Neurol.," 144, 321–337.

Bisiach, E. (1966) *Perceptual factors in the pathogenesis of anomia,* "Cortex," 2, 90–95.

Blackburn, H. L., & Benton, A. L. (1957) *Revised administration and scoring of the digit span test,* "J. Consult. Psychol.," 21, 139–143.

Critchley, M. (1953) *The Parietal Lobes.* Edward Arnold and Co., London.

De Renzi, E. (1960) *Un test semeiotico per l'afasia e per le funzioni connesse,* "Arch. Psicol. Neurol. Psichiat." 21, 17–64.

———, & Vignolo, L. A. (1962) *The token test: a sensitive test to detect receptive disturbances in aphasics,* "Brain," 85, 665–678.

Kok, E. P. (1964) *Modifications of speed of perception of pictures of objects in optic aphasia,* "Cortex", 1, 328–343.

Kreindler, A., & Fradis, A. (1961) *The Bucharest symposium on aphasia,* "World Neurol.," 2, 986–996.

Rochford, G., & Williams, M. (1962) *Studies in the development and breakdown in the use of names, I: the relationship between nominal dysphasia and the acquisition of vocabulary in childhood,* "J. Neurol. Neurosurg. Psychiat.," 25, 222–233.

Schuell, H. (1965) *Minnesota Test for Differential Diagnosis of Aphasia.* University of Minnesota Press, Minneapolis.

Spreen, O., Benton, A. L., & Fincham, R. W. (1965) *Auditory agnosia without aphasia,* "Arch. Neurol.," 13, 84–92.

———, & Van Allen, M. W. (1966) *Dissociation of visual and tactile naming in amnesic aphasia,* "Neurology," 16, 807–814.

Weigl, E. (1966) *On the construction of standard psychological tests in cases of brain damage,* "J. neurol. Sci.," 3, 123–127.

29.

Normative Observations on Neuropsychological Test Performances in Old Age*

INTRODUCTION

An ongoing clinical study of dementia and its relationships to neurologic, radiologic, and electroencephalographic findings in elderly patients necessitated the collection of a fairly extensive body of data on the neuropsychological test performances of normal older subjects. Since such data are relatively sparse, it was felt that the findings would be clinically useful and possibly also have a bearing on the more basic question of the nature of the decline of abilities with age. Data on the performances of 162 native-born subjects within the age range of 65–84 years will be presented.

METHOD

Subjects

The 34 men and 128 women who volunteered to be subjects in the study were

* A. L. Benton, P. J. Eslinger, and A. R. Damasio, *Journal of Clinical Neuropsychology*, 1981, 3, 33–42.

recruited from senior citizen organizations and retirement homes in Iowa City and surrounding communities. In each instance, the purposes of the parent project on dementia and the need for healthy control subjects were explained at an open meeting in the facility. The members of the audience were then invited to volunteer to participate. There was a marked predominance of women at these facilities, particularly in the senior citizens groups. About 40% of each group volunteered at the close of the meeting, the proportions of male and female volunteers being about equal. The residents of Iowa City were seen for neuropsychological examination at the Department of Neurology of the University of Iowa Hospitals, while the majority of the residents of the surrounding communities were examined at their homes. At the interview preceding examination, all the subjects stated that they considered themselves to be psychologically normal and in reasonably good health, and all denied a history of neurological disease or of psychiatric disorder requiring hospitalization. The distribution

Table 26. Number of men and women and mean education in the several age groups[a]

Age	Men	Women	Total
65–69 yrs.	2	26	28
	(13.5)	(13.6)	(13.5)
70–74 yrs.	20	42	62
	(13.6)	(13.8)	(13.7)
75–79 yrs.	'7	28	35
	(13.5)	(13.5)	(13.5)
80–84 yrs.	5	32	37
	(13.1)	(13.5)	(13.4)

[a] Mean years of education in parentheses.

of the sample in respect to age, sex, and educational level is shown in Table 26. As inspection of the table indicates, the educational background of the group was above average. The sample perhaps can be described as "normative" in the sense that it consisted of well-educated, healthy older persons either with time on their hands who volunteered to be subjects for altruistic motives or because they thought that the experience would be an interesting one.

Tests

1. *Temporal Orientation.* This test assessing the accuracy of identification of the year, month, day of month, day of week, and time of day was standardized on 180 control patients within the age range of 16–66 years and without evidence of history of brain disease, psychosis, or psychiatric illness requiring hospitalization (Benton, Van Allen, & Fogel, 1964; Levin & Benton, 1975). Perfect or near-perfect performances (scores of 99–100 by the adopted scoring system) were made by 92% and scores of 97–100 were made by 97% of the subjects. Performance level was not correlated with age, sex, or educational level. A comparable study by Natelson, Haupt, Fleischer, and Grey (1979) using the same test generated somewhat lower values, 85% making

scores of 99–100 and 94% making scores of 97–100. Natelson et al. found a small correlation ($r = .15$) between test scores and educational level, but no correlation between test scores and age, self-rated health status, or reported family income. A score of 96 or lower, corresponding to a performance level exceeded by 95% of the subjects in the combined studies, was classified as defective.

2. *Digit Span.* Administration and scoring differed from the WAIS Digit Span subtest in a number of respects. The subject is required to repeat both sets of digits of each length even when he has repeated the first set correctly; repetition or reversal of digits is terminated after three successive failures instead of two; credit is given for each set of digits correctly reproduced rather than in terms of the longest series correctly reproduced. As a consequence, a significantly more reliable estimate of performance level is obtained (Blackburn & Benton, 1957). The obtained raw score was transformed into the equivalent WAIS raw score and then into the equivalent WAIS scaled score for the 55–64 years age level (Wechsler, 1955, p. 107) Expected scaled scores were set at 10 for subjects with less than 12 years of education, 11 for those with 12–15 years of education, and 12 for those with 16 or more years of education.

Obtained scaled scores that were four or more points below expectation, corresponding to performance levels exceeded by approximately 94% of normal subjects, were classified as defective (cf. Hamsher, Benton, & Digre, 1980).

3. Digit Sequence Learning ("Digit Supra-span"). This test involves the presentation of a series of either eight or nine digits, depending upon the educational level of the subject, over repeated trials. The test is terminated after two correct repetitions on consecutive trials or after the 12th trial, whichever comes first. Details of scoring and normative standards are presented in Hamsher et al. (1980). This measure of short-term verbal retention has been demonstrated to be a more sensitive index of the presence of brain disease than digit span (Zangwill, 1943; Drachman & Arbit, 1966; Drachman & Hughes, 1971; Schinka, Note 1; Hamsher et al., 1980). Performance levels that were exceeded by 94–95% of contral patients within the age range of 16–64 years were classified as defective.

4. Controlled Oral Word Association ("Word Fluency"). This test in the Multilingual Aphasia Examination (Benton & Hamsher, 1978) requires the subject to produce as many words beginning with a given letter of the alphabet as he can recall over a one-minute period. Three letters are presented successively. The total number of acceptable words produced constituted a raw score, which was then corrected for the influence of educational level, sex, and age, the last correction being for the 60–64 year level. A corrected score of 22 or less was classified as defective, this performance level being exceeded by 97% of normal subjects.

5. Logical Memory (Wechsler Memory Scale). Raw scores on this test of para-graph recall were transformed into standard scores for the 60–64 years age group according to the method of Osborne and Davis (1978) whose sample had a mean educational level of 13.0 years, a mean WAIS Verbal Scale IQ of 104.4, and a mean Wechsler Memory Quotient of 102.2. Since our sample had a higher mean educational level and, from all indications, a higher mean Verbal IQ, a standard score of 11 (instead of 10) was set as the midpoint of the distribution. A subject's performance was classified as defective if his standard score was 6 or less (1.7 standard deviations or more below the mean).

6. Associate Learning (Wechsler Memory Scale). Raw scores on this verbal learning test also were transformed into standard scores for the 60–64 years age group as described by Osborne and Davis (1978). A subject's performance was classified as defective if his standard score was 6 or less, i.e., 1.7 standard deviations or more below the standard score of 11, corresponding to a performance exceeded by 95% of the standardization group.

7. Visual Retention Test. Error scores on this test of short-term visual memory were compared to expected scores for the 60–64 years age level and for the subject's educational background (Benton, 1974). Error scores that were four or more points above expectations, representing performance levels exceeded by approximately 96% of a normative sample, were classified as defective.

8. Facial Recognition. Performance on this test requiring the matching of unfamiliar faces has been found to be influenced to a moderate degree by age and educational level (Benton, Van Allen, Hamsher, & Levin, 1978). Raw scores were corrected for educational level (less

Table 27. Relative frequency of defective performances

Test	65–69 yrs. (n = 28)	70–74 yrs. (n = 62)	75–79 yrs. (n = 35)	80–84 yrs. (n = 37)
1. Temporal Orientation	0%	2%	6%	5%
2. Digit Span	4%	2%	6%	8%
3. Digit Sequence	18%	10%	14%	22%
4. Word Association	4%	2%	6%	11%
5. Logical Memory	4%	3%	3%	11%
6. Associate Learning	0%	0%	6%	11%
7. Visual Retention	7%	16%	40%	38%
8. Facial Recognition	0%	10%	14%	14%
9. Line Orientation	0%	2%	11%	8%

than 12 grades vs. 12 grades or more) and for age (56–65 years group). The median corrected score of the standardization group (equalled or exceeded by 58%) was 45. Corrected scores of 37 or less, corresponding to performance levels exceeded by 96.5% of normal adults were classified as defective.

9. Judgment of Line Orientation.

Performance on this test requiring the identification of the spatial orientation of lines in relation to a standard has been found to be influenced to a moderate degree by age and sex (Benton, Varney, & Hamsher, 1978). Failure is particularly closely associated with lesions of the right hemisphere in non-aphasic patients with brain disease. Raw scores (number of correct matches) were corrected for sex and the 50–59 years age level. Corrected scores of 18 or less, representing performance levels exceeded by 95% of the standardization sample, were classified as defective.

RESULTS

The proportion of defective performances by the subjects in each age group on each test is shown in Table 27. Inspection of the table shows that, with the exception of Digit Sequence Learning, failure on the verbal tests was quite infrequent. In contrast, the nonverbal tests generated a higher proportion of defective performances.

Temporal Orientation. There was no evidence of decline in performance level on this test. Score distributions were normal for all age levels. The same proportion of subjects (92%) made scores of 99–100 as in our standardization group.

Digit Span. There was no evidence of decline in performance on this test in subjects below the age of 80 years. The 80–84 years age group showed a slightly higher frequency of defective performances then the younger age groups. This lowering of performance level in the 80–84 years age group was also reflected in the finding that only 38% performed at or above the median score of the standardization group, as compared to 55% of the subjects in the age range of 65–79 years.

Digit Sequence Learning. Decline in performance level was shown by all the age groups. The decline was especially marked in the 80–84 years group where 22% of the subjects performed defectively as compared to the normative standards for subjects below the age of 65 years.

Controlled Oral Word Association. Subjects below the age of 80 years showed little evidence of decline in performance on this test in which scores are corrected for educational level as well as age and sex. In the 80–84 years group, 11% of the subjects made defective performances

Table 28. Distributions of scores on the test battery

No. of tests failed	65–69 yrs. (n = 28)	70–74 yrs. (n = 62)	75–79 yrs. (n = 35)	80–84 yrs. (n = 37)
0	18 (64%)	40 (65%)	14 (40%)	12 (32%)
1	9 (32%)	17 (27%)	11 (31%)	14 (38%)
2	1 (4%)	4 (6%)	7 (20%)	5 (14%)
3 or more	—	1 (2%)	3 (9%)	6 (16%)

(i.e., exceeded by 97% of subjects in the 60–64 years group).

Logical Memory and Associate Learning. Subjects below the age of 80 years showed no evidence of decline in performance on these tests. The subjects in the 80–84 years age group made a relatively high number of defective performances (11% vs. an expected 5%).

Visual Retention Test. All age groups showed a relatively high number of defective performances, the proportion of such performances increasing progressively with increasing age. This progressive decline in performance level was also evident in the proportions of subjects with scores at or above the median, which were 61%, 44%, 29%, and 16% for the 65–69, 70–74, 75–79, and 80–84 groups, respectively.

Facial Recognition. Subjects in the 70–84 years age groups showed a relatively high frequency of failing performance. The number of failures in the youngest age group (65–69 years) was not remarkable.

Judgment of Line Orientation. There was no evidence of early decline in level of performance on this test. The subjects in the 75–79 and 80–84 age groups showed a slightly higher frequency of failure than would be expected (11% and 8% vs. a theoretically expected 5%). The perfor-

mance of the 65–69 and 70–74 age groups were well within the normal range.

Overall Performance Level. The number of tests failed by each subject in each group was computed (Table 28). As will be seen, there was generally a progressive increase in the number of failures per subject with increasing age. However, very few subjects failed more than two tests in the battery of nine tests.

DISCUSSION

The performances of this sample of normal, well-educated, healthy older subjects showed little evidence of a generalized decline in mental ability below the age of 80 years. As Table 28 shows, only 4 subjects (3.2%) in the age range of 65–79 years performed defectively on three or more tests in the battery of nine tests. The overall relative frequency of failure among the 125 subjects in this age range was .07, as compared to a theoretical expectation of about .05. The 37 subjects in the 80–84 years range presented a different picture. The proportion of subjects performing defectively on three or more tests (16%) was still rather small but by no means negligible and the overall frequency of failure was .14.

It is evident that the diverse test performances are differentially vulnerable to the effects of ostensibly normal aging. Five of the nine performances stood up very well, at least until the age of 80 years. Among these were Temporal Orientation, Digit Span, and the memory-learning subtests of the Wechsler Memory Scale. The three tests that proved to be most sensitive to the effects of aging were Digit Sequence Learning, Visual Retention, and, to a somewhat lesser extent, Facial Recognition. In their study of digit sequence learning in patients with hippocampal lesions and older control subjects, Drachman and Hughes (1971) found the performance of the controls to be only slightly and nonsignificantly poorer than that of younger normal subjects. However, the mean age of their older subjects was 62 years, with a range of 51 to 69 years. It is clear from our results that many apparently healthy subjects over the age of 65 are significantly impaired in the capacity for auditory-verbal serial learning.

The finding that so many older subjects appear to suffer an almost precipitous decline in short-term visual memory or, more specifically, in reproducing visual designs from memory, is in excellent agreement with the results of the large-scale normative investigations of Poitrenaud and Clément (1965) and Arenberg (1978). Both studies found a substantial decline in Visual Retention Test performance in their carefully screened samples of normal subjects over the age of 60 years.

Occasionally, the idea is advanced that performances mediated by the right hemisphere show a more pronounced decline with age than do those mediated by the left hemisphere. The idea derives from the overall finding that older people are more likely to show impairment on nonverbal than on verbal tests. Our results offer little support for the idea. Of all the tests in the battery, Judgment of Line Direction is the one most closely associated with the integrity of the right hemisphere (Benton, Varney & Hamsher, 1978). Yet, the subjects in the 65–74 years age range showed a much lower frequency of failure on this test than they did on Digit Sequence Learning or Visual Retention.

The finding that, up to the age of 80 years, these older subjects showed no evidence of decline in performance on Controlled Oral Word Association was somewhat unexpected. This task is assumed to be a sensitive measure of verbal-associative fluency, which is often impaired in patients with diffuse or focal brain disease (cf. Milner, 1964; Benton, 1968; Ramier & Hécaen, 1970; Perret, 1974; Benton & Hamsher, 1978; Rosen, 1980) as well as in older normal subjects (Botwinick & Birren, 1963; Furry & Baltes, 1973). However, in a recent study Rosen (1980) found that her sample of subjects with a mean age of 84 years and a mean educational level of 12 years performed quite well on our Controlled Oral Word Association Test. They made an average of 9.2 acceptable associations per letter per minute while the subjects in our 80–84 years group (with a mean educational level of 13.5 years) made an average of 10.1 acceptable associations per letter per minute. In addition, Rosen's subjects made a mean score of 11.3 correct associations in the task of naming animals over a 1-minute period. Thus, both studies indicate that verbal-semantic associative functions do not necessarily suffer as significant a decline with age as the earlier literature might suggest.

From a clinical standpoint, both the test performances that did not decline and those that did decline with advancing age can be utilized to advantage in assessing the status of an older patient in whom the question of brain disease has been raised. The "stable" tests such as Temporal Orientation, Digit Span and Controlled Oral Word Association are of obvious value, since failure on these tasks suggests a pathological state of affairs of an organic or functional nature. The "sensitive" tests such as Digit Sequence Learning and Visual Retention can also be of value. Here, defective performance, which occurs so frequently among older normal subjects, is less informative than is adequate performance which, on the one hand, tends to exclude both amnesic syndromes and the presence of significant diffuse disease and, on the other hand, implies the preservation of a basic component of behavioral competence.

The traditional interpretation of the observed decline in mental abilities with advancing age is that it is a function of the normal aging process and that particularly severe decline represents either an acceleration of this process or the effects of concurrent disease which is associated with (but not an integral part) of aging. However, a somewhat different interpretation, based largely on longitudinal observation indicating that many elderly subjects do not show progressive decline in capacity over the course of years, holds that advancing age per se does not necessarily entail a decline in capacity and that observed decline, mild or severe, is determined by associated factors. For example, Jarvik and Falek (1963), retesting a sample of subjects who were 60 years of age or older (at initial testing) after an interval of eight years, found that varying proportions of them (ranging from 20% to 87%) showed either the same score or a better score on retest. The proportion of subjects maintaining or improving their performance level was lowest for the two speeded tests in the battery, the Wechsler-Bellevue Digit Symbol Substitution (20%) and a speed of tapping test (36%). In contrast, 87% of the subjects maintained or improved their performance on the repetition of digits and 73% maintained or improved their performance on the reversal of digits. The findings of the present study cannot provide critical evidence in favor or negation of this interesting hypothesis that normal aging does not necessarily produce impairment in cognitive functioning. However, the fact that so many of our subjects, including those in the 80–84 years age range, performed within normal limits on all nine tests in the battery is consonant with the hypothesis as well as with current conceptions that the neurological bases of the dementing diseases of the senium differ fundamentally in nature from central nervous system changes that occur in normal aging.

REFERENCE NOTE

Schinka, J. A. *Performance of brain damaged patients on tests of short-term and long-term verbal memory.* Unpublished doctoral dissertation, University of Iowa, 1974.

REFERENCES

Arenberg, D. Differences and changes with age in the Benton Visual Retention Test. *Journal of Gerontology,* 1978, *33,* 534–540.

Benton, A. L. Differential behavioral effects in frontal lobe disease. *Neuropsychologia,* 1968, *6,* 53–60.

Benton, A. L. *Revised Visual Retention Test: Clinical and experimental application.* 4th Ed. New York: Psychological Corporation, 1974.

Benton, A. L. & Hamsher, K. *Multilingual Aphasia Examination.* Iowa City: University of Iowa Hospitals, 1978.

Benton, A. L., Van Allen, M. W., & Fogel, M. L. Temporal orientation in cerebral disease. *Journal of Nervous and Mental Disease,* 1964, *139,* 110–119.

Benton, A. L., Van Allen, M. W., Hamsher K., & Levin, H. S. *Test of Facial Recognition.* Iowa City: University of Iowa Hospitals, 1978.

Benton, A. L., Varney, N. R., & Hamsher, K. Visuospatial judgment: A clinical test. *Archives of Neurology,* 1978, *35,* 364–367.

Blackburn, H. L., & Benton, A. L. Revised administration and scoring of the digit span test. *Journal of Consulting Psychology*, 1957, *21*, 139–143.

Botwinick, J., & Birren, J. E. Mental abilities and psychomotor responses in healthy aged men. In J. E. Birren et al. (Eds.) *Human aging: A biological and behavioral study*. Bethesda, National Institutes of Health, 1963.

Drachman, D., & Arbit, J. Memory and the hippocampal complex. *Archives of Neurology*, 1966, *15*, 52–61.

Drachman, D., & Hughes, J. R. Memory and the hippocampal complex. III. Aging and temporal EEG abnormalities. *Neurology*, 1971, *21*, 1–14.

Furry, C. A., & Baltes, P. B. The effect of age differences in ability-extraneous performance variables on the assessment of intelligence in children, adults and the elderly. *Journal of Gerontology*, 1973, *28*, 73–80.

Hamsher, K., Benton, A. L., & Digre, K. Serial digit learning: Normative and clinical aspects. *Journal of Clinical Neuropsychology*, 1980, *2*, 39–50.

Jarvik, L. F., & Falek, A. Intellectual stability and survival in the aged. *Journal of Gerontology*, 1963, *18*, 173–176.

Levin, H. S., & Benton, A. L. Temporal orientation in patients with brain disease. *Applied Neurophysiology*, 1975, *38*, 58–60.

Milner, B. Some effects of frontal lobectomy in man. In J. M. Warren & K. Akert (Eds.), *The frontal granular cortex and behavior*. New York: McGraw-Hill, 1964.

Natelson, B. H., Haupt, E. J., Fleischer, E. J., & Grey, L. Temporal orientation and education: A direct relationship in normal people. *Archives of Neurology*, 1979, *36*, 444–446.

Osborne, D., & Davis, J. L. Standard scores for Wechsler Memory Scale subtests. *Journal of Consulting and Clinical Psychology*, 1978, *43*, 115–116.

Perret, E. The left frontal lobe of man and the suppression of habitual responses in verbal categorical behavior. *Neuropsychologia*, 1974, *12*, 323–330.

Poitrenaud, J., & Clément, F. La détérioration physiologique dans le test de rétention visuelle de Benton: Résultats obtenus par 500 sujets normaux. *Psychologie Français*, 1965, *10*, 359–368.

Ramier, A. M., & Hécaen, H. Rôle respectif des atteintes frontales et de la latéralisation lésionelle dans les déficits de la "fluence verbale." *Revue Neurologique*, 1970, *123*, 17–22.

Rosen, W. G. Verbal fluency in aging and dementia. *Journal of Clinical Neuropsychology*, 1980, *2*, 135–146.

Wechsler, D. *Manual for the Wechsler Adult Intelligence Scale*. New York: Psychological Corporation, 1955.

Zangwill, O. L. Clinical tests of memory impairment. *Proceedings of the Royal Society of Medicine*, 1943, *36*, 576–580.

30.

Problems and Conceptual Issues in Neuropsychological Research in Aging and Dementia*

The neuropsychologist who is engaged in the study of normal aging, the assessment of cognitive functions in dementia, or the clinical evaluation of patients in whom the question of a dementia has been raised, faces a number of methodological and conceptual problems. Some of these apply to all behavioral studies of aging and are well known to gerontologists.

CROSS-SECTIONAL, LONGITUDINAL, AND CROSS-SEQUENTIAL DESIGNS

There is, for example, the question of the limitations and possibly misleading implications of cross-sectional study wherein subjects of different ages are compared with respect to cognitive test performance. The argument is a familiar one. When one compares representative samples of persons of different ages, one is also comparing persons of disparate educational backgrounds, with exposure to disparate environmental influences during their for-

mative years, and of disparate health status. As a consequence, observed differences in performance between the age groups may reflect the influence of these factors as well as the effects of the aging process per se, with the attendant risk of either overestimating or underestimating the differences attributable to aging.

Early investigators met the problem by equating different age groups for relevant determinants of performance, the most obvious of these being educational attainment. But this procedure introduced its own complications, the most important of which was that now one was comparing different segments of the population.

The educational statistics of the United States may be taken as an example (Dolmatch, 1979). In 1937, 18% of the adolescent population completed at least 1 year of postsecondary school training, i.e., university, college, or technical school. The comparable figures in 1957 and 1977 were 33% and 47%, respectively. No doubt a number of interrelated factors (including intellectual endowment) determined who did and did not enter post-

* A. L. Benton and A. B. Sivan, *Journal of Clinical Neuropsychology*, 1984, 6, 57–63.

secondary school training and one must assume that, in this respect, the youngsters who received this training in 1937 were a more select group than those in subsequent decades. Consequently, comparisons of different age groups with equivalent educational background run the risk of understimating the changes in performance attributable to aging per se. Conversely, to the extent that scholastic training does increase cognitive competence, comparisons of representative samples with differing educational backgrounds run the risk of overestimating performance differences attributable to the aging process.

In addition, there are practical difficulties in attempting to define "educational background" for the purpose of equating groups (cf. Krauss, 1980). Apprenticeship or on-the-job training is not ordinarily considered a part of educational background but the same training undertaken within the context of a technical school is. There is the question of how training experiences during the course of military service should be evaluated. Finally, there is the problem of the reliability of the basic information, which is usually obtained from the subject himself rather than from documentary sources.

Appreciation of the deficiencies of cross-sectional study has led to increasing utilization of longitudinal and sequential (or age-cohort) designs to investigate the effects of aging, The latter design, wherein samples of subjects of different ages are initially tested and then retested a few years later, is more practical than the strictly longitudinal design. Providing for a simultaneous comparison of cross-sectional and longitudinal data, it permits inferences regarding the rate of change in abilities from one age bracket to another.

The longitudinal design has been employed in clinical neuropsychology in studies of the relationship of age to rate

and extent of recovery from aphasic disorder, the length of the follow-up interval typically being 6 months to 1 year. But apart from these aphasia studies, there has been very little application of longitudinal or sequential designs in neuropsychological research when the age factor is the focus on interest. For example, studies of age-lesion interactions have generated results suggesting that older patients suffer more severe behavioral impairment than do younger patients as a consequence of presumably comparable brain lesions (Benton, 1977; Hamsher & Benton, 1978). But the findings were derived from cross-sectional comparisons of performance shortly after stroke or excision of a neoplasm and one does not know whether the observed differences were transient or long-lasting. Only longitudinal or cross-sequential study can provide the answer to this question.

Similarly, studies of the consequences of closed-head injury have shown that age is associated with a longer duration of posttraumatic coma (Wowern, 1966), a higher frequency of frank aphasic disorder (Heilman, Safran, & Geschwind, 1971), and a higher mortality rate (Jennett, Teasdale, Braakman, Minderhoud, & Knill-Jones, 1976). However, interpretation of these findings is complicated by the higher frequency of alcoholism as well as the greater likelihood of development of subdural hematoma in older patients (Levin, Benton, & Grossman, 1982). Again, only controlled longitudinal investigations can specify the relationship of age per se to the behavioral consequences of head trauma.

RATE OF DECLINE

The question of the rate of decline of abilities with age has proved to be a rather complicated one. Longitudinal and cross-sequential studies, which are considered to give a more valid picture of age-related (or ontogenetic) change than did the earlier cross-sectional studies, indicate that in general the decline of abilities with advancing age is less precipitous and occurs later in life than was thought to be the case. However, there are exceptions to this rule. For example, short-term visual memory has been found to show the same rate and pattern of decline whether measured cross-sectionally, longitudinally or cross-sequentially (Arenberg, 1978, 1982; Benton, Eslinger, & Damasio, 1981).

Of course, it has long been known that rate of decline is a function of the specific abilities being assessed. The drop in performance level is likely to be particularly marked on tasks in which speed of response is a component of performance level and on those that make demands on short-term memory. Thus, one finds clear evidence of slowing on reaction time tasks and of inefficiency in learning and retention with advancing age (Arenberg, 1978; Arenberg & Robertson-Tchabot, 1977; Birren, Woods, & Williams, 1980; Benton et al., 1981).

The observed rate of decline is also dependent upon the manner in which an ability is assessed. For example, verbal-associative fluency, as measured by the Thurstone Word Fluency test, shows a relatively early onset of decline with advancing age (Schaie & Labouvie-Vief, 1974). The test requires the subject to *write* as many words beginning with a given letter as he can think of over a 5-minute period and this is followed by a second task in which he writes as many four-letter words beginning with a given letter over a 4-minute period. However, an *oral* word fluency test, in which the subject utters (rather than writes) words beginning with a given letter and in which he is required to associate for only 1 minute at a time, has been found to give quite different results; here, performance

level shows no evidence of decline before the age of 75 years (Benton et al., 1981; Rosen, 1980). In this instance, it seems likely that the differences in mode of response (writing versus speaking) and in the length of the task (5 minutes versus 1 minute) are responsible for the discrepant findings with respect to age-related rate of decline.

The issue of the decline of abilities with age is further complicated by the observation that interindividual variability in performance tends to increase with advancing age (Anastasi, 1958; Botwinick, 1978; Dirken, 1972; Levin & Benton, 1973). The specific determinants of these individual differences in rate of decline have yet to be determined but the implications are obvious: although steady decline in abilities with age may be the rule, some persons show minimal decline or none at all.

Further, there is the observation that within a broadly defined normal population mental efficiency is correlated with health status. Subjects in excellent health tend to show somewhat superior cognitive performances than those with chronic (but not disabling) conditions such as hypertension or minor cardiovascular disease (Birren et al., 1980; Botwinick, 1978; Siegler, Nowlin, & Blumenthal, 1980). This holds for people in all age groups, not only the elderly, and indeed the differences between the healthy and not-so-healthy seem to be sharper for middle-aged than for older subjects. However, Wilkie and Eisdorfer (1971) found that elevated blood pressure in older subjects was predictive of a *subsequent* decline in level of cognitive function.

Finally, we have to be concerned about the significance of the psychological distress that may occur after retirement, loss of status, or bereavement. To the extent that such distress, as reflected in loss of morale and depression in mood,

deleteriously influences cognitive efficiency, it contributes to the picture of its
progressive decline with advancing age.
Yet these affective factors are not intrinsic
components of the aging process.

Neuropsychological research and
practice with older subjects face all these
problems of how to specify the rate and
nature of changes in behavioral capacities
with age, how to assess the trend toward
increased variability, and how to evaluate
the role of nonneurological disease and
motivational factors in performance.
There are no easy solutions but the problems cannot be ignored. They need to be
recognized in standardizing neuropsychological tests for clinical use and in utilizing
available norms in clinical practice. For
example, there is little doubt that the published norms for the WAIS are not a
sound basis for the interpretation of the
performances of older subjects (cf. Price,
Fein, & Feinberg, 1980).

NEUROPSYCHOLOGICAL RESEARCH AND DEMENTIA

Let us turn to another issue, namely, the
assessment and investigation of dementia.
With ever increasing frequency the clinical
neuropsychologist is called upon for help
in the early detection of dementia, in distinguishing between reversible and irreversible forms of the disorder, and in
differentiating "true" dementia from
"pseudodementia." At the same time,
neuropsychological study of dementia,
which was a rarity 10 years ago, has
become a major field of research.

What is "dementia?" It is simply a
nonspecific diagnosis of behavioral
incompetence referable to brain disease.
In essence, the diagnosis simply states that
the demented patient has suffered an overall decline in mental capacity that has rendered him unfit to meet the diverse
intellectual demands associated with the

obligations of everyday life. Some neurologists and psychologists have criticized
the concept as being too vague to be scientifically meaningful. They have urged that
it be abandoned on the grounds that it
conceals the wide individual differences in
patterns of cognitive disability shown by
patients diagnosed as demented and that
its employment tends to discourage analysis of the diverse defects shown by them
(cf. Stengel, 1964; Zangwill, 1964).

Neurologists and pyschiatrists have
long been aware that dementia is a catch-
all diagnosis and many classifications
have been offered. On clinical grounds,
different forms of dementia—global,
amnesic, aphasic, visuoperceptive—have
been identified. On anatomic grounds, a
distinction between cortical and subcortical types is made. On etiologic grounds,
reversible forms of dementia are differentiated from forms that are considered to
be irreversible, given the limitations of
current modes of treatment.

Moreover, in some respects, dementia
is a rather peculiar concept. If a patient
presents with a marked aphasic or amnesic disorder, he is often not classified as
"demented" even though he may also
show serious cognitive impairment
extending beyond his aphasia or amnesia
and even though he may be grossly incompetent from a behavioral standpoint. Evidently the specific disability takes
precedence over the general cognitive
impairment as a basis for diagnostic classification. Finally, it is worth pointing out
that the diagnosis of dementia carries with
it significant implications about the
patient's social, economic, and legal competence. Like the diagnosis of mental
retardation, it is a social, as well as a
medical or psychological classification.

Despite its scientific and theoretical
deficiencies, the concept of dementia is
not likely to be abandoned, at least not in
the immediate future. It is too useful from

a pragmatic standpoint precisely because it carries the social implications that were just mentioned. Hence, neuropsychologists have to work within the framework of the concept even if they may feel that it is scientifically dubious. But they need not take the concept too seriously in their investigative work. Certainly they should not restrict themselves to the study of older patients who have been diagnosed as demented. Rather they should undertake analyses of the patterns of cognitive deficit exhibited by older patients with or without demonstrable brain disease, whether or not they have been classified as "demented," and undertake the task of identifying the neural mechanisms underlying these patterns of cognitive deficit.

Investigative work along these lines is already being pursued, thanks to the opportunities for correlational study afforded by computed tomography, positron emission tomography and cerebral blood flow analysis. We think it is likely that the findings will lead to a radical modification of the concept of dementia.

REFERENCES

Anastasi, A. (1958). *Differential psychology* (3rd ed.). New York: Macmillan.

Arenberg, D. (1978). Differences and changes with age in the Benton Visual Retention Test. *Journal of Gerontology, 33,* 534–540.

Arenberg, D. (1982). Estimates of age changes on the Benton Visual Retention Test. *Journal of Gerontology, 37,* 87–90.

Arenberg, D., & Robertson-Tchabot, E. A. (1977). Learning and aging. In J. E. Birren & K. W. Schaie (Eds.), *Handbook of the psychology of aging* (pp. 421–449). New York: Van Nostrand Reinhold.

Benton, A. L. (1977). Interactive effects of age and brain disease on reaction time. *Archives of Neurology, 34,* 369–370.

Benton, A. L., Eslinger, P. J., & Damasio, A. R. (1981). Normative observations on neuropsychological test performances in old age. *Journal of Clinical Neuropsychology, 3,* 33–42.

Birren, J. E., Woods, A. M., & Williams, M. V. (1980). Behavioral slowing with age: Causes, organization, and consequences. In L. W. Poon (Ed.), *Aging in the 1980s* (pp. 293–308). Washington D.C.: American Psychological Association.

Botwinick, J. (1978). *Aging and behavior* (2nd ed.). New York: Springer.

Dirken, J. M. (1972). *Functional age of industrial workers.* Groningen: Wolters-Noordhoff.

Dolmatch, T. B. (Ed.) (1979). *Information please almanac, 1980.* New York: Simon & Schuster.

Hamsher, K. de S., & Benton, A. L. (1978). Interactive effects of age and cerebral disease on cognitive performances. *Journal of Neurology, 217,* 195–200.

Heilman, K. M., Safran, A., & Geschwind, N. (1971). Closed head trauma and aphasia. *Journal of Neurology, Neurosurgery, and Psychiatry, 34,* 265–269.

Jennett, B., Teasdale, G., Braakman, R., Minderhoud, J., & Knill-Jones, R. (1976). Predicting outcome in individual patients after severe head injury. *Lancet, 1,* 1031–1034.

Krauss, I. K. (1980). Between and within group comparisons in aging research. In L. W. Poon (Ed.), *Aging in the 1980s* (pp. 542–551). Washington D.C.: American Psychological Association.

Levin, H. S., & Benton. A. L. (1973). Age and susceptibility to tactile masking effects. *Gerontologia Clinica, 15,* 1–9.

Levin, H. S., Benton, A. L., & Grossman, R. G. (1982). *Neurobehavioral consequences of closed head injury.* New York: Oxford University Press.

Price, L. J., Fein, G., Feinberg, I. (1980). Neuropsychological assessment of cognitive function in the elderly. In L. W. Poon (Ed.), *Aging in the 1980s* (pp. 78–85). Washington D.C.: American Psychological Association.

Rosen, W. G. (1980). Verbal fluency in aging and dementia. *Journal of Clinical Neuropsychology, 2,* 135–146.

Schaie, K. W., & Labouvie-Vief, G. (1974). Generational vs. ontogenetic components of change in adult cognitive behavior: A fourteen year cross-sequential study. *Developmental Psychology, 10,* 305–320.

Siegler, I. L., Nowlin, J. B., & Blumenthal, J. A. (1980). Health and behavior: Methodological considerations for adult development and aging. In L. W. Poon (Ed.), *Aging in the 1980s* (pp. 599–612). Washington D.C.: American Psychological Association.

Stengel, E. (1964). Psychopathology of dementia. *Proceedings of the Royal Society of Medicine, 57,* 911–914.

Wilkie, F., & Eisdorfer, G. (1971). Intelligence and blood pressure in the aged. *Science, 172,* 959–962.

Wowern, F. von (1966). Posttraumatic amnesia and confusion as an index of severity in head injury. *Acta Neurologica Scandinavica, 42,* 373–378.

Zangwill, O. L. (1964). Psychopathology of dementia. *Proceedings of the Royal Society of Medicine, 57,* 914–917.

Bibliography

1934

Temporal factors in the formation of conditioned eyelid reactions in human subjects. *Journal of General Psychology*, *10*, 173–197.

1935

The interpretation of questionnaire items in a personality schedule. *Archives of Psychology*, No. 190.

With T. W. Forbes. The standardization of sixty-cycle electric shock for practical use in psychological experimentation. *Journal of General Psychology*, *12*, 436–442.

1936

Influence of incentives upon intelligence test scores of school children. *Journal of Genetic Psychology*, *49*, 494–497.

1937

With I. R. Stone. Consistency of response to personality inventory items as a function of length of interval between test and retest. *Journal of Social Psychology*, *8*, 143–146.

1938

Performances of school children on the Revised Stanford-Binet and the Kent EGY test. *Journal of Genetic Psychology*, *52*, 395–400.

The performance of pre-school children on the Kohs Block Design Test. *Journal of Genetic Psychology*, *53*, 231–233.

1939

Psychometric test results in two cases of precocious puberty. *Journal of Genetic Psychology*, *54*, 455–456.

1940

Mental development of prematurely born children: A critical review of the literature. *American Journal of Orthopsychiatry*, *10*, 719–746.

With J. D. Perry. A study of the predictive value of the Stanford Scientific Aptitude Test (Zyve). *Journal of Psychology*, *10*, 309–312.

1941

A study of the performances of young adults on the Kohs Block Design Test. *Journal of Applied Psychology*, *25*, 420–427.

With I. L. Howell. The use of psychological tests in the evaluation of intellectual function following head injury. *Psychosomatic Medicine*, *3*, 138–151.

With A. Weider & J. Blauvelt. Performances of

adult patients on the Bellevue Intelligence Scales and the Revised Standford-Binet. *Psychiatric Quarterly*, 15, 802–806.

1942

With J. D. Perry. Short method of administering the Kohs Block Design Test. *American Journal of Orthopsychiatry*, 12, 231–233.

1945

A visual retention test for clinical use. *Archives of Neurology and Psychiatry*, 54, 212–216.
Rorschach performances of suspected malingerers. *Journal of Abnormal and Social Psychology*, 40, 94–96.
The Minnesota Multiphasic Personality Inventory in clinical practice. *Journal of Nervous and Mental Disease*, 102, 416–420.

1946

A visual retention test for clinical use. New York: Psychological Corporation.
With K. A. Probst. A comparison of psychiatric ratings with Minnesota Multiphasic Personality Inventory scores. *Journal of Abnormal and Social Psychology*, 41, 75–78.

1947

With S. S. Ackerly. Report of a case of bilateral frontal lobe defect. *Proceedings of the Association for Research in Nervous and Mental Disease*, 27, 479–504.

1948

With S. I. Kornhauser. A study of "score faking" on a medical interest inventory. *Journal of the Association of American Medical Colleges*, 23, 57–60.

1949

With N. T. Collins. Visual Retention Test performance in children: Normative and clinical observations. *Archives of Neurology and Psychiatry*, 62, 610–617.
With L. M. Schultz. Observations on tactual form perception (stereognosis) in preschool children. *Journal of Clinical Psychology*, 4, 359–364.

1950

A multiple choice type of the Visual Retention

Test. *Archives of Neurology and Psychiatry*, 64, 699–707.
The experimental validation of the Rorschach Test. *British Journal of Medical Psychology*, 23, 45–58.
With M. D. Fite. The psychological examination. In D. H. Fryer & E. R. Henry (Eds.), *Handbook of applied psychology*. New York: Rinehart.

1951

El test de Rorschach como prueba perceptiva. *Revista de Psicologia General y Aplicada*, 6, 443–457.
With P. Alden. Relationship of sex of examiner to incidence of Rorschach responses with sexual content. *Journal of Projective Techniques*, 15, 231–234.
With J. F. Hutcheon & E. Seymour. Arithmetic ability, finger-localization capacity and right-left discrimination in normal and defective children. *American Journal of Orthopsychiatry*, 21, 756–766.

1952

The experimental validation of the Rorschach Test II. The significance of Rorschach color responses. *American Journal of Orthopsychiatry*, 22, 755–763.
La signification des tests de rétention visuelle dans le diagnostic clinique. *Revue de Psychologie Appliquée*, 2, 151–179.
With L. S. Abramson. Gerstmann symptoms following electroshock treatment. *Archives of Neurology and Psychology*, 68, 248–257.

1953

Manuel pour l'application clinique du Test de Rètention Visuelle. Editions du Centre de Psychologie Appliquée, Paris.
With A. Bandura. "Primary" and "secondary" suggestibility. *Journal of Abnormal and Social Psychology*, 48, 336–340.

1954

Diagnostic des maladies cérébrales par les méthodes psychologiques. *Encéphale*, 43, 54–72.

1955

The Revised Visual Retention Test: Clinical

and experimental applications. New York: Psychological Corporation. (3rd ed., 1963; 4th ed., 1974).

Development of finger-localization capacity in school children. *Child Development, 26,* 225–230.

Right-left discrimination and finger-localization in defective children. *Archives of Neurology and Psychiatry, 74,* 383–389.

Cerebral disease in a child. In A. Burton & R. E. Harris (Eds.), *Clinical studies in personality.* New York: Harper.

Aspects psychométriques de la debilité mentale. *Revue de Psychologie Appliquée, 5,* 81–95.

With H. L. Blackburn. Simple and choice reaction time in cerebral disease. *Confinia Neurologica, 15,* 327–338.

With B. D. Cohen. Right-left discrimination and finger-localization in normal and brain-injured subjects. *Proceedings of the Iowa Academy of Science, 62,* 447–451.

With C. H. Hartman & I. G. Sarason. Some relations between speech behavior and anxiety level. *Journal of Abnormal and Social Psychology, 51,* 295–297.

With R. Swanson. Some aspects of the genetic development of right-left discrimination. *Child Development, 26,* 123–133.

1956

Jacques Loeb and the method of double stimulation. *Journal of the History of Medicine and Allied Sciences, 11,* 47–53.

The concept of pseudofeeblemindedness. *Archives of Neurology and Psychiatry, 75,* 379–388.

The Rorschach test in epilepsy. *American Journal of Orthopsychiatry, 26,* 420–426.

The Rorschach test and the diagnosis of cerebral pathology in children. *American Journal of Orthopsychiatry, 26,* 783–791.

With R. Meyers. An early description of the Gerstmann syndrome. *Neurology, 6,* 838–842.

1957

With H. L. Blackburn. Practice effects in reaction-time tasks in brain-injured patients. *Journal of Abnormal and Social Psychology, 54,* 109–113.

With H. L. Blackburn. Revised administration and scoring of the digit span test. *Journal of Consulting Psychology, 21,* 139–143.

With F. L. Menefee. Handedness and right-left discrimination. *Child Development, 28,* 237–242.

1958

Significance of systematic reversal in right-left discrimination. *Acta Psychiatrica et Neurologica Scandinavica, 33,* 129–137.

Le temps de réaction chez les malades présentant des lésions cérébrales. *Revue de Psychologie Appliqué, 8,* 103–119.

1959

Right-left discrimination and finger localization: Development and pathology. New York: Hoeber-Harper.

Finger localization and finger praxis. *Quarterly Journal of Experimental Psychology, 11,* 39–44.

With R. C. Jentsch & H. J. Wahler. Simple and choice reaction times in schizophrenia. *Archives of Neurology and Psychiatry, 81,* 373–376.

With R. J. Joynt. Reaction time in unilateral cerebral disease. *Confinia Neurologica, 19,* 247–256.

1960

Motivational influences on performance in brain-damaged patients. *American Journal of Orthopsychiatry, 30,* 313–321.

With R. C. Jentsch & H. J. Wahler. Effects of motivating instructions on reaction time in schizophrenia. *Journal of Nervous and Mental Disease, 130,* 26–29.

With R. J. Joynt. Early descriptions of aphasia. *Archives of Neurology, 3,* 205–222.

With J. D. Kemble. Right-left orientation and reading disability. *Psychiatria et Neurologia* (Basel), *139,* 49–60.

1961

The fiction of the "Gerstmann syndrome." *Journal of Neurology, Neurosurgery and Psychiatry, 24,* 176–181.

With M. L. Fogel. Test de rétention visuelle: Normes revues et complétées. *Revue de Psychologie Appliquée, 11,* 75–77.

With A. L. Sahs. Application de la psychologie aux problémes de la neurologie. *Revue de Psychologie Appliquée, 11,* 95–101.

With O. Spreen. Visual memory test: The simulation of mental incompetence. *Archives of General Psychiatry, 4,* 79–83.

1962

The Visual Retention Test as a constructional praxis task. *Confinia Neurologica, 22,* 141–155.

Behavioral indices of brain damage in children. *Child Development, 33,* 199–208.

Dyslexia in relation to form perception and directional sense. In J. Money (Ed.), *Reading disability: Progress and research needs in dyslexia.* Baltimore, Md.: Johns Hopkins University Press.

Clinical symptomatology in right and left hemisphere lesions. In V. Mountcastle (Ed.), *Interhemispheric relations and cerebral dominance.* Baltimore, Md.: John Hopkins University Press.

With H. P. Bechtoldt & M. L. Fogel. An application of factor analysis in neuropsychology. *Psychological Record, 12,* 147–156.

With H. M. Burian & R. C. Lipsius. Visual cognitive functions in patients with strabismic amblyopia. *Archives of Opthalmology, 68,* 785–791.

With M. L. Fogel. Three-dimensional constructional praxis: A clinical test. *Archives of Neurology, 7,* 347–354.

With R. J. Joynt & M. L. Fogel. Behavioral and pathological correlates of motor impersistence. *Neurology, 12,* 876–881.

With M. McGavren. Qualitative aspects of visual memory test performance in mental defectives. *American Journal of Mental Deficiency, 66,* 878–883.

With R. Meyers & G. J. Polder. Some aspects of handedness. *Psychiatrica et Neurologia* (Basel), *144,* 321–337.

With S. Sutton, J. A. Kennedy, & J. R. Brokaw. The crossmodal retardation in reaction time of patients with cerebral disease. *Journal of Nervous and Mental Disease, 135,* 413–418.

1963

With J. W. Bird. The EEG and reading dis-

ability. *American Journal of Orthopsychiatry, 33,* 529–531.

With H. L. Blackburn. Effects of motivating instructions on reaction time in mental defectives. *Journal of Mental Subnormality, 9,* 81–84.

With A. Elithorn, M. L. Fogel, & M. Kerr. A perceptual maze test sensitive to brain damage. *Journal of Neurology, Neurosurgery and Psychiatry, 26,* 540–544.

With R. J. Joynt. Three pioneers in the study of aphasia. *Journal of the History of Medicine and Allied Sciences, 18,* 381–383.

With O. Spreen. The simulation of mental deficiency on a visual memory test. *American Journal of Mental Deficiency, 67,* 909–913.

1964

Developmental aphasia and brain damage. *Cortex, 1,* 40–52.

Contributions to aphasia before Broca. *Cortex, 1,* 314–327.

The psychological evaluation and differential diagnosis. In H. A. Stevens and R. Heber (Eds.), *Mental retardation: A review of research.* Chicago: University of Chicago Press.

With J. C. Garfield & J. C. Chiorini. Motor impersistence in mental defectives. *Proceedings, International Congress on the Scientific Study of Mental Retardation.* Copenhagen, Denmark.

With R. J. Joynt. The memoir of Marc Dax on aphasia. *Neurology, 14,* 851–854.

With O. Spreen. Visual memory test performance in mentally deficient and brain-damaged patients. *American Journal of Mental Deficiency, 68,* 630–633.

With M. W. Van Allen & M. L. Fogel. Temporal orientation in cerebral disease. *Journal of Nervous and Mental Disease, 139,* 110–119.

1965

Johann A. P. Gesner on aphasia. *Medical History, 9,* 54–60.

The problem of cerebral dominance. *Canadian Psychologist, 6,* 332–348.

Some aspects of mental retardation. *American Journal of Orthopsychiatry, 35,* 830–837.

With S. Muehl & J. R. Knott. EEG abnormality and psychological test performance in reading disability. *Cortex*, *1*, 434–440.

With O. Spreen. Comparative studies of some psychological tests for cerebral damage. *Journal of Nervous and Mental Disease*, *140*, 323–333.

With O. Spreen & R. W. Fincham. Auditory agnosia without aphasia. *Archives of Neurology*, *13*, 84–92.

1966

Problemi di neuropsicologia. Florence: Editrice Universitaria.

Language disorders in children. *Canadian Psychologist*, *7*, 298–312.

With J. C. Garfield & J. C. MacQueen. Motor impersistence in brain-damaged and cultural-familial defectives. *Journal of Nervous and Mental Disease*. *142*, 434–440.

With O. Spreen & C. G. Miller. The phi-test and measures of laterality in children and adults. *Cortex*, *2*, 308–321.

With O. Spreen & M. W. Van Allen. Dissociation of visual and tactile naming in amnesic aphasia. *Neurology*, *16*, 807–814.

With M. W. Van Allen & M. C. Gordon. Temporal discrimination in brain-damaged patients. *Neuropsychologia*, *4*, 159–167.

1967

Problems of test construction in the field of aphasia. *Cortex*, *3*, 32–58.

Constructional apraxia and the minor hemisphere. *Confinia Neurologica*, *29*, 1–16.

Psychological tests for brain damage. In A. M. Freedman & H. I. Kaplan (Eds.), *Comprehensive textbook of psychiatry*. Baltimore, Md.: Williams & Wilkins.

With J. G. Borkowski & O. Spreen. Word fluency and brain damage. *Neuropsychologia*, *5*, 135–140.

With D. Jones & J. C. MacQueen. Hand preference and manipulative dexterity in normal and retarded children. *Journal of Mental Deficiency Research*, *11*, 49–53.

With O. Spreen, M. W. Fangman & D. L. Carr. Visual Retention Test, Administration C: Norms for children. *Journal of Special Education*, *1*, 151–156.

1968

Differential behavioral effects in frontal lobe disease. *Neuropsychologia*, *6*, 53–60.

Right-left discrimination. *Pediatric Clinics of North America*, *15*, 747–758.

La praxie constructive tri-dimensionnelle. *Revue de Psychologie Appliquée*, *18*, 63–80.

With D. Jones. Reaction time and mental age in normal and retarded children. *American Journal of Mental Deficiency*, *73*, 143–147.

With A. L. Sahs. Aspects of developmental dyslexia. *Journal of the Iowa Medical Society*, *58*, 377–383.

With M. W. Van Allen. Impairment in facial recognition in patients with unilateral cerebral disease. *Cortex*, *4*, 344–358.

1969

Development of a multilingual aphasia battery: Progress and problems. *Journal of the Neurological Sciences*, *9*, 39–48.

Disorders of spatial orientation. In P. J. Vinken & G. W. Bruyn (Eds.), *Handbook of clinical neurology* (Vol. 3). Amsterdam: North-Holland; New York: Wiley-Interscience.

Constructional apraxia: Some unanswered questions. In A. L. Benton (Ed.), *Contributions to clinical neuropsychology*. Chicago: Aldine.

With A. Carmon. Tactile perception of direction and number in patients with unilateral cerebral disease. *Neurology*, *19*, 525–532.

With A. Carmon. Patterns of impaired sensitivity and unilateral cerebral disease: Reexamination of Head's theory. *Journal of the Israeli Medical Association*, *77*, 287–290.

With A. Carmon & D. Bilstrom. Thresholds for pressure and sharpness in the right and left hands. *Cortex*, *5*, 27–35.

1970

Hemispheric cerebral dominance. *Israel Journal of Medical Sciences*, *6*, 294–303.

Neuropsychological aspects of mental retardation. *Journal of Special Education*, *4*, 3–11.

Interactive determinants of mental deficiency. In H. C. Haywood (Ed.), *Social-cultural aspects of mental retardation.* New York: Appleton-Century-Crofts.

With H. L. Dee. A cross-modal investigation of spatial performances in patients with unilateral cerebral disease. *Cortex, 6,* 261–272.

With H. L. Dee & M. W. Van Allen. Apraxia in relation to hemispheric locus of lesion and aphasia. *Transactions of the American Neurological Association, 95,* 147–150.

With E. E. Ellis. Test de praxie tri-dimensionnelle: Observations normatives. *Revue de Psychologie Appliquée, 20,* 256–258.

With H. Hécaen. Stereoscopic vision in patients with unilateral cerebral disease. *Neurology, 20,* 1084–1088.

With R. J. Joynt. Anatomical determinants of behavioral change. In A. L. Benton (Ed.), *Behavioral change in cerebrovascular disease.* New York: Harper & Row.

1971

Psychologic testing. In A. B. Baker & L. Baker (Eds.), *Clinical neurology.* New York: Harper & Row.

A biblical description of motor aphasia and right hemiplegia. *Journal of the History of Medicine and Allied Sciences, 26,* 442–444.

With O. Abramsky & A. Carmon. Masking of and by tactile pressure stimuli. *Perception and Psychophysics, 10,* 353–360.

With A. Carmon. Parametric aspects of tactile resolution. *Perception and Psychophysics, 10,* 331–334.

With D. J. Fontenot. Tactile perception of direction in relation to hemispheric locus of lesion. *Neuropsychologia, 9,* 83–88.

With M. C. Gordon. Correlates of facial recognition. *Transactions of the American Neurological Association, 96,* 146–150.

With J. Sauguet & H. Hécaen. Disturbances of the body schema in relation to language impairment and hemispheric locus of lesion. *Journal of Neurology, Neurosurgery and Psychiatry, 34,* 496–501.

1972

The "minor" hemisphere. *Journal of the History of Medicine and Allied Sciences, 27,* 5–14.

Hemispheric cerebral dominance and somes-thesis. In M. Hammer, K. Salzinger, & S. Sutton (Eds.), *Psychopathology: Essays in honor of Joseph Zubin.* New York: Wiley-Interscience.

With D. J. Fontenot. Perception of direction in the right and left visual fields. *Neuropsychologia, 10,* 447–452.

With H. S. Levin. An experimental study of "obscuration." *Neurology, 22,* 1176–1181.

With K. C. Smith & M. Lang. Stimulus characteristics and object naming in aphasic patients. *Journal of Communication Disorders, 5,* 19–24.

With M. W. Van Allen. Prosopagnosia and facial discrimination. *Journal of the Neurological Sciences, 15,* 167–172.

With M. W. Van Allen. Aspects of neuropsychological assessment in patients with cerebral disease. In C. M. Gaitz (Ed.), *Aging and the brain.* New York: Plenum Press.

1973

Visuoconstructive disability in patients with cerebral disease: Its relationship to side of lesion and aphasic disorder. *Documenta Ophthalmologica, 34,* 67–76.

The measurement of aphasic disorders. In A. Cáceres Velasquez (Ed.), *Aspectos patológicos del lenguaje.* Lima, Peru: Centro Neuropsicologico del Lenguaje.

With H. S. Levin. A comparison of the effects of ipsilateral and contralateral tactile masking. *American Journal of Psychology, 86,* 435–444.

With H. S. Levin. Age and susceptibility to tactile masking effects. *Gerontologia Clinica, 15,* 1–9.

With H. S. Levin. Age effects in proprioceptive feedback performance. *Gerontologia Clinica, 15,* 161–169.

With H. S. Levin & N. R. Varney. Tactile perception of direction in normal subjects: Implications for hemispheric cerebral dominance. *Neurology, 23,* 1248–1250.

1974

With H. S. Levin & M. W. Van Allen. Geographic orientation in patients with unilateral cerebral disease. *Neuropsychologia, 12,* 183–191.

1975

Developmental dyslexia: Neurological aspects. In W. J. Friedlander (Ed.), *Advances in neurology.* (Vol. 7) New York: Raven Press.

Psychological tests for brain damage. In A. M. Freedman, H. I. Kaplan, & B. J. Sadock (Eds.), *Comprehensive textbook of psychiatry* (2nd ed.). Baltimore, Md.: Williams & Wilkins.

Hemispheric dominance and visual perception. *Neurological Medicine* (Tokyo), *2,* 143–161.

Neuropsychological assessment. In D. B. Tower (Ed.), *The nervous system.* New York: Raven Press.

With H. J. Hannay & N. R. Varney. Visual perception of line direction in patients with unilateral brain disease. *Neurology, 25,* 907–910.

With H. S. Levin. Temporal orientation in patients with brain disease. *Applied Neurophysiology, 38,* 56–60.

With D. M. Pierce. Relationship between monocular and binocular depth acuity. *Ophthalmologica, 170,* 43–50.

With A. Tartaglione & D. P. Goff. Reaction time to square-wave gratings as a function of spatial frequency, complexity and contrast. *Brain Research, 100,* 111–120.

With N. R. Varney. Tactile perception of direction in relation to handedness and familial handedness. *Neuropsychologia, 13,* 449–454.

1976

Historical development of the concept of hemispheric cerebral dominance. In S. F. Spicker & H. T. Engelhardt (Eds.), *Philosophical dimensions of the neuromedical sciences.* Dordrecht, The Netherlands: Reidel.

With H. J. Hannay & N. R. Varney. Visual localization in patients with unilateral brain disease. *Journal of Neurology, Neurosurgery and Psychiatry, 39,* 307–313.

With H. S. Levin. Proprioceptive feedback performance in patients with focal brain lesions. *Journal of Neurology, 212,* 117–121.

1977

Historical notes on hemispheric dominance. *Archives of Neurology, 34,* 127–129.

Reflections on the Gerstmann syndrome. *Brain and Language, 4,* 45–62.

Interactive effects of age and brain disease on reaction time. *Archives of Neurology, 34,* 369–370.

The amusias. In M. Critchley & R. A. Henson (Eds.), *Music and the brain.* London: William Heinemann Medical Books.

With K. Hamsher. The reliability of reaction time determinations. *Cortex, 13,* 306–310.

With H. S. Levin. Facial recognition in "pseudoneurological" patients. *Journal of Nervous and Mental Disease, 164,* 135–138.

1978

Some conclusions about dyslexia. In A. L. Benton & D. Pearl (Eds.), *Dyslexia: An Appraisal of Current Knowledge.* New York: Oxford University Press.

The interplay of experimental and clinical approaches in brain lesion research. In S. Finger (Ed.), *Recovery from brain damage.* New York: Plenum Press.

The cognitive functioning of children with developmental dysphasia. In M. Wyke (Ed.), *Developmental dysphasia.* London: Academic Press.

With K. de S. Hamsher. *Multilingual Aphasia Examination.* Iowa City: University of Iowa Hospitals.

With K. Hamsher. Interactive effects of age and brain disease on cognitive performance. *Journal of Neurology, 217,* 195–200.

With M. W. Van Allen, K. de S. Hamsher, & H. S. Levin. *Test of Facial Recognition.* Iowa City: University of Iowa Hospitals.

With N. R. Varney & K. Hamsher. Lateral differences in tactile directional perception. *Neuropsychologia, 16,* 109–114.

With N. R. Varney & K. Hamsher. Visuospatial judgment: a clinical test. *Archives of Neurology, 35,* 364–367.

1979

The neuropsychological significance of finger recognition. In M. Bortner (Ed.), *Cognitive*

Growth and Development. New York: Brunner/Mazel.

Body schema disorders: Finger agnosia and right-left disorientation. In K. M. Heilman & E. Valenstein (Eds.), *Clinical neuropsychology.* New York: Oxford University Press.

Visuoperceptive, visuospatial and visuoconstructive disorders. In K. M. Heilman & E. Valenstein (Eds.), *Clinical neuropsychology.* New York: Oxford University Press.

With A. R. Damasio. Impairment of hand movements under visual guidance. *Neurology,* 29, 170–178.

With K. Hamsher & H. S. Levin. Facial recognition in patients with focal brain lesions. *Archives of Neurology,* 36, 837–839.

With N. R. Varney. Phonemic discrimination and aural comprehension among aphasic patients. *Journal of Clinical Neuropsychology,* 1, 65–75.

1980

Dyslexia: evolution of a concept. *Bulletin of the Orton Society,* 30, 10–26.

The neuropsychology of facial recognition. *American Psychologist,* 35, 176–186.

Psychological testing of brain damage. In H. I. Kaplan, A. M. Freedman, & B. J. Sadock (Eds.), *Comprehensive textbook of psychiatry,* 3rd Ed. Baltimore, Md.: Williams & Wilkins.

Psychological testing of children. In H. I. Kaplan, A. M. Freedman, & B. J. Sadock (Eds.), *Comprehensive textbook of psychiatry,* 3rd Ed. Baltimore: Williams & Wilkins.

✓ With S. D. Lindgren. Developmental patterns of visuospatial judgment. *Journal of Pediatric Psychology,* 5, 217–225.

With K. de S. Hamsher & K. Digre. Serial digit learning: normative and clinical aspects. *Journal of Clinical Neuropsychology,* 2, 39–50.

1981

Aphasia: Historical perspectives. In M. T. Sarno (Ed.), *Acquired aphasia.* New York: Academic Press.

Focal brain damage and the concept of localization of function. In C. Loeb (Ed.), *Studies in cerebrovascular disease.* Milan: Masson Italia Editore.

With P. J. Eslinger & A. R. Damasio. Normative observations on neuropsychological test performances in old age. *Journal of Clinical Neuropsychology,* 3, 33–42.

With A. Tartaglione, L. Cocito, G. Bino, & E. Favale. Point localisation in patients with unilateral brain damage. *Journal of Neurology, Neurosurgery and Psychiatry,* 1981, 44, 935–941.

With A. Tartaglione, U. Raiteri, A. Seneghini, L. Cocito, & E. Favale. Visual localization of points in a plane. *Journal of General Psychology,* 1981, 104, 133–143.

1982

Child neuropsychology: retrospect and prospect. In J. de Wit & A. L. Benton (Eds.), *Perspectives in Child Study.* Lisse: Swets and Zeltlinger.

Significance of nonverbal cognitive abilities in aphasic patients. *Japanese Journal of Stroke,* 4, 153–161.

Spatial thinking in neurological patients: Historical aspects. In M. Potegal (Ed.), *Spatial abilities: Developmental and physiological foundations.* New York: Academic Press.

With H. S. Levin & R. G. Grossman. *Neurobehavioral consequences of closed head injury.* New York: Oxford University Press.

With N. R. Varney. Qualitative aspects of pantomime recognition in aphasia. *Brain and Cognition,* 1, 132–139.

1983

With P. J. Eslinger. Visuoperceptual performances in aging and dementia. *Journal of Clinical Neuropsychology,* 5, 213–220.

With K. Hamsher, N. R. Varney, & O. Spreen. *Contributions to Neuropsychological Assessment.* New York: Oxford University Press.

With M. C. Masure. Visuospatial performance in left-handed patients with unilateral brain lesions. *Neuropsychologia,* 21, 179–181.

1984

Visuoperceptual, visuospatial and visuoconstructive disorders. In K. M. Heilman and

E. Valenstein (Eds.), *Clinical Neuropsychology*, 2nd Edition. New York: Oxford University Press.

Hemispheric dominance before Broca. *Neuropsychologia*, 22, 807–811.

Constructional apraxia. *Seminars in Neurology*, 4. 220–222.

Dyslexia and spatial thinking. *Annals of Dyslexia*, 1984, 34, 69–86.

With L. Ewing-Cobb & H. S. Levin. Age and recovery from brain damage: A review of clinical studies. In S. W. Scheff (Ed.), *Age and recovery in the central nervous system*. New York: Plenum Press.

With A. B. Sivan. Problems and conceptual issues in neuropsychological research in aging and dementia. *Journal of Clinical Neuropsychology*, 6, 57–63.

Index